50 Great Activities for Children Who Stutter

50 Great Activities for Children Who Stutter

Lessons, Insights, and Ideas for Therapy Success

by
Peter Reitzes

pro·ed
An International Publisher
8700 Shoal Creek Boulevard
Austin, Texas 78757-6897
800/897-3202 Fax 800/397-7633
www.proedinc.com

pro·ed
An International Publisher

8700 Shoal Creek Boulevard
Austin, Texas 78757-6897
800/897-3202 Fax 800/397-7633
www.proedinc.com

ISBN 1-4164-0125-3

This product was developed by Imaginart International, Inc., in cooperation with the publisher, PRO-ED, Inc.

Illustrations by Rick Menard

Printed in the United States of America
1 2 3 4 5 6 7 8 9 10 10 09 08 07 06

Dedication

I would like to dedicate this book to Phillip Schneider—my colleague, my mentor, and my friend. I have learned from Dr. Schneider that stuttering is allowed and that people who stutter may do anything they want to do in life and may do so while stuttering. Thank you, Phil.

Contents

Foreword

Peter Reitzes has learned from life that the most painful and debilitating aspect of stuttering is not the presence of speech interruptions, it is the tendency to give up the right to express oneself out of the fear of stuttering. Peter's book guides you to sensitively work with children so they do not choose silence over self-expression.

Awareness is the key to change. This book offers wonderful activities that help children get to know themselves, their feelings, and what it is they do when they stutter. This process is the key to meaningful, long-term change.

Peter's book is a powerful and supportive companion that will enable you to smile more often and enjoy your days as you work with children who stutter. It will show you how to replace the darkness of shame and isolation, which often accompany stuttering, with the joys of freedom of speech and self-acceptance.

As speech professionals we often feel alone and frustrated by our limited power to erase stuttering from our clients' lives. This book places Peter, as a personal mentor, by your side. The ideas are presented so clearly and warmly that you feel Peter's presence in the therapy room with you. He guides you with his wisdom and experience from years of dealing with stuttering in his own life and as a speech–language pathologist in the schools and in private practice.

Children have a right to express themselves. That right is not restricted to those people who speak smoothly. It is for all people. This is the powerful and positive message that is the underlying theme of Peter's book. The book gathers ideas and information from many sources and collects them into one practical, effective resource for those of us who work in the schools and in private practice.

I personally thank Peter for sharing his work with us. Know that through you, Peter's ideas and activities will bring joy and fulfillment into the lives of children who stutter.

Phillip Schneider, PhD
Associate Professor of Communication Disorders, Queens College, CUNY
National Stuttering Association's Speech Pathologist of the Year, 2004

Preface

As a stutterer, as a speech–language pathologist, and as a listener, I have grown to understand that stuttering is the absolute worst thing in this world . . . *if we do not talk about it.* When I speak with stutterers, to parents of children who stutter, and to professionals, I offer the following advice: Talk about stuttering. My experience has been that when you talk about stuttering, stuttering just is not that bad.

Growing up, I quickly realized that stuttering was not something I was supposed to be doing or talking about. When I spoke, people often looked away from me or laughed uncomfortably, and some people mocked and teased me. Like many, I frequently chose to avoid talking rather than risk stuttering. This meant not raising my hand in class; avoiding social situations, such as attending parties or joining sports teams; and missing many opportunities because of the fear that my stuttering would be heard. In many ways I did not grow up stuttering—I grew up trying not to stutter.

When I was in elementary school, a teacher wrote on one of my educational progress reports, "Peter looks like a stutterer trying to hide his stuttering." The professional advice given to my parents was, "If you talk about stuttering with your child, the stuttering will get worse." No one knew to tell us that *stuttering is allowed* and that talking about stuttering is the key to managing stuttering.

Many adult stutterers, reflecting on their childhood, report hearing the word *stutter* only when they were teased or when adults whispered it to each other in another room. Things we whisper about are shameful and bad. A major goal of this book is to demonstrate to clinicians the many ways that they may talk openly about stuttering with children who stutter. Clinicians are shown how to engage stuttering honestly, openly, and productively.

Only after meeting hundreds of people who stutter did I realize that many other people grew up just like me—feeling alone and isolated because of the way they talk. Only as an adult, after years of support from fine speech–language pathologists and self-help organizations, did I learn that by discussing stuttering much of the fear and desperation inherent in the disorder disappears. Something very interesting happens when people who stutter, their clinicians, and family members begin an open engagement and discussion of stuttering—stuttering becomes normal, and managing and talking about stuttering also becomes normal.

In this book the thoughts and experiences of people who stutter are presented in the form of quotes, stories, and poems. They were reprinted from newsletters, books, Web sites, electronic mailing lists, electronic discussion forums, and radio programs. Also, many stories and poems presented throughout this text were written specifically for inclusion in this book and appear here for the first time. I know of no better way to define and explain stuttering than to allow people who stutter to do so for themselves.

Peter Reitzes, MA, CCC-SLP

Acknowledgments

I would like to acknowledge the assistance of colleagues and friends who offered valuable suggestions and comments during the writing of this book. Thanks to John Ahlbach, Dorvan Breitenfeldt, Charlie Diggs, Joseph Donaher, Ken Drolet, Leslie Furmansky, Stephen Hood, Elizabeth Mendez, Bob Quesal, Phillip Schneider, Gregory Snyder, Kenneth St. Louis, and Woody Starkweather. I would also like to thank Bill Murphy, Peter Ramig, and Scott Yaruss for offering research-related suggestions.

Very special thanks to my brother, David Reitzes, who edited the earliest versions of my manuscript and continued to make valuable suggestions on later drafts. My parents, Marc and Barbara, and my sister, Becky, have always supported me and have been a source of strength during this project. I would also like to thank Patty Walton for suggesting that I write this book and for introducing me to my editor, Cindy Drolet. Cindy encouraged and supported me and helped me stay focused. I am very fortunate to have worked with such a determined and organized editor. David Cohen offered continuous support and encouragement throughout this project.

Many people contributed personal stories about stuttering, specifically written for children who stutter. They are Yelena Averbukh, Alan Badmington, David Brandau, John Coakley, Mark De Biasio, Andy Floyd, Leslie Furmansky, Elizabeth Kapstein, Ken St. Louis, Nora A. O'Connor, Jason W. Pearson, Lucy Reed, Lee Reeves, Jeff Shames, Gregory Snyder, Junior Tereva, Anthony Troiano, Bernie Weiner, Barry Yeoman, and several authors who wish to remain anonymous. Thank you.

The Stuttering Foundation of America (SFA) has allowed me to include an adapted version of the brochure *The Child Who Stutters: Notes to the Teacher.* The National Stuttering Association (NSA) has granted permission to reprint the stories and poem "Climbing to the Top," "I know How You Feel," "Stuttering Poem," and "What Letting Go Means to Me," and FRIENDS: The National Association of Young People Who Stutter has allowed us to reprint "Cerena" and "My Name Is Christian and I Wish It Wasn't." I am very grateful to these fine organizations for their generosity.

Introduction and How To Use This Book

Elizabeth Kapstein, co-founder of the first self-help group for people who stutter in New York City, has described her experience growing up stuttering by saying, "I always felt that communication and speaking were for others" (as cited in Caggiano, Kapstein, & Reitzes, 2003). One of the main goals of this book is to demonstrate to children who stutter that communicating and speaking is for them. The therapy approach and activities focus on enabling students to identify and explore stuttering, talk about stuttering, and modify and reduce their stuttering so that communication is easier.

The activities included are intended for children who are 7 to 12 years of age. Many of the lessons may also be used with younger students and junior high school students and are appropriate for group and individual therapy. This book includes 50 lessons with detailed directions and reproducible handouts. With the exception of a few inexpensive items, such as Silly Putty, small balls, and an abacus, everything you need to conduct therapy is included.

This activity book was designed to be *fun.* Children cannot be expected to have the same level of motivation that many adults bring to therapy. By creating a situation in which working on stuttering is enjoyable, students will want to continue returning to speech class (Van Riper, 1973).

At stuttering workshops and speech pathology conferences across the country, I have heard many clinicians and graduate students ask the question, "What do I do with children who stutter?" The cry of the speech–language pathologist is, "Tell me what to do Monday morning." The activities and discussions in this book answer these concerns. This book was written with the belief there is always something productive and fun to do in therapy with children who stutter.

Organization of This Book

The book is divided into two parts: The first is Insights and Ideas for Therapy Success, and the second is 50 Great Activities: How-To, Handouts, and Homework. Comprehensive appendixes follow these two divisions. A brief description will follow.

Insights and Ideas for Therapy Success

Two sections are included in this part of the book:

- What You Need To Know About Stuttering
- Your Tools for Successful Stuttering Therapy

What You Need To Know About Stuttering contains facts, data, first-hand descriptions, and discussions about stuttering that seek to define and explain this often puzzling disorder. Important topics such as the growth and maintenance of stuttering, primary and secondary stuttering behaviors, and the effects of teasing are discussed. You will be provided with a solid foundation for understanding people who stutter that supports the therapy approach and activities used in this book.

Your Tools for Successful Stuttering Therapy provides the basic tenets of working successfully with children who stutter. Important treatment topics are discussed, including the importance of creating a "stutter friendly" therapy environment, keeping therapy fun, teaching speech strategies or "tools," teaching the difference between productive and unproductive speaking strategies, and writing goals. This section prepares you to confidently begin using the activities that are in the second part of the book.

50 Great Activities: How-To, Handouts, and Homework

Five sections of activities are offered:

- Identifying and Exploring Stuttering
- Practicing Speech Tools
- Learning the Facts
- Uncovering Feelings
- Targeting Language and Stuttering Goals

The activities focus on helping students identify aspects of their stuttering, talk about stuttering, use speech tools to manage and control stuttering, learn about stuttering, and work on stuttering while also working on concomitant language delays. Speech–language pathologists use many terms to describe physical and motoric speech management skills, such as pull-outs, bouncing, and cancellations. It is common for these to be called speech helpers, techniques, strategies, controls, or tools. In this book the term *speech tools* is preferred.

The majority of activities in this manual may be used for multiple purposes and to achieve multiple goals. Just as the human body uses primary and secondary muscle groups when lifting heavy objects, the activities in this book have primary as well as secondary goals.

Appendixes

The appendixes include reproducible forms that are used across multiple activities, such as the Stuttering Homework form, Speech Class Guest Passes, the Scorecard, and Stuttering Awards. Also included are the following: an adapted handout of a brochure for teachers published by the Stuttering Foundation of America; a collection of stories and poems written by adults who stutter that is specifically for children who stutter; and a discussion about Altered Speech Feedback (ASF). The altered speech feedback discussion was included because its most notable forms, Delayed Auditory Feedback (DAF) and Frequency Altered Feedback (FAF), are currently "hot topics" in the stuttering community and in the field of speech–language pathology. The appendixes also offer information about several stuttering organizations that are valuable resources for you to have.

Homework and Handouts on CD

For your convenience, a CD is included with this manual, containing all of the handouts and homework assignments. When preparing a lesson, you may choose to use the CD to print out the pages you wish to give to sudents, or you may photocopy the pages from the book if you prefer.

Successfully Using the Activities

The majority of the activities in this book may be repeated many times. Each student or group of students will have favorite activities, and you will also have favorite activities. Repeat and modify these popular lessons to achieve the desired goals.

This book should not be treated like a recipe in which you start at the beginning and work toward the end. When preparing a lesson plan, it is appropriate to choose from different sections of the activities to find the ones that best meet the current needs of your students. Although some activities, such as making a stuttering bulletin board (see Post It–Activity 37), may take several sessions to complete, many other activities take considerably less time.

You will want to come to speech class prepared with goals and activities, but be flexible so that you can address and meet the timely needs of students (Ramig & Bennett, 1997). For example, if a student comes to speech class and is upset about his teacher interrupting him when he stutters, this would be a good day to introduce Do You Read Me?–Activity 35 (from the Uncovering Feelings section) in which students write a letter to their teacher about stuttering. If a student comes to class anxious about an upcoming class presentation, this would be a good time to review speech tools, such as voluntary stuttering and pausing, presented in the Practicing Speech Tools section.

The five sections of activities in this book will be useful for different children at different times. For example, if a student is unable to discuss stuttering or work on speech tools because she is unaware that she is stuttering, you will initially want to focus on the activities in Identifying and Exploring Stuttering. If a student is unable to work on using speech tools because she is ashamed of stuttering, you will want to spend time focusing on the activities in the Uncovering Feelings section and the Learning the Facts section.

The Why and How of Homework

Many activities include homework assignments that support or expand upon the specific goals of the activity. These homework assignments may also be used during speech class as additional therapy activities. You may use the homework activities exactly as presented or as models for writing your own homework assignments.

You are not expected to use all of the homework assignments that follow an activity. Look through the homework and choose the assignment or assignments that best meet the needs of your students. Homework can also be used to reinforce an activity that was previously covered. For example, several sessions or weeks after students first do Stuttering Interviews–Activity 30, assign Stuttering Interviews homework so that students continue to practice talking openly about stuttering. Throughout the therapy process, assign homework from different speech tool activities so that students are constantly practicing what they have already learned. Homework is a good way to "bring the clinic into the real world" by encouraging students to practice skills outside of the therapy room with a variety of people (Yaruss & Reardon, 2003, p. 38).

Some activities, such as 20 Questions–Activity 40, do not have specific homework assignments because these activities may be used to practice any of the four speech tools covered in the book. In this case you may use the reproducible homework form located in Appendix A to write your own assignments, or you may also assign homework from a previous lesson. This allows students to use and practice skills taught earlier in the therapy process.

Most important, be sure to review homework assignments in speech class with students before the assignments are taken home. Children should clearly understand what is expected of them before leaving speech class; this helps to avoid unnecessary frustration.

Working with Parents

It is typically viewed as ideal to consider parents an integral and essential part of speech therapy. This book offers numerous homework assignments that offer parents and other caregivers opportunities to become involved in their child's therapy. For more information on counseling parents and engaging parents in the therapy process, see Dell (2000), Gregory and Gregory (1999), Hill (2003), Manning (2000), Ramig (1993), and Starkweather and Givens-Ackerman (1997). Workshops and conferences held by organizations such as the Stuttering Foundation of America, FRIENDS: The National Association of Young People Who Stutter, and the National Stuttering Association often focus on parent counseling and working with families (see Appendix E for contact information).

Part 1

Insights and Ideas for Therapy Success

What You Need To Know About Stuttering

Basic hallmarks of stuttering, such as the complex nature of its variability and the desire for people who stutter to hide and conceal the disorder, are difficult for many to grasp. In this section the disorder of stuttering is discussed and demystified for you as a clinician. These discussions are intended to separate facts from fiction—to give you a firm grasp of what stuttering is and is not.

Separating Fact from Fiction

When entering into therapy, many stutterers and families hold misperceptions about the disorder. For example, it is not uncommon to hear a child or a parent say that stuttering was caused by an occurrence such as receiving a bump on the head or watching a scary movie. One adult in his late 20s was convinced that his father caused and maintained his stuttering as the result of insensitive parenting. By understanding stuttering, you are able to begin the process of replacing such misperceptions about the disorder with essential facts and knowledge. Walter Manning (2000), a speech–language pathologist who stutters, wrote about the positive experience he had working with clinicians who understood the nature of stuttering:

> I [have] encountered clinicians who not only knew about the surface features of the problem but also showed me that they had insight about how this problem influenced my responses to my predicament. They understood something about the deep structure and the intrinsic nature of the problem. They knew that at the center of my decision making was the fact that I often felt helpless. I had little or no sense of being able to control my speech. Sometimes I had what felt like "lucky fluency," which, at the time, I regarded as a good thing. But a moment later I would be unable to communicate even my most basic thoughts. Even when I wasn't overtly stuttering, I experienced the problem as I constantly altered my choices and constricted my options due to even the possiblitiy of stuttering. (p. 116)

What Is Stuttering?

To put it simply, stuttering is two things: Stuttering is a disorder of talking, and stuttering is also a disorder of not talking. Stutterers not only struggle to speak, they often struggle to avoid speaking. Stutterers struggle to get the words out, and they struggle to move forward from one sound or syllable to the next. But many people who stutter, to varying degrees, struggle to avoid talking. A survey conducted by the National Stuttering Association, a self-help organization, found that out of 544 adult stutterers, 81% reported avoiding speaking situations (McClure, 2003; McClure & Yaruss, 2003). In other words, this study found that more than 8 out of 10 stutterers avoid speaking situations because they may stutter.

Common avoidance behaviors include word substitutions (i.e., saying "automobile" instead of "car"), circumlocutions (speaking around the words you really want to say), postponements (waiting or pausing before a feared word or sound in the hope that the stuttering moment will pass), and simply not talking. Jezer (1997) wrote in his autobiography, "There isn't a person who stutters who hasn't gone into a restaurant and ordered something he didn't like because it was preferable to ordering something he did like but couldn't say" (p. 10).

Many stutterers are able to anticipate when they will stutter. This is similar to being at the gym, working out on a stair climber or an exercise bike, and being able to view the hills on the screen before they arrive. Van Riper (1982) wrote, "[Stutterers] scan approaching speech situations and certain words with an alertness almost inconceivable to the normal speaker. Their radars are constantly revolving" (p. 131).

Although some stutterers may be entirely "overt" or entirely "covert" in their stuttering, most stutter overtly at times and also attempt to hide their stuttering at other times. By 5 years of age, it is common for many children who stutter to avoid speaking situations, especially at school (Bloodstein, 1995). Some preschool children avoid stuttering in a variety of environments, such as in the classroom and even at home (Gottwald & Starkweather, 1995). A study by Hayhow, Cray, and Enderby (2002) found that people who stutter were most adversely affected by their stuttering while at school. This study noted, "The most commonly cited response to stammering at school was to avoid such difficult situations as reading aloud and asking or answering questions in class" (pp. 5–6).[1] Although stuttering is raising your hand in class and getting stuck on sounds and words, stuttering is also knowing the answer but refusing to raise your hand in class because of the possibility that you may stutter. In an essay presented on a popular Web site, the Stuttering Homepage, one stutterer explained:

> On numerous occasions I felt as though being mute would be easier than speaking and stuttering. In elementary school the class would be taking turns reading aloud. When I knew that my turn was approaching, I would ask to go to the bathroom. But even that was difficult because I would have to raise my hand and ask loudly for permission. Also within the classroom, I would spend most of my day looking down at the floor in hopes that the teacher would not call on me. When I was called on, I would often reply with a shrug or "I don't know." This seemed safer

[1] In England the term *stammering* is used instead of stuttering.

> than trying to say the answer I had in my head since I would probably get stuck in a block or prolongation on the first sound. I often shied away from joining a group of people and dreaded having to say my name when being introduced to a group of people. Looking back now, I missed out on so many experiences as a child and denied myself and others a relationship because of my stuttering. (Donohue, 2003, para. 1)

When discussing children who are 7 and 8 years of age, Starkweather and Givens-Ackerman (1997) wrote, "It becomes important at this age to do anything but stutter in front of people" (p. 68). It is commonly reported that children as young as 2 and 3 years of age avoid stuttering by changing and substituting words and by refusing to speak. One mother shared with me that her 3-year-old will ask for ice-cream flavors other than chocolate, even though chocolate is his favorite, because he wishes not to stutter. Coping mechanisms, such as this one that are learned in childhood, frequently continue into adulthood. For example, after finding out that I am a speech–language pathologist, a man I had played softball with for several years confided in me that he had a "little speech problem." He shared, "Nobody knows that I stutter. When I feel a stutter coming on, I either stop talking or change what I want to say." This man most certainly learned to avoid stuttering in these ways during childhood.

Most stutterers report that speaking in public during tasks such as ordering food at a restaurant or talking to a salesperson are very stressful and difficult situations. Stutterers have reported walking around stores for hours looking for merchandise rather than risking the chance of stuttering by asking a salesperson. For example, in New York City it is common for expensive razors to be kept behind the registers in drugstores. I worked with one stutterer who reported walking into many different drugstores until he found one store with his brand of razors that could be pointed to without his having to ask for them by name. Nonproductive coping strategies such as this one typically begin in childhood.

There are some stutterers who hide their stuttering and avoid speaking to such a degree that many close friends and family members are not even aware that they stutter. An adult explained, "I have been a popular and successful university teacher for more than 30 years. . . . I have also been a covert stutterer all my life. I am so covert that I didn't discuss my stuttering with anyone until I was more than 30 years old" (Dartnell, 2003).

Although many stutterers avoid speaking because of their fear of stuttering, avoidance behavior may also be a reaction to the physical struggle of speaking. A 13-year-old girl described the physical component of stuttering as feeling "like climbing a steep hill" (Schofield, 2001). An adult described her feeling of being in a "bad stutter." She explained, "Make a fist with one hand and put the other hand over [the] top of the [the] fist. Now push one against the other" (Klumb, 2002, p. 7). When stutterers experience this much struggle with their speech, it seems only normal to want to avoid stuttering.

It is very common for stutterers to make major life decisions based on the possibility of stuttering (Manning, 2000). Stuttering is growing up making lists of jobs you cannot do because it is often assumed that professionals, such as attorneys, politicians, police officers, and teachers are not allowed to stutter. At a workshop I recall meeting a high school senior who was being scouted by several colleges and universities for a football scholarship. When asked if he enjoyed football, this young man stated, "I stutter, I can't do anything else." One teenager wrote, "When I was in elementary school, I anticipated that as an adult I would have a job that did not require talking to other people" (Cepler, 2003, p. 3).

It is important to note that the fears that many children and adults hold of not being accepted into a certain profession because they stutter are not unfounded. For example, an adult reported that a professor in college advised him to, "Get out of education. You are a stutterer; you will never make a good educator. You will be an embarrassment in the classroom." (Caseman, 2001, p. 118). While working on my master's degree in speech pathology, I was informed that the only way I would be able to graduate from my department and become a speech–language pathologist was if my speech was 100% free of stuttering (see Reitzes & Starkweather, 1999). Even though most professionals in the field of speech–language pathology would ardently disagree, the message I received was loud and clear—stuttering was not allowed.

On the Covert-S[2] electronic mailing list[3], one stutterer shared that when he was a freshman in college he chose to major in finance even though he wanted to be an architect. He made this major life decision because he felt unable to say "architect" without stuttering (Roach, 2003). Stories such as these are exceedingly common among people who stutter. Manning (2000) stated, "Herein lies the basis of the handicap for many individuals who stutter: the life choices they make or fail to make, based on the fact that they are people who stutter" (p. 130).

Stuttering Variability

Stuttering is a highly variable disorder (Cooper, 2000; Starkweather, 1987). Although there are many characteristics that define the disorder of stuttering, perhaps variability is the most striking. Dell (1993) explained, "I contend that if there is a universal truth about stuttering, it is that the disorder is intermittent and variable and often eludes our attempts at categorization" (p. 46). Carlisle (1985) has pointed out that stuttering is not a "continual handicap" (p. 5) as is being blind or deaf. That is, it is normal for stutterers to go minutes, hours, days, weeks, months, and even years without stuttering, and then, all of a sudden, the stuttering comes back.

---

[2] Covert-S is an electronic mailing list specifically created to discuss issues pertaining to people who identify as current or former covert stutterers.

[3] An electronic mailing list is an e-mail–based discussion group in which members send an e-mail to the group address (such as stutteringchat@yahoogroups.com), and that e-mail is automatically sent to every member of the list for discussion.

The variability of stuttering is one of the most frustrating aspects of the disorder to grasp for both the clinician and the stutterer (Yaruss, 2002). Van Riper (1982) quoted a former client as saying, "I can't get used to it. I can't get used to it. I wish I were blind or deaf or crippled. Then I'd always be that way, and though it would be hard, I could finally accept it. But the way it is, I talk all right for a bit and then get clobbered" (p. 2).

Stuttering variability often corresponds to the level of communicative pressure and communicative stress that the speaker feels (Kalinowski, Stuart, Wamsley, & Rastatter, 1999). This may explain why a significant reduction of stuttering tends to occur when people who stutter speak without any listeners present (Bergmann, 1987; Hood, 1975). It is normal for the frequency of stuttering to vary greatly depending on a host of situational speaking factors, such as the size of the audience, the level of communicative pressure, time pressures, the reactions of listeners, and the speaker's concerns about social approval (Bloodstein, 1995).

Sheehan (1975) inserted an interesting angle to the topic of variability by suggesting that whereas stuttering is variable, moments of not stuttering were also variable. He stated, "A stutterer is one who does not know where his next word is coming from" (p. 104). Similarly, people who stutter often view moments of not stuttering as being lucky, also known as *lucky fluency* (Breitenfeldt, 2003; Manning, 2000), and moments of stuttering as being unlucky. These feelings are most certainly attributable, at least in part, to the variable nature of the disorder. Williams (1979) wrote, "Stutterers come to believe that an instance of stuttering just 'happens' in spite of everything they do to prevent it" (p. 243). It is very common to hear stutterers describe feeling helpless; this most certainly has something to due with the whimsical and capricious nature of the disorder.

The variability of stuttering may inadvertently lead some to think that a person who stutters does not have a "real" stuttering problem. For example, a mother of a 3-year-old has shared with me that every time her son went a few days or more without much stuttering, the grandmother or grandfather informed the family, "You see, he really isn't stuttering—you are just overreacting." This refusal to validate the grandson's stuttering and the therapy he was receiving was extremely hurtful and negative for the mother.

Although stuttering variability is frustrating for stutterers and their families, it can also be frustrating for teachers. Some have been reluctant to refer students to me for screening because they assume that real stuttering should occur regularly, without periods of remittance. Teachers often assume that if a student is not stuttering every time that student speaks, I will not take that teacher's concerns seriously. I worked with a teacher who suggested that it might not be a good idea to provide speech therapy to her student during days in which the child was not demonstrating stuttering behaviors. The teacher said to me, "She hasn't stuttered at all this week—I don't think she needs speech class." In this situation I informed the teacher that these "reduced stuttering days" are therapeutically helpful because students have the opportunity to work on speaking strategies and to work on talking openly about stuttering without the stress and emotions that often accompany "high frequency stuttering days."

Adding to the complexity of stuttering variability is the fact that many stutterers are able, to varying degrees, to hide and conceal their stuttering. There are days when a child may be able to easily substitute words or easily avoid speaking tasks in class. But there are other days the student just cannot find that elusive synonym and, instead of changing his answer, takes a chance at saying the exact word he wants to say only to find himself caught in a stutter. The child who is tired from a sleepless night or sick may not have the energy to scan ahead for possible stuttering moments. For some children, the variability and complex nature of stuttering is only compounded by the variability and unreliable nature of avoidance strategies.

The Cause and Growth of Stuttering

The bad news is that authorities on stuttering really do not know what causes stuttering (Conture, 2003; Culatta & Goldberg, 1995; Gregory, 1995; Van Riper, 1982; Wingate, 1997). The good news is that speech–language pathologists typically know what makes stuttering grow (become more frequent and more struggled) and are able to offer helpful approaches and strategies to treat and support people who stutter.

Starkweather and Givens-Ackerman (1997) have aptly noted, "There are as many causes as there are people who stutter because the real cause is the pattern of reactions that the person brings to it" (p. 58). They suggest, "There is no single etiology, but as many etiologies as there are stories of development" (p. 24). Conture (2003) explained, "We still haven't found the 'knife' that causes stuttering. However, we do know something about the 'salt' that keeps it going, aggravates [it], or makes it worse" (p. 10).

In the vast majority of situations, stuttering is not the result of a psychological or social problem. Manning (2000) has stated that the pain arising from stuttering is "a normal reaction to an unwanted situation" (p. 247). People who stutter have been reported to demonstrate significantly greater feelings of anxiety and social discomfort during socially demanding speaking situations (Cable, Colcord, & Petrosino, 2002; Craig, 1990; Kraaimaat, Vanryckeghem, & Van Dam-Baggenc, 2002; Messenger, Onslow, Packman, & Menzies, 2004). Conture (2001) suggested, "It is a sign of psychological intactness for a child to become concerned about and hesitant to do what he or she cannot do well." Stuttering is often considered a disorder of reactions or, as Starkweather and Givens-Ackerman (1997) stated, "The disorder creates the disorder" (p. 70). Starkweather (1999) explained:

> We have all met the stutterers who began with what seemed like the innocuous avoidance device of changing a word from one that is perceived to be difficult to one that will be easier to say. Sometimes, indeed, the new word is produced more fluently, but alas sometimes it isn't. Gradually, this strategy typically leads to more and more word changing, to changing sentence structure to accommodate a different sentence. Eventually the person is talking in a most roundabout way and

> is in fact difficult to understand. (p. 239)

Stuttering, for many, has become a vicious circle of struggle and avoidance in which the disorder maintains and exacerbates itself (Breitenfeldt & Lorenz, 2000). An adult stutterer suggested, "Stuttering is a like a mushroom; it grows best in the dark." What he meant was that the more people try to hide stuttering, the more difficult their problem becomes. Guitar (2000) suggested, "The more you don't want to stutter, the more you do stutter" (p. 52). This is why a popular phrase in the stuttering community is: Avoid avoidance.

Van Riper (1948) described how stuttering often grows through sound and word fears. He wrote:

> Sounds themselves become fear. A child remembers his brother laughing at his stuttering on the word *potatoes.* He gets a similar penalty on *paper.* What is he to deduce but that words beginning with *p* are more likely to bring stuttering than a word beginning with *s,* on which he has never remembered having difficulty? These feared sounds spread. Not only *p* words but *b* words soon look difficult. Both of these words require tight lip contact. Then the fear spreads to include the *m* and *w* consonants. (p. 32)

The Emergence of Stuttering

Stuttering typically emerges between the ages of 2 and 5 (Andrews, Craig, Feyer, Hoddinott, Howie, & Neilson, 1983; Shapiro, 1999), 2 and 6 (Breitenfeldt & Lorenz, 2000), or 4 and 6 (Starkweather & Givens-Ackerman, 1997). In Facts–Activity 24, students are informed that most people begin stuttering between the ages of 2 and 8. Although this may be considered inaccurate by researchers, many stutterers do not actually recall noticing their stuttering until 7 or 8 years of age. This may be because for some children, their stuttering grows more noticeable to them as they grow older. By slightly widening the age range of when stuttering develops, many children's personal memories and experiences are taken into account.

It is very rare for adults or teens to begin stuttering without having stuttered during early childhood. When I hear of a 10- or 11-year-old child who has "just started stuttering," my first thought is that she probably stuttered as a younger child and is therefore undergoing a relapse. Or her stuttering is simply becoming more noticeable.

The Relationship Between Age and Severity of Stuttering

In addition to chronological age, the time a child has spent stuttering is an important variable and component to the disorder (Conture & Guitar, 1993). Manning (2000) suggests, "Although a child's chronological age is a factor influencing the behavioral features and severity of the stuttering syndrome, age is not as meaningful as the length of time stuttering has been taking place" (p. 318). Conture (2001) explains, "It is *not* our experience that chronological age is significantly related to the frequency, duration, or severity of stuttering in preschool/early school-age stuttering" (p. 143).

As an example, a student who is 6 years old and has been stuttering for almost 4 years may react very differently toward his stuttering than a student who is 7 years old and has been stuttering for only one year. It is not safe to assume that the 7-year-old has a more debilitating stuttering problem. Perhaps the 6-year-old has built up tremendous feelings of guilt and shame around his stuttering and has many avoidance behaviors and secondary reactions, whereas the 7-year-old child demonstrates fairly easy moments of stuttering with little fear or embarrassment.

The Linguistic Location of Moments of Stuttering

Stuttering typically occurs on the first sounds or phonemes of words (Andrews et al., 1983) and at the beginning of utterances (Peters & Hulstijn, 1987; Van Riper, 1973). In one study of 22 preschool children, it was found that "97.8% of stuttering events occurred on the first syllables of words and 76.5% on the first sounds of syllables" (Natke, Sandrieser, van Ark, Pietrowsky, Kalveram, 2004, p. 109). Stuttering also commonly occurs within words (i.e., "Septttember") but is extremely rare at the end of words (i.e., "Septemberrr"). Some people may occasionally stutter on final vowel sounds (i.e., saying "soooo" for "so") but not on final consonants (i.e., saying "soapppp" for "soap"). Van Riper (1982) recognized that

> first words, or words that come early in the sentence, seem to be stuttered upon more often that those that follow. For once the research is almost unanimous in this regard. It clearly shows that stutterers have more trouble "getting started" in their utterances. (p. 179)

The location of stuttering moments within sentences and within words is an important factor to keep in mind during therapy. Because most moments of stuttering occur at the beginning of words and at the beginning of sentences, most speech therapy strategies typically focus on helping the client to initiate the first sounds of sentences and the first sounds of words and syllables.

Primary and Secondary Stuttering Behaviors

Primary stuttering includes repetitions, prolongations, and blocks of speech. Secondary behaviors, also known as coping behaviors and "tricks," are unproductive reactions to primary stuttering behaviors. Secondary symptoms include a vast array of behaviors, such as foot tapping, arm swinging, eye blinking, deep breathing, eyebrow raising, nasal snorting or flaring, and speaking with a low-pitched or quiet voice. Most simply, secondary behaviors are extra movements, such as finger snapping or tongue clicking, that are in addition to, or in place of, primary stuttering behaviors. Starkweather (1987) wrote, "Most, probably all, of the accessory features of stuttering are designed to postpone, avoid, terminate, escape from, hide, disguise, or diminish the impact of stuttering" (p. 125). Some research has suggested that secondary behaviors begin developing near the onset of primary stuttering (see Yairi & Ambrose, 2005).

Secondary behaviors are used either before a moment of stuttering to avoid or postpone the impending stutter or during a moment of stuttering to escape from the stutter. For example, if a person who stutters fears saying his own name, he might get in the habit of loudly clearing his throat before introducing himself in an attempt to ward off, wait out, or struggle through the impending stuttering moment. This throat clearing is secondary to the primary stuttering and typically becomes louder and more pronounced over time. If stuck in the middle of a block, the stutterer may get in the habit of rocking her head in an attempt to release from the stutter.

Many people who stutter use interjections, such as "um" and "uh," to postpone moments of stuttering or to aid them in initiating speech. One fifth-grade student entered into therapy using the phrases "for example" and "because" in an attempt to release himself from moments of stuttering. The student would use either phrase, often up to five or six times, until he was released from his stuttering. At other times this student would use these phrases before stuttering as a way to postpone or "wait out" an anticipated moment of stuttering. Michael Sugerman (2001), a co-founder of the National Stuttering Association, explained:

> Throughout my school years, I recall using tricks to enable me to get through class presentations. . . . These strategies were many and varied: talking in a low voice, talking very fast, nodding my head, and using filler words. I remember doing a talk on Copernicus in eighth grade. That day the word *okay* was my prop [starter]; I inserted it after almost every word. (p. 79)

Many secondary behaviors appear quite bizarre. A teenager often spoke with a fake French accent when he anticipated stuttering. For example, when he would go shopping, he would speak to salespersons while using this French accent. The fake accent was secondary to his primary stuttering. Sometimes the fake accent would help him speak without stuttering, but other times he would stutter while using the accent. The more he came to rely upon the French accent, the more he stuttered when using it. When this happened he would then incorporate additional secondary behaviors into his speech, such as repeating the word *well* and waving his hands until he felt able to move forward with his speech. Instead of simply repeating, prolonging, or blocking on a word, this young man would often get stuck using an array of three or more secondary behaviors.

One fourth-grade child would anticipate stuttering and immediately begin to use several secondary behaviors that made it look like he was thinking about his answer. This student would tap his chin, say "hmm," raise his eyebrows, and direct his eye gaze upward, all in an attempt to pretend he was formulating an answer. These four secondary behaviors were repeated numerous times until he was able to get the word out or change his answer. Many times the student simply gave up trying to speak and said, "I don't remember" or "Skip me." Murphy (1997a) described his secondaries in this way:

> As far back as I can remember and until my mid-30s, I vigorously attempted to hide my stuttering at all costs. My bag of tricks was full. Word substitutions, circumlocutions and other avoidances were my mainstay. . . . If these preventatives failed and stuttering began, I was prepared with many disguise behaviors: pretending to have a coughing spasm, a sudden sneeze, or letting all of my air out and trying to talk with what is called expiratory air reserve. (para. 1)

Secondaries develop because a stutterer discovers that, initially, behaviors such as coughing, foot tapping, nasal snorts, or any other accessory movements help her move through or avoid moments of stuttering. The stutterer begins to rely on the trick, and the secondary behavior becomes part of the stuttering. Pretty soon, though, the secondary behavior ceases to release the stutterer from her struggle. The stutterer may then respond by increasing the range or strength of the secondary behavior. For example, if one eye blink ceases to work, the stutterer will often blink harder and more frequently in an attempt to escape from stuttering. When a speech–language pathologist observes a person who stutters lifting her foot up high and stamping down, it is safe to assume that this secondary behavior probably began in a much less exaggerated way, such as a little toe tap or little foot tap. It is no wonder that Van Riper (1982) was convinced that "much of the behavior that goes under the name of stuttering is learned" (p. 312).

Stuttering, Breathing, and Misarticulations

It is not uncommon to hear clinicians say they work on retraining the speaking mechanism because people who stutter "learned how to speak incorrectly" or "learned how to breathe incorrectly." In my opinion, people who stutter produce all of the sounds of speech as well as anyone else, and stutterers breathe as correctly as anyone else (Reitzes & Starkweather, 1999). The problem is that sometimes while people who stutter are talking, they get stuck. As a consequence of getting stuck or of attempting to avoid getting stuck, many stutterers may misarticulate sounds or demonstrate irregular breathing behaviors, such as shallow breathing, irregular or aperiodic respiratory cycles, audible exhalations, gasping, talking on exhausted breath, and thoracic tension.

Atypical breathing patterns in response to stuttering are secondary symptoms. These breathing behaviors are similar to when a stutterer may tap her foot or blink her eyes. Suggesting that stuttering is a breathing problem is similar to suggesting that stuttering is a blinking problem. Different stutterers simply demonstrate different secondary behaviors in response to their stuttering.

Stutterers' Negative Attitudes

Negative attitudes toward stuttering are prevalent in both children and adults who stutter (Andrews & Cutler, 1974; DeNil & Bruten, 1991; Guitar, 1998; Silverman, 2004). It is common for stutterers to have feelings of "unworthiness," "inadequacy," and "inferiority" (Ainsworth, 1968, pp. 12–14). Murphy (1997b) wrote, "Common emotions that are paired with stuttering include anxiety, fear, and sometimes anger. Underlying these feelings are the two emotions shame and guilt" (p. 1). People who stutter may develop low self-esteem and feel "defective," "dumb," or "incompetent" (Williams, 2003, p. 58). Starkweather & Givens-Ackerman (1997) wrote that children who stutter often feel "that they are simply not very good as people" (p. 68). Van Riper (1982) noted that a person who stutters often comes to view himself "not only as an inefficient speaker but as an undesirable and reprehensible one" (p. 233). Sugerman (2001) explained:

> [Until I was 21] my stuttering represented my entire self-image. I was dominated by stuttering. It was difficult for me to express my wants and feelings. I stuttered and worried about what the listener would think of me as a person who stuttered. I struggled to push words out and felt helpless, anxious, afraid, ashamed, and guilty. (p. 78)

Another adult said: "Stuttering is a deep feeling of not being able to survive because we cannot speak. As a kid my whole body was affected; I saw my whole future crumble. That was not reality, but just a feeling that seemed a reality" (Guerin, 2003, para. 2).

Some stutterers are reported to use negative self-talk (Chmela & Reardon, 1997; DeNil & Bruten, 1991; Ramig & Bennet; 1995). For example, I worked with a teenager who repeated, "I'm stupid" in her head every time she stuttered. One stutterer explained, "Negative thinking, which was very common in my life, centered around my speaking. [I thought] I can't do this because I stutter. I'm so stupid because I stutter" (Floyd, 1999, p. 129).

Stutterers may hold negative feelings for various reasons, including social or familial disapproval and self-imposed or imagined disapproval. One 12-year-old stutterer explained:

> Ever since I could talk I stuttered. This always gave me the feeling that my parents were somehow let down by my speech dysfluency. When I first got these feelings, I used to sit alone and cry and wish to be normal. (Carabetta, 1999. p. 55)

An adult woman, looking back at her childhood, wrote:

> Stuttering has a stigma about it that people who stutter must have something wrong with them. I always felt that it was shameful for my father. . . . As a very little girl, I didn't talk much around him because I was afraid of stuttering. (Summerlin, 2001, pp. 31–32)

Teasing and Bullying

Teasing is frequently reported by stutterers to be one of the worst, if not the worst, aspect of stuttering. Whereas somewhere between 49% and 56% of all school-age children are bullied or teased in school at some time, the incidence increases to 81% for children who stutter (Langevin, 2001). Nearly half of parents and teachers report being unaware of the bullying and teasing that children who stutter endure (Hugh-Jones & Smith, 1999). The two most common forms of teasing were found to be imitation and name-calling (Langevin, Bortnick, Hammer, & Wiebe, 1998). Children who stutter have been found to be significantly more likely to be rejected by their peers and viewed as less popular than children who do not stutter (Davis, Howell, & Cooke, 2002). It is not surprising that stutterers report feelings of exclusion. In addition to causing negative feelings and emotions, teasing and bullying may also have the effect of triggering stuttering behaviors (Murphy, 2000; Murphy & Quesal, 2002). An 11-year-old stutterer described her own experience with teasing when she wrote:

> "Stupid!" "Stuttermouth!" These are some of the names you get called when you stutter. When I try to speak, people laugh at me, stare at me, and even try and imitate me. People do this because they do not understand that stuttering is a disability, almost the same as needing a wheelchair. (Young, 1998, p. 14)

Listed below are four quotes describing teasing situations by school-age children who stutter. They are from the Stuttering Homepage (2005, www.stutteringhomepage.com).

> People make fun of me because I *stutter*, and now they do it because I go to speech therapy. They say, "If you t-t-t-talk like th-th-th-this, then you weren't born r-r-r-right." (Rebecca)

> They tease me and talk about me because I stutter. They make fun of me because of how I look when I stutter because sometimes I tap my leg or stomp. (Lewis, age 11)

> My cousin Tim teases me about my stuttering by saying I "act like a retard." I was teased by a boy in my class when I was answering a question and I stuttered. He whispered, "You look stupid when you talk." (Michelah, age 8)

> Once while I was talking to an adult, I was stuttering on the "a" sound and the adult mocked me. I felt very angry. I didn't say anything to her; I just walked away. From that moment on my trust for that person changed. She is the adult; she should know better. I used to think she was a really kind person and a caregiver that was there for me. Now my feelings have changed about her. (Kyle, age 10)

As just demonstrated, teasing and bullying is not the sole domain of children. Some stutterers report being bullied or teased by adults. When discussing an experience in college, one adult wrote, "A teacher once said in exasperation that I was depriving a village somewhere of an idiot" (Hopewell, 2000, p. 3). Another stutterer wrote, "I was given all sorts of nicknames by my schoolmates and even at times by the teachers themselves" (Lukong, 2003, p. 5).

Dealing with the topics of emotions and feelings, teasing and bullying situations, and negative attitudes is as therapeutically significant to the treatment of stuttering as teaching strategies to control moments of stuttering (Chmela & Reardon, 2001; Guitar, 1998; Sheehan, 1970; Starkweather & Givens-Ackerman, 1997; Yaruss & Reardon, 2002). This book provides numerous activities, such as You Feel That Way Too?–Activity 31, It's Showtime–Activity 32, Do You Read Me?–Activity 35, and Questions and Answers–Activity 33 (from the Uncovering Feelings section), that help students express their feelings and talk about teasing and negative feelings. For more information on bullying and teasing, see the text *Bullying and Teasing: Helping Children Who Stutter* (Yaruss, Murphy, Quesal, & Reardon, 2004).

Feeling Alone

Feeling alone and isolated is a hallmark of stuttering for school-age children (Guitar & Reville, 2003). Many children enter their teenage years without ever having met another stutterer (Zebrowski, 2003). Most families are uncomfortable talking about stuttering and avoid doing so. In a story titled "Am I the Only One?" a teenager shared a very common experience for children who stutter:

> [Am I the only one?] That is the question I ask over and over in my head every day at school. You look around and you see handicapped people in wheelchairs, people who are blind and deaf, and, of course, people with braces. You never see a kid who stutters. (Cochran, 1998, p. 33)

In a story titled "I Thought I Was the Only One," an adult woman writing about her childhood explained:

> I didn't know there was anything you could do about stuttering. I came from a small town, and no one stuttered around me, so I didn't know. I mean, heck, I just did not know that there were other people who stuttered besides me. (Sliger, 2001, p. 76)

The previous story reminds me of a workshop I co-facilitated in Hayes, Kansas, on the Stutter Across America tour in 2002. This FRIENDS sponsored tour was billed as a "mobile support group" in which we drove across the country and brought stuttering awareness and stuttering support to towns and cities in America. An adult stutterer in his 30s showed up at the workshop and agreed to speak on a panel of local residents who stuttered. His audience was a group of speech–language pathologists and graduate students. During his impromptu presentation, this man started crying and shared that he had never met another stutterer until that night. He stated that he had many preconceived notions about how another stutterer might appear and that he was pleasantly surprised to find that stutterers were just "normal" people, like everybody else.

In a personal account written for this book, Yelena Averbukh explained:

> When I got a little older and turned 12, I became more self-conscious and my stuttering started to bother me. I started to avoid all possible speaking situations, such as phone conversations and chatting with my friends. I did not return phone calls and did not respond to birthday party invitations. I was feeling very lonely. (See Appendix C.)

In addition to not knowing other stutterers, it is commonly reported that family members, teachers, and significant adults in a child's life are reluctant to acknowledge stuttering. People who stutter have often described stuttering as their "dirty little secret" in which no one uses the word *stuttering* or talks openly about stuttering. This has been referred to as the "conspiracy of silence." An adult stutterer explained:

> I never did mind talking about stuttering when or if it came up; it just never seemed to come up and I rarely brought it up myself. Most people don't know how to handle it so they just leave it alone and pretend it isn't there. (Johnson, 2003, p. 1)

One teenager described stuttering as a big pink elephant that sat on his shoulder. He explained that everyone saw the elephant and everyone, including himself, pretended that the elephant was not there. In a remarkably similar vein, an adult described the covert aspects of his stuttering as ignoring "the elephant in the living room" (Linton, 2003, p. 2). Guitar (1998) warned that when adults do not talk to children about stuttering, "children often begin to think that their speech is so terrible that even their mother and father are too ashamed to talk about it. This is an awful message to give a child" (p. 355).

One year I worked in an elementary school with five boys who were in group therapy together. These boys were extremely fortunate to have other stutterers within the same age range available for group therapy. Yet, at times, even these students felt alone and abnormal because of their stuttering. During one session we read a poem written by a woman who stutters. One of the boys asked, "Do girls really stutter?" Even though the group had spent many sessions learning about stuttering and had researched Annie Glenn and other famous women who stuttered, they did not actually believe that women stuttered because they had never met a girl or woman who did. In response, I set up a visitation with a clinician from a local school and a female student she worked with who stutters. I also arranged to have an adult woman who stutters visit the group. These experiences helped my students to feel less isolated and alone and was one more step in "normalizing" their stuttering (see Murphy, 1999, 2000, for information on normalizing stuttering).

Stuttering: A Disorder of Listening

Many people who stutter spend so much time and energy worrying about stuttering and trying to hide and avoid stuttering that they often demonstrate difficulty listening. In an e-mail sent to the Stutt-L electronic mailing list titled "Poor Listeners," an adult who stutters discussed the difficulty of attending to others:

> We are so concerned with our own speech that we never hear the other person. . . . I never heard one word anyone else said because I was so worried that I would not be able say my name. Moreover, I would interrupt a lot because I would speak whenever I had that feeling that I could finally get something out, regardless of the fact that someone else was talking. (Steiner, 2002)

In a story contributed to this book called "My Turn," Jeff Shames discussed worrying about the possibility of stuttering while sitting in class and waiting to be called on to read. Shames wrote:

> I would get more and more nervous as my turn drew closer. I hoped that my reading would be short and not have too many sounds that I would stutter on. I became so worried that I didn't hear anything that was said by the other kids. (See Appendix C.)

To prevent stuttering from being heard, many stutterers attempt to search ahead to anticipate how they will respond to various questions and requests. For example, one stutterer wrote, "When my teacher used to ask questions of the class, I would mull long and hard over the perfect reply, anticipating any and all potential counter questions" (Vinjamoori, 2004). Spending this much time attempting to weed out and avoid potential stuttering moments makes it very difficult to concentrate on what other students and the teacher are actually saying.

Many stutterers also become confused and are unable to think while caught in a moment of stuttering. This state has been described as a "kind of a trance" (Carlisle, 1985, p. 4) or an "out of body experience" (see Starkweather & Givens-Ackerman, 1997, p. 34). Van Riper described this as "le petit mort" or the little death (as cited in Starkweather & Givens, 2003, para. 11). Heite (2001) referred to this as a form of dissociation, meaning that stutterers were attempting to distance themselves from a difficult situation.

Stuttering and Language

Studies have shown that as the length and grammatical complexity of utterances increase, there is a corresponding increase in the frequency of stuttering behaviors (Gaines, Runyan, & Meyers, 1991; Logan & Conture, 1995; Ratner & Sih, 1987; Riley & Riley, 1983; Yaruss, 1999; Zackheim & Conture, 2003). Starkweather and Gottwald (1990) explained, "Stuttering is likely to occur at locations that are linguistically demanding," such as on "long words and [on] long and complex sentences" (p. 144). Disfluencies among both children who stutter and children who do not stutter are commonly associated with language formulation and may be heard at the beginning of noun phrases and at clausal boundaries (see Trautman, Healey, Norris, 2001).

Researchers have also pointed out that the more complex the utterance becomes, the more complex the motor plan for producing it becomes (Amster & Starkweather, 2000; Peters, Hulstijin, & Starkweather, 1989). As the length and grammatical complexity of speech increase, so do the motoric and linguistic demands put upon the speaker (Starkweather & Gottwald, 1990). To put it simply, as the length and complexity of language and spoken utterances increase, so does the potential for stuttering.

Stuttering with Concomitant Speech and Language Disorders

It is frequently reported that a sizable proportion of children who stutter demonstrate other concomitant speech or language difficulties (Anderson & Conture, 2000; Bloodstein, 2002; Logan & Lasalle, 2003). A study of 2,628 children who stutter found that almost 63% demonstrated other, concomitant disorders (Blood, Ridenour, Qualls, & Hammer, 2003). One survey found that 44% of children who stutter also met their state's criteria for phonological and/or language impairment (Arndt & Healey, 2001). Another survey of over 1,000 children who stutter found that 68% were reported to have at least one or more co-existing problem, such as a speech and language disorder or a neurological or emotional problem (Blood & Seider, 1981). Although it is clear that many children who stutter demonstrate other difficulties and impairments, it is unclear if this group is more likely to demonstrate phonological and language disorders than children who do not stutter (see Nippold, 1990, 2001, 2002, 2004a; Paden, 2005; Ratner & Hakim, 2004). Children who stutter are certainly as susceptible to language delays and disorders as their nonstuttering peers (Nippold, 2004b). It is commonly noted that existing concomitant disorders, such as language, learning, and emotional disorders, could "exacerbate" a person's stuttering (Yairi & Ambrose, 2005, p. 354).

Many clinicians and researchers believe that, under the right circumstances, it is appropriate to work concurrently on stuttering and other speech and language disorders. Logan and Lasalle (2003) suggest a framework for when to treat stuttering with concomitant disorders. To summarize, they suggest the following:

- When stuttering is demonstrated to be the primary communication problem, stuttering should be the primary focus of therapy.
- When stuttering and the concomitant articulation or language impairment are demonstrated to be of near equal priority, a cyclic method of therapy is recommended.
- When stuttering is demonstrated to be a low level of priority, the concomitant articulation or language problem should be the primary focus of therapy.

Some clinicians hesitate to treat students who stutter for co-existing articulation errors. Dell (2000) has warned that treating a child with articulation delays while also treating him for stuttering may, in some circumstances, be unproductive. Dell stated, "Putting too much pressure on his articulation errors may bring on more stuttering by creating fears of certain sounds" (p. 17). It has been noted that some children begin stuttering in response to receiving articulation therapy (Van Riper, 1982). Starkweather and Givens-Ackerman (1997) explain, "When stuttering appears it is often in concert with the exact same sounds on which the child has been working" (p. 56). In light of this, Conture (2001) suggests that clinicians use "low-key" therapeutic strategies when working with children who stutter (p. 94).

Many authorities in the field believe that stuttering and articulation disorders may be treated concurrently when the clinician feels it is appropriate (Campbell, 2003; Conture, 2001; Gregory, 1986, 2002; Guitar, 1998; Logan & Lasalle, 2003; Ramig & Bennett, 1995; Wall & Meyers, 1995; Wolk, 1998). Some advocate treating stuttering while *indirectly* working with a child on phonological difficulties (Conture, Louko, & Edwards, 1993; Louko, Conture, & Edwards, 1999). Ratner (1995) and Wolk suggest treating concomitant phonological delays in an indirect manner in order to avoid exacerbating the child's stuttering.

Not only do many children who stutter demonstrate other impairments, but stutterers often receive therapy in small group settings that include students who are working on other speech and language difficulties (Manning, 2000; Williams & Dugan, 2002; Yaruss, 2002). Caseload sizes are a prominent concern of clinicians working in the schools (American Speech-Language-Hearing Association, 2000). A study by Brisk, Healey, and Hux (1997) found that 38% of school clinicians treat children who stutter in groups that include students with other speech and language disorders. Clinicians in public schools are often unable to form therapy groups that consist solely of children who stutter because of high caseload considerations and because many speech pathologists have few, if any, stutterers on their caseloads (Ramig & Bennett, 1995).

Clearly there is a need for activities that target stuttering goals while also targeting language goals. In this book the activity section titled Targeting Language and Stuttering Goals focuses on simultaneously treating stuttering and receptive, expressive, and pragmatic language needs. For further information regarding treating children who stutter with concomitant speech and language impairments, see Conture, 2001; Conture, Louko, and Edwards, 1993; Guitar, 1998; Logan and Lasalle, 2003; Louko, Conture, and Edwards, 1999; Nippold, 1990, 2001, 2002, 2004a, 2004b; Manning, 2000; and Ratner, 1995.

Understanding Stuttering Leads to Better Treatment

To treat children who stutter to the best of our abilities, we need to command a basic understanding of the disorder (Ramig & Bennett, 1997). A clinician's therapeutic plan is guided by his understanding of the nature of stuttering (Van Riper, 1975). Yaruss & Reardon (2002) explained, "A key principle underlying all aspects of treatment for school-age children who stutter is the idea that students—and their clinicians—must always understand why they are doing the things they are doing in therapy" (p. 198). This section has laid the foundation for treating school-age children who stutter.

Your Tools for Successful Stuttering Therapy

At a stuttering workshop I once attended, the keynote speaker informed the audience, "Stuttering is only what you hear." The speaker explained that speech–language pathologists should only work with children on their overt stuttering behaviors by teaching them to use speaking strategies. The speaker's belief was that clinicians should avoid talking openly to children about stuttering. She stated that children who avoid stuttering by using word substitutions or by avoiding certain speaking situations should be encouraged to continue using these strategies. She explained that using avoidance techniques were preferable to having overt moments of stuttering.

This book takes a much different view of therapy for children who stutter because of the widespread understanding that *the dominant maintaining factors of the disorder are the symptoms you do not hear.* So many of the problems surrounding stuttering are the result of avoidance, shame, and fear. Getting stuck while saying sounds and words is certainly a problem, but the disorder becomes more debilitating the more children try not to stutter and try not to talk about or acknowledge their stuttering.

The *stuttering iceberg* has become a popular and often quoted analogy in the stuttering community. Joseph Sheehan (1970), a speech–language pathologist who stuttered, explained, "Stuttering may be linked to an iceberg, with the major portion below the surface. What people see and hear is the smaller portion; much greater is that which lies below the surface, experienced as fear, guilt, and anticipation of shame" (p. 13). Stutterers like this analogy because it offers a clear, vivid description of the stuttering behaviors and feelings that are often kept concealed and hidden away. One stutterer suggested that 10% of the stuttering problem is the visible tip of the iceberg, which is made up of "audible stuttering," whereas 90% of the stuttering problem is the area below the waterline that is composed of "fear, shame, guilt, anxiety, hopeless[ness], isolation, denial" and other feelings (Hicks, 2003, para. 2).

Although it is important to help school-age children learn and use tools to move forward in their speech and to stutter less often, working on identifying and changing attitudes for the school-age child is often considered the most important aspect of therapy (Dell, 2000; Murphy, 1999; Starkweather & Givens-Ackerman, 1997). For children who demonstrate negative feelings surrounding their stuttering, it is crucial that you focus on the emotions that often hold stutterers back. Negative thinking needs to be replaced with positive thinking (Ramig & Bennett, 1995). It is important to keep in mind that speech tools are only one aspect of therapy and far from a cure-all.

This section offers much more than speaking strategies. Whereas speech tools are thoroughly explained, you are also guided through all of the vital components of successful therapy, including creating a stutter-friendly therapy environment, talking about stuttering and feelings, being open and having fun during all aspects of therapy, setting goals, and measuring progress. This section fully prepares you to use the activities that comprise the major portion of the book.

Creating a Motivating and Safe Environment

Therapy Must Be Fun

Van Riper (1973) pointed out, "The child is brought to therapy; he seldom seeks it" (p. 426). You need to keep in mind that *children who stutter are children with an adult problem.* Children are not coming to therapy to work on stuttering; they are coming to have fun. It is the speech–language pathologist's job to make therapy fun for children while creating rich opportunities for reflection, growth, and change; this will ensure that students will want to come back to therapy.

Stuttering Must Be Allowed

Your first duty when working with stutterers is to create an environment in which stuttering not only is allowed but encouraged. As described earlier, stuttering is often maintained by the child's attempts to speak without stuttering. By permitting, allowing, and encouraging stuttering, you create an environment in which stuttering may be dealt with openly, productively, and in a nonpunitive manner. Hood has appropriately suggested that the clinician's slogan could be, "Stuttering is permitted here" (S. B. Hood, personal communication, September 4, 2003).

To change and modify how a person stutters, stuttering has to be allowed. For example, when learning how to ski, I was taught to fall before I was taught to go forward. This approach was explained to me very simply: "If you do not know how to fall safely, you will never enjoy skiing and you will choose not to ski." Likewise, you cannot learn to stutter less often and with less struggle if you do not allow yourself to stutter.

When working with a student who is demonstrating shame about stuttering, you may lighten the situation with humor by making a comment such as, "If you come to speech class and do not stutter, then we do not have anything to work with!"

Stuttering Must Not Be Punished or Discouraged

You must not punish stuttering in any way. Students should be rewarded and praised for participating in and attending to therapy activities regardless of the child's level of stuttering or control. Some clinicians make the mistake of praising a child only when she is not stuttering. The nature of stuttering is that many children who stutter will attempt to hide and avoid their stuttering. By praising only the absence of stuttering, you unwittingly send the message that moments of stuttering are to be avoided and feared. This negative message only leads to more avoidance and more stuttering. By punishing moments of stuttering you are maintaining, not alleviating, the problem.

You need to reward students for their participation and attempts, not for decreases in the frequency or severity of stuttering. For example, if a student is practicing a speech tool, instead of commenting on the reduction of stuttering behaviors, you might say, "I like how you are remembering to use your speech tools today." If a child comes to speech class and is stuttering a lot with little control, reward the student for speaking openly instead of sitting silently. You may say, "I can tell that speaking is hard for you today, and I am so proud of you for not giving up."

Sometimes clinicians may accidentally punish a child for stuttering by responding in nonverbal ways, such as looking away from the child when she is stuttering. It is important to react to stuttering calmly. Maintain eye contact when a student is stuttering and never verbally or nonverbally reprimand a student for stuttering. Looking away from a child when she is stuttering sends the message that the student is doing something wrong.

Feelings Need To Be Validated

Any feelings that students express about stuttering are allowed (Sheehan, 2003). In his book on counseling, Luterman (2001) explained that feelings just exist and that there are no right or wrong feelings. If a student is angry, frustrated, sad, or happy about stuttering, you need to validate these feelings by listening and responding in a noncritical manner (Schneider, 2003). For example, it is not uncommon for students who are teased to voice anger; some may make comments such as, "I can't wait to beat that guy up." Instead of telling a student that these feelings are the wrong feelings to have, make a point of listening and exploring the situation. In this situation, instead of making a blanket statement such as, "Fighting is wrong" or "Hitting won't solve this problem," help the student explore all of his options. Engage students in discussing many of the options that he has at his disposal, such as speaking to a teacher. And remind students that by simply coming to their speech teacher and asking for help, they are showing courage and taking responsibility when faced with a difficult situation.

Students Need To Know Other Children Who Stutter

To help prevent and counteract negative feelings associated with the stuttering, you need to create many opportunities for students to meet other children who stutter. By doing so you ensure that students will not grow up feeling alone and isolated with their stuttering. Children who grow up playing together, stuttering together, talking about stuttering together, and managing their stuttering together, grow up understanding that stuttering is allowed and that managing it is possible. Donaher has stated, "The best role models for children who stutter are other children who stutter" (as cited in Reitzes & Caggiano, 2003, p. 27).

If there are several students who stutter in the same school, these children should be given plenty of opportunities to get to know each other and attend speech class together. Also, invite speech–language pathologists from local schools and their students who stutter to visit and meet your students. Arrange for your students to visit other children who stutter. On my students' Individualized Education Programs (IEPs), I mandate goals that require students to participate, at least several times a year, in activities with other children who stutter. This ensures that, legally, my students must be provided opportunities to interact with other children who stutter. For example, an IEP goal may read, "Brian will interview 3 children who stutter, on 3 separate occasions during the school year, about stuttering." After having met other children who stutter, students then communicate via telephone, e-mail, or mail. Homework assignments are one way to encourage children who stutter to stay in contact and learn from one another. I also inform parents about local stuttering workshops in which they can expect their child to meet other children and adults who stutter.

When arranging intervisitations and therapy sessions, it is recommended that clinicians attempt to group children by "similar stuttering behaviors and attitudes" (Ramig & Bennett, 1995, p. 144). Grouping by age ranges is also an important consideration. It is also helpful to occasionally schedule sessions in which teenage or adult stutterers come and speak with younger students and parents about their stuttering experiences.

Inviting Guests to Speech Class "Normalizes" Stuttering

Normalizing speech class and speech therapy should be a priority for all clinicians. You and your students should encourage guests to come to speech class throughout the therapy process. Guests learn a lot about stuttering and often go back to class and tell everyone how much they enjoyed speech class. Students learn to speak casually about stuttering and get practice using speech tools in front of their friends. Students of all ages tend to respect their friends who stutter even more when they see how hard they are working on their speech. *Speech class guests help take the stigma out of stuttering and the stigma out of going to speech class.* It is very powerful and motivating for a student who stutters to hear a nonstuttering peer say, "Speech class is cool; can I come back?"

There are several ways to go about inviting guests to therapy. In a school setting, inform teachers that it is helpful for students to bring friends and classmates on occasion to therapy. Explain that students perform better and work harder when they know that their problem is accepted and understood by their peers. Tell teachers that the more comfortable students become with their stuttering, the more likely they are to participate in class.

If you are in private practice, discuss with family members the benefits of including guests in the therapy process. Ask the family to bring with them, on occasion, the child's friends or siblings. For clients who are seen in their homes, include babysitters, relatives, friends, and neighbors in therapy. This helps to normalize stuttering and speech therapy for people who come into regular contact with the child.

When guests are included in therapy, you need to ensure that stuttering is treated respectfully and with dignity. For example, during the Stuttering Awards activity, guests are encouraged to compete with children who stutter for different awards, such as the Longest Stutter, the Shortest Stutter, and the Coolest Stutter. Students and guests may tease one another in a friendly way during this activity, thus you need to make sure that friendly banter does not turn into hurtful or mean-spirited teasing. Only guests who can participate in a friendly manner should be included in therapy. If inappropriate behaviors (i.e., interruptions or teasing) occur, engage the group in a discussion about appropriate speech class behaviors (Guitar & Reville, 2003).

Reproducible Speech Class Guest Passes are included in Appendix A. Using these passes is optional. They are included to give children the opportunity to officially invite their friends and peers to speech class. Students enjoy the formality of these passes and using them helps to build anticipation for speech class. There are two versions of the Speech Class Guest Pass: One is an open invitation and one asks guests to come with three written questions about stuttering. When guests arrive with their questions, engage students in openly discussing the questions. Doing so often leads to meaningful, thoughtful, and open conversations about stuttering.

Self-Help Groups Are an Important Component of Therapy

Self-help organizations, such as FRIENDS and the National Stuttering Association, bring together people who stutter, their families, and professionals to share experiences and information. Lee Caggiano (1998), the mother of a person who stutters, a speech–language pathologist, and director of FRIENDS, explains:

> I know what a tremendous impact support groups can have on the lives of children who stutter and their families and am deeply troubled that so many young people continue to live in isolation and shame. It is critical that we begin to provide all children with this support and sense of empowerment. (para. 2)

After the 2002 FRIENDS convention, a teen wrote to the FRIENDS Internet discussion board:

> Every year I look forward to [the] FRIENDS [convention] and it's so sad when it's over. . . . I have learned that I am not the only one who stutters and that there are

> people out there who are just like me. Also, that there are many people who care so much about stuttering that they are willing to give up a weekend and go talk to all of us about it.

Support groups like FRIENDS and the NSA have national conventions and local workshops that are held in different cities throughout the year. You may check to see if there is a workshop you, your students, and family members may attend (see Appendix E).

Measuring Successful Therapy

The field of speech–language pathology has long debated the treatment of stuttering. Clinicians and researchers have sharp disagreements concerning what constitutes successful therapy.

In this book the act of stuttering itself is a fundamental component of a successful therapy process. After all, how can a child change how she stutters if she comes to speech class and refuses to stutter? How can you help students change how they stutter and how they feel about stuttering if they do not feel that stuttering is allowed? When a child demonstrates shame or guilt when he stutters, you may simply say, "I am so glad that you are stuttering today; now we have something to work with!"

When the goal of speech therapy is the total absence of stuttering, therapy is destined to fail. There is no cure for stuttering, and as a consequence of this fact, speech–language pathologists and other professionals should not promise or imply that a cure is possible. Jezer has written about the pitfalls of striving for the absence of stuttering. He (1997) wrote:

> The only cure for stuttering is silence. Because stutterers who don't speak don't stutter, my usual response to failure at therapy was to stop talking. If total fluency is the goal in speech therapy (as it is in many but not all kinds of speech therapy), then being silent—or avoiding speaking situations in which I feared that I might stutter—was a way to assure myself that I was making progress. (p. 3)

Reardon (2000) wrote:

> Just counting dysfluencies does not address the complexity of stuttering. The overall goal of therapy is not fluent speech but more effective communication. Success can come in small steps of increased self-esteem, increased acceptance of stuttering, and decreased fear and avoidance behaviors. These gains are vital in managing stuttering but do not show up on fluency counts. (p. 19)

Success occurs when students express how they feel about stuttering with their clinicians, teachers, parents, family, and peers. For example, success is having students take responsibility for their own stuttering by doing things like writing letters and talking openly to their teachers about stuttering. Successful therapy has also been defined as follows:

> Gaining sufficient confidence to be comfortable about communication and to be able to speak easily in most situations. However . . . the child and the parents should realize that there will be some variation in fluency and that therapy focuses on the management of these variations. (Campbell, 2003)

Williams and Dugan (2002) wrote that the major goal of therapy may be expressed as "saying whatever you want to say, whenever you want to say it, even if you sometimes stutter" (p. 2). At times during the therapy process, clients may even stutter more rather than less (Manning, 2000; Starkweather & Givens-Ackerman, 1997).

Manning (1999a) discussed how increased moments of stuttering are often a positive aspect of therapy. He wrote, "Increased stuttering usually occurs with decreased avoidance. So, under certain circumstances, one sign of progress could very well be an increase in the frequency of your stuttering" (para. 37).

A less struggled form of stuttering is also a major sign of success. This often occurs when students who have grown to rely on secondary and avoidance behaviors begin to revert back to primary stuttering behaviors. For example, after working several months with a 4-year-old, the child greatly reduced his use of secondary behaviors to break free of moments of stuttering. Instead of raising his vocal pitch to break free of a stutter, he replaced this secondary behavior with what his mother described as "easy repetitions." The child was in the process of returning to primary stuttering—a very positive step. The parents recognized that although their son certainly was not cured, he was now stuttering in an easier manner and was beginning to productively move through dysfluencies. He no longer needed to rely upon secondary behaviors.

Walton and Wallace (1998) recognize that changes in a child's pattern of stuttering are a sign of success. They wrote the following:

> One or more of the following changes are early indications of progress: advanced stuttering behaviors (that is, blocks and prolongations) change to more repetitive behavior; individual stuttering moments are less severe; the duration of core behaviors (that is, repetitions, prolongations, and laryngeal blocks) decreases; secondary behaviors decrease in frequency or severity; or the nature of the child's fluency cycle changes (increased periods of fluency and shorter cycles of stuttering). (p. 7)

This has been a general discussion about what constitutes success. Specific IEP goals are provided in the Writing Goals section presented later in this section of the book that allow you to document and measure therapeutic progress. For example, one sign of success is a decrease in fear and avoidance behaviors. There are many goals offered in the Writing Goals section that address this. One goal calls for the student to "Complete 5 stuttering interviews during the school year with teachers, staff members, neighbors, or relatives and review them during speech class." This goal allows students to decrease their fear and avoidance of stuttering by talking with others in an open and productive way about the disorder.

Learning the Therapy Approach

An important aspect of managing stuttering is learning and using speech tools. Speech tools (or strategies) are used to move forward through sounds, words, and sentences and to stutter less frequently. Speech tools fall into one of the following two broad therapy approaches that clinicians use to treat people who stutter:

- Stuttering modification (also referred to as *stuttering easily*)
- Fluency shaping (also referred to as *stuttering less often*)

Stuttering modification tools are used to help the student stutter in a smoother, easier, less struggled manner. The final outcome of stuttering modification is not to cure the client of stuttering but to provide the child with tools that he feels confident in using to move forward through moments of stuttering. *The goal of stuttering modification is not the total absence of stuttering.* Rather, the goal is to stutter in smoother, less abnormal ways (Bloodstein, 1995; Dell, 2000). Clients are taught how to modify or mend moments of stuttering as they are occurring. For example, if a stutterer is repeating the /d/ sound in the word *dog*, he would smooth out the repetition, as it is happening, by easily stretching the /d/ and saying "ddddog." Traditionally, clinicians using a stuttering modification approach feel it is also important to work with clients on the negative feelings and attitudes that often accompany their stuttering.

Fluency shaping is a therapy approach that has different meanings for different clinicians (St. Louis, 2001). Typically, fluency-shaping approaches are based on the belief that people who stutter learned how to speak or breathe incorrectly. The final goal or outcome of fluency-shaping approaches is the total absence of stuttering. Fluency-shaping therapies commonly reward fluency and punish stuttering behaviors (Shapiro, 1999). Clinicians often start with helping students slow the articulation rate (the within word rate) of syllables to a full second or more before working on producing more natural sounding speech. Traditionally, clinicians using a fluency-shaping approach focus on speech production and do not address the negative feelings and emotions that often coincide with the disorder.

Donaher (2001) stated that although the speaking strategies or tools are similar in both stuttering modification and fluency-shaping therapy approaches, the fundamental difference is found in their goals. For example, both therapy approaches may ask a student to prolong the first sound of a word in a smooth or easy manner. *Whereas a stuttering modification approach would use this prolongation to promote easy stuttering, a fluency-shaping approach would use the prolongation to promote nonstuttered speech.*

To meet the communication needs of their students, many clinicians practice an integrated treatment approach in which aspects of stuttering modification and fluency-shaping therapies are used together (Conture, 2001; Cooper & Cooper, 1985; Guitar, 1998; Guitar & Peters, 2003; Healey, Scott, & Ellis, 1995). This book advocates a similar position. Stuttering modification tools are used in conjunction with pausing, a progressive fluency-shaping tool, to offer students a comprehensive, effective, and nonpunitive course of therapy. Using this book, you will be able to confidently offer students speech tools that will help them stutter more easily and less often.

For more information on stuttering modification and fluency-shaping therapies, see Guitar (1998), Guitar & Peters (2003), Manning (2000), and Shapiro (1999).

The Four Speech Tools

You need to present speech tools that are basic and easy to remember so that students will be able to use them during stressful speaking situations. The four speech tools used in this book allow the clinician to keep therapy simple, effective, and fun. They are listed here and described in this section:

- Stretching
- Bouncing
- Voluntary stuttering
- Pausing

As mentioned earlier, the major therapy approaches for treating people who stutter are stuttering modification (easy stuttering) and fluency shaping (stuttering less often). Stretching, bouncing, and voluntary stuttering are stuttering-easily tools, and pausing is a stuttering less often tool. As well as being a speech tool, voluntary stuttering is also a favorite desensitization strategy used to help students face their stuttering fears and avoidances. Stretching, bouncing, and voluntary stuttering may be traced back to Van Riper (1973). Pausing is derived from the work of Schneider (1994, 1998). All four speech tools are described here.

Stretching

Stretching allows students to initiate a word or a sentence in a smooth, prolonged, controlled manner. Stretching also allows students to smooth-out or stretch-out of a sound or a word while stuttering. For example, if a stutterer is blocking on the /m/ sound in *mother,* he would stretch-out of the stutter by smoothly stretching the /m/ and then gently opening his mouth to initiate the vowel sound ("mmmmother"). The student is modifying the moment of stuttering in an attempt to move forward to the next sound and to then complete the word. As described in detail later, stretching is demonstrated to students using Silly Putty. As you, the clinician, slowly stretch the Silly Putty, simultaneously stretch (prolong) the first sound of the word you are saying in an easy and smooth manner.

Bouncing

Like stretching, bouncing allows students to initiate a word or a sentence in a smooth, controlled manner. Students do so by gently bouncing or repeating the first sound or syllable of a word. For example, to bounce on the word *tiger,* the student would bounce the first sound a few times by saying "ti-ti-ti-tiger" in an easy and smooth manner. Bouncing also allows students to smoothly bounce-out of a sound or a word while stuck in the middle of a stutter. Stutterers repeat dysfluencies at a faster rate or tempo than normal speakers repeat normal disfluencies (Van Riper, 1982). By practicing bouncing at a slower rate, the stutterer is able to slow her repetitions to approximate more normal-sounding speech. Also, another hallmark of stuttering behavior is replacing the correct vowel with the schwa vowel, thus saying "tu-tu-tu-table" instead of "tay-tay-tay-table." By practicing bouncing on the correct vowel, children are learning to stutter in a way that is more typical of normal speech. As described in detail later, bouncing is initially demonstrated by using a bouncy ball (the kind of rubber ball you get from a gumball machine). Each time the ball hits the ground, the child repeats the first syllable. Because balls bounce slower than stuttered repetitions, the student is learning to change or alter her stuttering pattern to approximate normal, nonstuttered disfluencies in other's speech.

Voluntary Stuttering

Voluntary stuttering is the polar opposite of hiding and concealing stuttering and, for many stutterers, is the single most important tool at their disposal. Voluntary stuttering (also known as *stuttering on purpose, pseudo stuttering, fake stuttering,* and *negative practice*) is used for at least four different purposes in therapy:

- To desensitize people who stutter to their fears and anxieties about stuttering
- To practice easy stuttering by using stretching and bouncing
- To help stutterers listen to themselves and others by staying focused and attentive instead of worrying about the possibility of stuttering
- To demonstrate to listeners and oneself that stuttering is not shameful or bad

Desensitizing Oneself to Fears and Anxieties About Stuttering. Through voluntary stuttering, students enter into speaking situations as stutterers instead of as people trying to hide or avoid stuttering. Students use voluntary stuttering to reduce their fear of stuttering by getting their stuttering immediately out in the open so that they do not have to worry and fear the possibility of stuttering. For example, students may be assigned the task of asking a question at a store while stuttering noticeably (on purpose) on the first word they say. A student may ask a clerk, "Eeeeexcuse me, when do you close today?" For many, the reduction of speaking fears resulting from voluntary stuttering makes focusing on speaking easier.

Because of the variability of the disorder, many stutterers do not know when their stuttering will occur. As a consequence many people who stutter spend entire conversations waiting in dread for their stuttering to first appear. It is common for stutterers to think, "When will my stuttering finally be heard?" By stuttering on purpose at the beginning of a conversation, the speaker is able to get his stuttering immediately out into the open. This helps to reduce the fear of talking and the fear of stuttering. "Voluntary stuttering neutralizes the variable and intermittent nature of the disorder" (Reitzes, 2005, para. 7).

When students stutter on purpose in an easy manner, it will sound very similar to stretching and bouncing. Some students will recognize this and comment that "fake stuttering sounds the same as when we do stretching and bouncing." You may want to say, "Stuttering on purpose is just like stretching or bouncing on purpose—all of our speech tools are related."

Practicing Easy Stuttering Using Stretching and Bouncing. Asking a student to use stretching or bouncing to initiate speech is a form of voluntary stuttering. Through voluntary stuttering, people who stutter set themselves an example or model for how they want to stutter. If they enter into a speaking situation and voluntarily stutter gently and smoothly on several words while maintaining good eye contact, then when a real stutter comes along, they will be better able to stutter easily, in a forward-moving manner, with good eye contact.

Staying in the Moment While Listening to Oneself and Others. By entering into a speaking situation as a stutterer and not as someone attempting to conceal her problem, many find a way to analyze and respond to their speech during stuttering moments. Voluntary stuttering allows students to "stay grounded in the moment" and think while they are stuttering. Students will find it easier to concentrate on what they are saying instead of worrying about the possibility that they may stutter. Students are better equipped to listen to and consider what is being said to them. Also real moments of stuttering tend to carry with them stress and emotional baggage. By stuttering on purpose, students are able to practice speech tools in a calm and thoughtful manner without the negative emotions that typically accompany real stuttering.

Demonstrating That Stuttering Is Not Shameful or Bad. When stuttering on purpose, stutterers also set a tone for how other people should react to their stuttering. By voluntarily stuttering while maintaining eye contact, stutterers project to listeners that they are not ashamed or troubled by their stuttering and that the listeners need not be either.

Many adults and children have gained much from using voluntary stuttering. In a message titled "You Can Run but You Can't Hide," sent to the electronic mailing list "Stutt-L," an adult stutterer wrote:

> I quit running from blocks when I discovered the power of voluntary stuttering. I feel comfortable with it because its purpose is not fluency but an easier, more relaxed way to stutter, without those dreaded secondaries. I know I communicate better when using it. (Troiano, 2002, para. 3)

In a message sent to Stutt-L titled "Pseudo-Stuttering," an adult stutterer discussed the positive and empowering experience of watching his speech–language pathologist model voluntary stuttering during therapy. He wrote the following:

> When she did her fake stuttering in front of store clerks, she wasn't embarrassed in the least. That amazed me at first, but what I didn't realize at the time was the impact it had on me internally, in what my inner voice told me about my own stuttering. It helped reduce that speech monster to a little mouse. . . . [The] fear of stuttering is the thing that holds many of us back. (Harkavy, 2002)

Pausing

Pausing (as indicated here by commas), briefly, for a, *fraction of a second,* between words, has the effect, of reducing, the frequency of stuttering. Pausing, should not occur, within words, but, between words. Students, are not, expected, to pause, for several seconds, at a time. Ideally, each pause, should be brief, and last, no more, than a second.

Pausing may be effective for decreasing stuttering frequency because it

- reduces time pressure constraints felt by the speaker, and
- reduces the speaker's muscle tension before moments of stuttering.

Stuttering behaviors tend to increase in response to time pressure felt by the speaker. For example, when speaking to people who frequently interrupt them or appear impatient, stutterers often feel the need to speak quickly, thus creating more opportunities for struggle. Schneider explained:

> Stuttering is a time-pressure issue. Just as some drivers always have to speed even though they get into lots of accidents when they do, many stutterers feel a need to rush through their speech to make up for the time they spend stuttering. Many fluency sensitive speakers seem to prefer a rapid, forward-force speaking style. This style may be adopted because of the fear of being stopped and the need to "make up for lost time." Or, maybe the speaker is just pre-wired to speak at a tempo that drives the system beyond its fidelity of control. (P. Schneider, personal communication, August 20, 2004)

The increase in rate resulting from time-pressure stressors often results in more stuttering and causes the muscles involved in speech to become "stiff, slow-moving, uncoordinated, and tremulous" (Starkweather, 1987, p. 76). Various studies and researchers have found that people who stutter typically speak using higher levels of muscular tension than nonstutterers (see Starkweather, 1987; Starkweather & Givens-Ackerman, 1997; van Lieshout, Peters, Starkweather, & Hulstijin, 1993). Also, Starkweather and Givens (2003) point out that when stutterers attempt not to stutter, this struggle to avoid "tends to increase muscular tension, which makes smooth, easy talking more difficult" (para. 16). It is my belief, shared by others, that the use of pausing may allow the muscles involved in speech production to avoid becoming overly tense or contracted, thus reducing the potential for stuttering.

Some speech–language pathologists and researchers do not advocate the use of pausing. Some clinicians warn that teaching students a strategy to reduce the frequency of stuttering unintentionally demonstrates that the act of stuttering is unacceptable. Some specialists, even those in the area of fluency, have never been exposed to pausing, whereas others know very little about it. As this book advocates, as long as pausing is presented within a therapy approach that also engages children in talking about stuttering, learning about stuttering, and identifying and exploring stuttering, students will clearly understand that stuttering is allowed.

Assembling a Stuttering Kit

For several decades variations of stuttering kits, stuttering toolboxes, and stuttering tool belts have been used by speech–language pathologists to teach children speech tools and speaking strategies. The toys and items kept in these kits are used to help students learn speech tools and identify stuttering behaviors.

When working with elementary school students, you will need to assemble a stuttering toolbox that contains Silly Putty, a bouncy ball, toy eyeglasses, a mirror, bubbles, and a child's abacus. You may collect these items for each child or for each therapy group. Each item is briefly discussed below; you will learn how they are used in the activity section titled Practicing Speech Tools.

Silly Putty. Silly Putty is used to teach stretching. Silly Putty may be purchased for approximately $2.00 at most toy stores and drugstores. It comes in many different colors inside a small plastic egg (about the size of a plastic Easter egg). The putty is the consistency of tough taffy, the size of an adult thumb, and it can be easily stretched.

Bouncy Balls. Bouncy balls are used to teach bouncing. Bouncy balls come in many different colors and may be purchased at most toy stores and party stores and from candy or bubblegum dispensers for approximately 25 cents. A bouncy ball is typically the size of a golf ball or smaller and bounces high (much higher then a tennis ball) after being dropped on a hard surface.

Toy Eyeglasses. Toy eyeglasses are used to emphasize the importance of eye contact. Toy eyeglasses may be purchased at dollar stores, party stores, and toy stores and come in many designs and styles.

Mirrors. Handheld mirrors are used to help students identify, describe, and label primary and secondary stuttering behaviors.

Bubbles. Bubbles are used to demonstrate to students that stuttering gently, without pushing or struggling, is helpful for stuttering easily. Bubbles may be purchased at drugstores, party stores, toy stores, and dollar stores.

Abacus (children's size). Caggiano has noted that an abacus is an excellent demonstration tool for teaching students the concept of pausing (L. Caggiano, personal communication, March, 14, 2004). An abacus, also known as a Chinese calculator, is often used to teach beginning math skills and may be purchased at toy stores and teacher supply stores. Whereas an adult's abacus may be as small as a person's palm, a child's abacus is much larger and will not fit in a Stuttering Kit. A child's abacus features easily movable colored beads and is usually made of wood.

Deciding Which Speech Tools Are for Which Students

If a student does not respond well to all of the four speech tools, it is often wiser to focus on the ones that are proving to be most effective and most successful. For example, if a student really enjoys using stretching to smooth-out of a stutter and enjoys bouncing much less, you may wish to focus on stretching while occasionally revisiting bouncing. This ensures that a student's individual needs are taken into account while also showing him that he has other options.

Ideally, it is best to expose students to all four speech tools and then to focus on the ones that prove to be the most helpful. There are, however, exceptions. For example, one fourth-grade student did not like using pausing, yet was able to use this technique quite effectively. This student stuttered on approximately 50% of the words he said and was often misunderstood by his classmates and teachers. On days in which his stuttering was very frustrating for him, I would say something like, "Avi, I know that you might not be crazy about using pausing, but let's practice it for a few minutes today while playing a game." Although I knew that Avi did not like using pausing, I also knew that when he did use pausing, his frustration level significantly decreased because his speech became much more intelligible. When working with Avi, I made a point to focus on stretching, a tool Avi wanted to use, while also practicing pausing, a tool I felt would offer him immediate relief.

Modeling All Assignments

You need to model all behaviors that you wish students to practice and use (Breitenfeldt & Lorenz, 2000; Ramig & Bennett, 1995; Walton & Wallace, 1998). You cannot expect students to stutter openly and use their speech tools if you are not willing to do the same. As Dell (2000) has pointed out, "We never make a child do anything that we haven't done first" (p. 40). You need to model stuttering and speech tools casually and frequently throughout the therapy process. It has been said that good clinicians stutter as much as their clients. You also should be willing to model and demonstrate any assignment; this ensures that the assignment is reasonable (Breitenfeldt & Lorenz, 2000). For example, if you assign students the task of stretching the first sound of a sentence while asking a question at a local store, you need to be the first to demonstrate this assignment in public for students to observe. If you are unwilling to use a speech tool in public, then how can a student feel safe doing so?

Some clinicians worry that their voluntary or modeled stuttering will not sound "real." A study using 40 graduate and undergraduate speech and hearing science students found that listeners were not able to distinguish between real or authentic stuttering and simulated stuttering (Fucci, Leach, Mckenzie, & Gonzales, 1998). Rest assured that your modeled stuttering *will* sound real. When using voluntary stuttering, never say to the person you are speaking with, "I really don't stutter; I am just using fake stuttering." Doing so sends the message to students that stuttering is something in need of an apology. Never apologize for stuttering or for using voluntary stuttering.

Taking a Break from Speech Tools

During therapy give students breaks from using and practicing speech tools. Speech tools help students reduce the severity and frequency of their struggle but are only one element of a comprehensive treatment approach that emphasizes exploring, talking about, and learning about stuttering.

There will be many speech sessions in which you will want to focus on learning and talking about stuttering without focusing on speech tools. For example, if I am spending one or more speech classes helping students search the Internet for stuttering-related information, our focus will not be to practice speech tools.

By having breaks students may begin comparing speaking while using speech tools to speaking without tools. They begin to see that using speech tools actually makes a difference. Also, using speech tools often takes a lot of mental and physical effort. Taking breaks helps to ensure that speech class stays fun and enjoyable, and you can show students that their clinician is not a sergeant constantly drilling them.

There are several ways to take breaks from speech tools. You may start class by not using speech tools for 5 to 10 minutes and then focus on tools for the next 5 to 10 minutes. At other times you may go without using speech tools for one session or even several sessions. During these sessions, therapy should focus on identifying, learning about, and discussing stuttering.

Recognizing That Speech Tools Are Not a Cure

Many clinicians discuss speaking strategies with other professionals and students as if they were 100% effective and foolproof. Remember that *sometimes children are just going to stutter.* By presenting speech tools as infallible, the clinician makes the mistake of creating a situation in which when the child stutters, it is her fault because she did not try hard enough. Speech tools are not perfect, and stutterers cannot or should not be expected to use them all the time. You need to present speech tools as helpful skills that offer children options to manage their stuttering; never present speech tools as a perfect solution to solve stuttering.

Although many students will be motivated to practice their speech tools, some express frustration when they are not able to use their tools as well as they would like. It is common for stutterers to tell their clinician that, at times, it is easier to stutter than it is to use speech tools. One stutterer explained:

> I do utilize some of the techniques I have learned in therapy, but many times it's just too much to think about. It's a lot of work to think about what I want to say, how to say it, and then to put it all together. (Klumb, 2002, p. 7)

It is not rare for a student to say, "Sometimes my speech tools don't work." If a student mentions this, be pleased that he trusts you enough to be honest and is open to seeking guidance. The student's feelings need to be validated. For example, say, "I understand that you are very frustrated because your speech tools do not always work. Sometimes no matter how hard you practice and work, you still stutter, and that is okay."

Treating Secondary Stuttering Behaviors

When stutterers stop avoiding and hiding stuttering, secondary behaviors such as eye blinking, foot tapping, and nasal snorting tend to go away by themselves. Instead of asking or encouraging stutterers to stop using secondary behaviors or "tricks," you need to offer students better options for managing their stuttering. Speech tools demonstrate to students that there are productive ways to move forward with their speech.

Secondary behaviors are the result of trying to avoid, postpone, or escape from moments of stuttering. Once stuttering is not only allowed but encouraged, and once a student has productive ways to move through moments of stuttering, there is no reason for the student to continue swinging her arms or blinking her eyes. Secondary behaviors typically go away, or are greatly reduced, once the stutterer begins stuttering openly and using productive tools to move forward through difficult speaking situations. An adult explained:

> I do not even work on "getting rid" of my stuttering but mainly focus on stuttering in a relaxed forward-moving pattern. The idea is to navigate around those hard blocks and stutter easily, without much effort. The secondaries melt away when I am able to do this. (Troiano, 2004, para. 2)

I once worked with a student whose mother was extremely concerned about his frequent eye blinking. This student was diagnosed by his pediatrician as being nervous and as having unusually large eyelashes. Even though the doctor never tried to cut this child's eyelashes, the doctor was convinced that the eyelashes were the root of his eye-blinking behavior. I explained to the mother that the eye blinking was probably a reaction her son was having to his stuttering and that he was using it both to avoid and to "break free" from moments of stuttering. After a year in speech therapy, the eye blinking stopped, and the mother asked me how this happened. I explained that by offering her son a better way to control his stuttering, he no longer needed to blink his eyes.

Activities in this book, such as Stuttering Private Eye–Activity 7, encourage students to describe their primary as well as their secondary stuttering behaviors. This allows them to become aware of the effort and struggle they put into avoiding stuttering.

Preventing Speech Tools from Becoming Secondary Behaviors

A speech tool, if used correctly, is a strategy or skill that reduces the struggle and avoidance behaviors inherent in stuttering. However, if a speech tool is used and practiced incorrectly, it has the potential to become a secondary behavior. For example, I worked with an eighth-grader who was taught as a young girl to smoothly stretch her speech during moments of stuttering. She was shown to clasp her hands together and to slowly pull her hands apart while simultaneously prolonging her speech. Although this clasping and pulling of the hands may serve well as a demonstration tool to be used initially or occasionally in therapy, this child believed that she was supposed to incorporate these hand movements permanently into her speech. The hand movements were never phased out. This student was taught to rely on extra behaviors and movements that only added to her stuttering problem.

When I use Silly Putty, bouncy balls, or other props to demonstrate speech tools, I make a point of referring to these props as "training wheels." I explain to students that once they "get the hang of" how to use speech tools, it is time to "take the training wheels off." It is important to explain to students that the props are only a demonstration tool. For example, after showing students the concept of stretching while using Silly Putty, I put the prop away and explain, "We should be stretching only with our mouths now."

The ultimate goal of speech tools is to lessen the struggle of stuttering by reducing extraneous movements and behaviors. Although you need to teach tools and strategies that are aimed at decreasing struggle behaviors, you also need to monitor students closely to ensure that they do not use speech tools in unproductive ways. When a stuttering tool is used in a way that makes stuttering grow and become more debilitating, it is in fact functioning as a secondary. Make sure that any speaking tool or strategy taught is used productively to lessen the struggle of stuttering.

Using Stuttering Inducers

Just as conditions such as talking in unison and singing often increase fluency or prohibit stuttering, many conditions trigger stuttering. At times you may want to introduce what Conture (2001) referred to as "barbs" or "fluency inhibitors" to trigger or precipitate moments of stuttering (p. 230). These stuttering triggers include asking students to repeat themselves, speak faster, tell jokes, and tell complicated stories. You may also trigger stuttering by interrupting students, creating challenging expressive language demands, hurrying or rushing the speaker, and turning or looking away from students while they are speaking.

You may wish to trigger stuttering to challenge students to use their speech tools. For example, there are many times during therapy when a student may stutter very little or not at all. This is a good time to gently challenge the student's ability to stay in control of his speech by including several stuttering triggers. Do so by initiating a conversation in which the student is asked to use a speech tool such as a stretch-out to move forward through moments of stuttering. Then introduce a stuttering trigger, such as pretending not to hear a student. You may say, "I'm sorry, I didn't catch that. Please say it again." In this example, because the student is asked to repeat himself, there is a good likelihood that he will stutter when responding. This provides the student with an ideal opportunity to use the assigned speech tool.

As mentioned earlier, formulating and organizing language often leads to increased stuttering behaviors. You may ask a student to complete a task that is linguistically challenging for him, such as explaining the plot of a favorite movie. When the student is faced with a moment of stuttering, ask him to stretch-out or bounce-out of the block. Nippold (2004b) has pointed out that clinicians may consider increasing the difficulty of conversational tasks while students work on fluency strategies. She explained, "Once the client is ready, the clinician should determine how much challenge can be tolerated. This means that the client should experience successful communication most of the time" (p. 41). Nippold explained that for some children who stutter, conversing with unfamiliar speaking partners is more likely to trigger stuttering than speaking with familiar partners. She stated that discussing unfamiliar topics is more likely to cause moments of stuttering than discussing familiar topics.

I recall my own speech therapy in which my clinician would occasionally look away from me while I was talking, or he would pretend to occupy himself with paperwork as I spoke. By doing so he was purposefully creating situations in which I was more likely to stutter. Because speech tools are most difficult to use when they are most needed (Starkweather & Givens-Ackerman, 1997), the clinician was wise to challenge me to use them during stuttering inducing situations. The King of Pausing–Activity 22 is one example of how clinicians may use stuttering triggers during therapy.

Helpful Tips for Communicating with Children Who Stutter

It is important to remember that your style of speaking and listening may have an effect on your students' speech and stuttering. Schneider has suggested that clinicians make attempts to speak with "an energy level (loudness, tempo, animation, and complexity) that is lower than the child's" (P. Schneider, personal communication, March 1, 2005). One way to achieve this is to focus on speaking with a reduced rate, a soft and gentle voice, and a calm demeanor. When students ask you a question, pause briefly before responding. This helps to control the rate of the conversation and of the entire session. In response to this style of speaking, students typically show a corresponding decrease in struggle behaviors. Also by speaking in such a style, Schneider has noted that you make it clear to your students that you are available to listen.

Taking New Skills into the Real World

Successful therapy focuses on helping the student function outside of the therapy room. The therapy room is a familiar environment in which students grow to feel safe when discussing stuttering and working on their speech. Children need to be able to talk about stuttering outside of the therapy room with family members, teachers, and friends. Speech tools learned within the safe confines of the therapy room need to be regularly practiced in real-life situations, such as classrooms, homes, and public places. It may never occur to children to use their speech tools outside of the therapy room if you do not lead the way.

In this book speaking strategies and activities that help students talk openly about stuttering are first worked on in the therapy room and then transferred to more challenging environments. For example, in Stuttering Interviews–Activity 30, students practice interviewing each other about stuttering in the therapy room before interviewing others, such as parents and school staff members. Students practice using speech tools first in the therapy room before doing so in public locations, such as stores and local establishments.

Stuttering Is Hard Work

This is a phrase that I heard often while working as a student clinician at the Successful Stuttering Management Program (SSMP) in Salt Lake City, Utah. Although you do not want to push children who stutter too hard, bear in mind that being a stutterer is hard and changing how one stutters is also hard. Speech therapy needs to be fun for school-age children, but it cannot always be easy because being a stutterer is not easy. Because stuttering is often difficult, you must be able to gently push and challenge children when they are scared of trying activities, such as talking about stuttering, voluntary stuttering, or speaking in front of a class. Manning (1999b) wrote, "We must nudge them [young people who stutter] every so often and force them to extend, both physically and mentally, well beyond the limit they have come to expect for themselves" (p. 162). Starkweather (2002) noted, "Therapy is not all about making your clients feel good. Sometimes it is vital that they feel uncomfortable, afraid, embarrassed, sad, or angry. Therapy consists of providing support and challenge. Support should always come first" (para. 4).

Choosing Your Terminology

To help counteract and reverse the negative feelings that often coincide with stuttering, you need to consistently use positive language and positive terminology to describe stuttering. For example, instead of saying, "Michael stutters badly," say, "Michael stutters well." Using positive terminology helps to "de-awfulize" and normalize stuttering by creating a productive, safe, and stutter-friendly environment.

Shapiro (1999) explained, "How we talk with children, particularly children who stutter, is critically important to helping children establish or maintain positive feelings about communication and themselves" (p. 331). Manning (1996) pointed out, "By changing the way we describe a problem, we can often change the problem itself" (p. 195). Starkweather and Givens-Ackerman (1997) have noted, "Language can be a window through which the clinician can model an attitude toward the disorder that is nonavoidant and unafraid" (p. 8).

Below is a discussion concerning some commonly used terms in the field of speech–language pathology. This discussion will guide you in carefully considering your use of language when working with children who stutter, their families, and teachers.

Stuttering Badly Versus Stuttering Well

Many people who stutter and many speech–language pathologists are beginning to replace the expression *stuttering badly* with *stuttering well.* Although some people who stutter, teachers, and parents may describe a moment of stuttering by saying, "That sure was a bad stutter," you may chime back, "That sure was a good stutter" (Donaher, 2003a, p. 1). Terminology should always lean toward the positive. There is nothing to be gained by describing stuttering as "bad." Using positive terms, such as stuttering well, creates a situation in which stuttering is not punitive and may be worked on openly, without shame.

Stuttering Mildly, Moderately, and Severely

Using terms such as *mild, moderate,* or *severe* with parents and teachers does little to describe how the disorder affects a child and may only confuse the matter. For example, I worked with a fourth-grader who used several avoidance strategies—often speaking in a whisper to avoid stuttering and frequently substituting words and using circumlocutions. Referring to this child as a mild stutterer because she could seldom be heard to stutter would not have acknowledged the constant fear and stress this child felt surrounding speaking situations. Instead of using a label to categorize this student, I sat down with the teacher and mother to fully explain the grip that stuttering had taken on this girl's ability to speak openly and freely.

Manning (2000) pointed out, "Speakers who substitute words, circumlocute portions of sentences, or avoid words and speaking situations may be stuttering severely but simply do not demonstrate their problem in an overt manner" (p. 132). There are people who stutter who are considered by many to be severe stutterers, yet their speech is only a minor inconvenience to them. Luper & Mulder (1964) wrote:

> It is well to remember that the amount of stuttering a child displays may not correlate with his feelings about it. A child may show only little stuttering and be deeply concerned, or he may have speech that is marked by frequent moments of stuttering and only be intrigued—not disturbed by the way he sounds. (pp. 89–90)

Instead of describing a person who stutters or moments of stuttering as mild, moderate, or severe, use terminology and language that precisely describes the stuttering. For example, instead of saying, "Lisa stutters severely" or "Lisa stutters badly," say, "Lisa stutters frequently, often for a full second or more in duration, with concomitant secondaries including eye blinking, tongue thrusting, and open mouth blocks."

Fluency, Disfluency, Dysfluency, and Stuttering

In general, *fluency* is used to indicate smooth, nonstruggled, forward-moving speech in relation to both its production and content; fluency is perceived as nondisordered, nonstuttered speech (Starkweather, 1987). *Disfluency* is used to describe the normal speech disruptions that most speakers, including stutterers, demonstrate, and *dysfluency* is used to describe atypical, stuttered speech disruptions.

I advocate using the terms fluency, disfluency, and dysfluency as infrequently as possible. Teachers, parents, school administrators, and students often become confused when the term fluency is used to describe stuttering behaviors. Often causing this confusion is the fact that the term fluency is widely used throughout educational systems to describe a child's level of reading proficiency. Some teachers, other professionals, and parents believe that there is a direct link between stuttering and reading ability. For example, one third-grade teacher I worked with was certain that her student's stuttering was caused by his inability to read fluently. This teacher was convinced that as soon as the student could read at his grade level, the stuttering would disappear. By using the terms fluency, disfluency, and dysfluency, you risk strengthening the misperceptions surrounding reading and stuttering.

In schools with high English-as-a-Second-Language (ESL) populations, the term fluency is used to describe a child's level of English language proficiency. Using the term fluency to describe stuttering behaviors risks confusing the matter with ESL issues.

Additionally, by using the term fluency, you risk setting the child up for unrealistic goals, frustration, and failure. For example, at a stuttering workshop I once heard a mother say to her son, "If you work hard, then one day you can be a fluent speaker." What the child undoubtedly heard was, "If you work hard then one day you will not stutter."

Many clinicians and parents are fearful of using the term *stuttering*. They often believe that by saying the word stutter they would somehow be hurting the child. By avoiding the term stuttering and using dysfluency in its place, clinicians and families may be unintentionally demonstrating to children that stuttering is shameful and to be avoided and feared. If the only people who use the term stuttering are teasers and bullies, then people who stutter will grow to regard stuttering as shameful. Starkweather and Givens-Ackerman (1997) warn:

> Children who grow up with a stuttering problem in a family where the problem is not mentioned come to believe that it is an unspeakable thing. This categorizes stuttering with topics such as bathroom behavior or sex, which are genuinely private matters. Stuttering does not belong in such a category. (p. 113)

Because the terms fluency, disfluency, and dysfluency are prevalent in the stuttering community and in speech–language pathology, they should not and cannot be ignored. It is certainly appropriate to use these terms if doing so helps to explain stuttering, but make a point to use the term stuttering.

In general, I use the term stuttering to describe moments of stuttering, and I also use the term stuttering to describe avoiding stuttering. For example, if a student shares a story in which he did not raise his hand in class because of his fear of stuttering, I would describe this as avoiding stuttering. When a student uses a speech tool such as stretching to stretch-out of a stutter, I refer to this as smooth stuttering, not as fluent speech.

One fourth-grade student often referred to her stuttering as her "mouth traffic." She explained that stuttering made her feel like her mouth was stuck in a long traffic jam. In this situation the student was not avoiding talking about stuttering but had simply found a term that she felt was more descriptive. Many younger children, such as those in the first or second grades, may probably not understand the term stuttering. One first grader used the terms *bumps* and *sticks* to describe his own stuttering (see Tatarniuk, 1998). Other children may refer to their *sticky speech* or *bumpy talk.* The point is, *talk openly about stuttering* and avoid using euphemisms and nondescriptive terms, such as dysfluency. If a child is too young to understand the term stuttering, help her generate her own labels and descriptors. Several activities in this book focus on these goals.

Stutterer Versus Person Who Stutters

Within the stuttering community there is a fierce debate that is frequently repeated and expanded upon but never settled. Some people who stutter speak of themselves as *stutterers,* whereas others like being referred to as *people who stutter* or the acronym PWS (the acronym CWS is used for *children who stutter*). Some even use a creative solution such as *people living with stuttering.*

The term stutterer is viewed by some to be offensive, distasteful, or inappropriate because they view people who stutter as much more than disordered people. Shapiro (1999) wrote, "Referring to a person as a stutterer establishes that the disorder captures the essence of the person" (p. 15).

Due to the combined efforts of the self-help movement, supportive friends and relatives, and speech therapy, many have come to view the term stutterer to signify a positive and active engagement of stuttering. Some of its proponents use the term stutterer because they believe that you cannot work on a problem until you admit to having a problem.

Starkweather and Givens-Ackerman (1997) explain that the term person who stutters and the acronym PWS are viewed by some stutterers as "a kind of euphemism—a softening of the harsh reality of the disorder and, as such, a form of avoidance that does not serve the person well" (p. 8). In a detailed study St. Louis (1999) found that using the term people who stutter over stutterer or stammerer did not reduce, in any way, negative beliefs held by the public toward the disorder of stuttering.

Most importantly, when working with stutterers, choose terminology based on the needs and sensitivities of your clients. For example, when working with a 5-year-old kindergarten student, the terms stutterer or person who stutters may mean nothing to the child, and the terms bouncy or bumpy speech may be more conducive for initiating discussion of the child's behaviors. When working with a teen or adult who has decided that the term stutterer makes them feel empowered and strong, it would be inappropriate to use the term person who stutters with this person. When working with a family that is accustomed to using the term stutterer instead of person who stutters, it may be inappropriate to try to change their choice of terminology. Such a recommendation by the clinician may unintentionally suggest to parents that using the term stutterer over person who stutters in some way has harmed their child. For the purposes of this book, both the terms person who stutters and stutterer are used.

Writing IEP Goals

Below is a sample list of goals that you may use as a reference for your own goal writing. Goals are listed under the activity section to which they pertain. You will need to individualize these goals for your students. In the Targeting Language and Stuttering Goals section, only examples of stuttering goals are listed. For the sake of brevity, no language goals were included.

There is an extra section of goals titled "Participating in Speech Class with Other Children Who Stutter." This section was included because there are many children who stutter who attend speech therapy who have not had the opportunity to work with other children who stutter. By including goals from this section on a child's Individualized Educational Program, you are requiring that a child who stutters interact several times a year with other children who stutter. This requires clinicians to talk to schools or clinics in their area to schedule intervisitations with other children who stutter.

Identifying and Exploring Stuttering

Student will

- Identify primary and secondary stuttering behaviors, in clinician-modeled stuttering, with 80% accuracy.

- Identify moments of stuttering in himself or herself with 80% accuracy.
- Identify the point of constriction during moments of stuttering (such as lips or vocal folds) with 80% accuracy.
- Identify his or her own feared sounds and words with 80% accuracy.
- Identify his or her own 3 feared speaking situations with 80% accuracy.
- Identify 3 ways in which he or she avoids stuttering.

Practicing Speech Tools

Student will

- Identify clinician-modeled speech tools (stretching, bouncing, pausing, voluntary stuttering) with 80% accuracy.
- Stretch (or bounce) on the first sounds of targeted words with 80% accuracy.
- Stretch-out (or bounce-out) of moments of stuttering, during 5-minute conversations, with 80% accuracy.
- Use the voluntary stuttering speech tool on targeted words, in the therapy room, with 80% accuracy.
- Use voluntary stuttering during role-playing situations, in the therapy room, with 80% accuracy.
- Use voluntary stuttering on targeted words in public by voluntarily stuttering, holding the stutter, and then bouncing-out of the stutter, 3 times during the school year, with 80% accuracy.
- Pause after the first word in a sentence, for 5-minute intervals, with 80% accuracy.
- Use pausing (or another speech tool) during 3 stuttering interviews with 80% accuracy.
- Explain and demonstrate speech tools to speech class guests, on 3 occasions, with 80% accuracy.
- Practice stretching the first word of every sentence, when talking on the phone with a speech class partner, for 5 minutes.
- Identify moments of poor eye contact during conversation with the clinician, for 5-minute intervals, with 80% accuracy.

Learning the Facts

Student will

- Demonstrate comprehension of 8 facts about stuttering with 80% accuracy.
- Name 5 famous people who stutter, and 2 facts about each person, with 80% accuracy.
- Research a famous person who stutters and write a one-paragraph summary about this person.
- Research stuttering and explain 5 facts or opinions about stuttering, with 80% accuracy.
- Research 2 theories of the cause of stuttering and present these 2 theories in speech class (or other classes).
- Research 2 organizations dedicated to stuttering and present information about these organizations to speech class (or other classes).

Uncovering Feelings

Student will

- Participate in 3 stuttering plays during the school year.
- Write a stuttering play to express a personal stuttering experience.
- Write 1 stuttering story and 1 stuttering poem describing personal stuttering experiences, and then read these works to the class or to guests for discussion.
- Complete 5 stuttering interviews during the school year with teachers, staff members, neighbors, or relatives, and review these during speech class.
- Write a stuttering letter to inform a teacher about 3 general facts about stuttering and 3 specific facts about student's own stuttering, with 80% accuracy.
- Show his or her drawing about what stuttering feels like to speech class guests and discuss how the drawing relates to stuttering, on 2 occasions.
- Invite guests to speech class to participate in stuttering plays, followed by a discussion on teasing, on 2 occasions.
- Read 2 Dear Abby stuttering questions and discuss how he or she feels about the difficulties people who stutter faced in these situations.

- Read his or her own stuttering story or stuttering poem to a relative, teacher, or staff member and discuss it.
- Discuss 5 stuttering questions with peers and guests during the school year.
- Write one Dear Abby question asking others for advice and present it to speech class.

Targeting Language and Stuttering Goals

Student will

- Use pausing during joke telling after the first word in every sentence, with 80% accuracy.
- Use stretching (or bouncing), on the first word of the punch line of a joke, with 80% accuracy.
- Practice voluntary stuttering during the activity 20 Questions, by stuttering on targeted words, with 80% accuracy.
- Bounce-out (or stretch-out) of moments of stuttering when playing the activity Barrier Games, with 80% accuracy.

Participating in Speech Class with Other Children Who Stutter

Student will

- Participate in speech class activities with other children who stutter at least 3 times during the school year.
- Share a stuttering poem and a stuttering story with another child who stutters.
- Teach stretching, bouncing, and pausing to 2 different children who stutter and answer their questions about these tools.
- Write a stuttering play with another child who stutters and act out the play during therapy.
- Choose one speech class activity to teach another child who stutters.
- Complete 3 homework assignments that involve calling another student who stutters.
- Write 3 questions to ask a child or adult who stutters about that person's stuttering, and present these questions during therapy to that child or adult who stutters.

- Practice voluntary stuttering, with one or more children who stutter, in the therapy room.
- Practice voluntary stuttering, with one or more children who stutter, during a role-playing activity.
- Practice voluntary stuttering, with one or more children who stutter, in public.

Using the Activities

You are now ready to begin using the 50 therapy activities to meet the needs of your students. This section will guide you in using the activities and the therapy approach that are the focus of this book.

From the onset of therapy, each student should have an easily accessible speech file or folder to hold his completed work. The file will allow you to review completed assignments and assess student progress and growth. Speech files will become particularly important during activities such as creating bulletin boards and newsletters about stuttering (see Big News–Activity 36 and Post It–Activity 37), which require students to use previously completed assignments.

A Description of the Activities

The activities are grouped into five sections. They are as follows:

- Identifying and Exploring Stuttering
- Practicing Speech Tools
- Learning the Facts
- Uncovering Feelings
- Targeting Language and Stuttering Goals

Identifying and Exploring Stuttering

In this section activities are offered that help students identify and explore many aspects of their stuttering, including when and how they stutter; primary and secondary stuttering behaviors; articulator placement during moments of stuttering; and feared sounds, words, and speaking situations. For example, in Stutter Tag–Activity 1, you model moments of stuttering for the students. They compete to be the first to identify a moment of stuttering by raising their hands. Students are then called upon to identify the word stuttered on. During several activities in this section, students are given opportunities to create self-generated labels for stuttering behaviors. For example, instead of referring to a moment of stuttering as a "repetition," the student may call it bumpy speech or sticky speech. These self-generated labels are just one way that children begin to actively engage stuttering. As with all the lessons in this book, the activities in this section also help reduce the shame of stuttering while promoting trust in you and camaraderie among peers.

Practicing Speech Tools

In this section students learn and practice four speech tools: stretching, bouncing, voluntary stuttering, and pausing. These tools help students stutter with less struggle and stutter less often. Students also use voluntary stuttering to help reduce their fears of stuttering. Students practice speech tools in a hierarchical fashion—first in the therapy room; then during role-playing situations; and then in stressful situations, such as speaking in class or in a public location (i.e., a store or restaurant). Using appropriate eye contact is also taught in this section.

Learning the Facts

Most children know very little about stuttering or have only a vague idea of why they stutter (Williams, 2003). In this section children learn basic information and facts about stuttering. These activities educate students about stuttering so that the disorder becomes normalized, "de-awfulized," and demystified (see Dell, 1993; Murphy, 1996, 1999, 2000; Ramig & Bennet, 1995). For example, in Famous Role Models–Activity 6, students research famous people who stutter, such as James Earl Jones and Marilyn Monroe, and then create a poster giving some highlights of their lives. By learning about successful people who stutter, children grow to understand that they may also be successful and talented people who stutter. Students display the stuttering poster in a school cafeteria or classroom to advertise their stuttering and to educate others about stuttering.

Uncovering Feelings

Stutterers hold numerous negative feelings and self-perceptions about stuttering. Many speech–language pathologists believe that these negative feelings are a major factor that maintains the disorder. Some authorities on stuttering believe that working on attitudes is the most important component of speech therapy. The activities in this section help students express how they feel about stuttering; discuss stuttering openly with their peers, teachers, and family; and consider productive responses to teasing and bullying situations. The activities also help students feel that they are not alone or isolated with their stuttering. For example, in Stuttering Interviews–Activity 30, students interview friends, teachers, and family members about stuttering by asking questions such as, "What do you think causes stuttering?" and "Do you feel that stutterers could be classroom teachers?" This activity opens up dialogue about stuttering with people students come into regular contact with and demonstrates to all involved that talking about stuttering is not only acceptable but also beneficial. By focusing on feelings and emotions about stuttering, students are often more able and more willing to work directly on speaking strategies.

Targeting Language and Stuttering Goals

Because of high caseloads and other conditions facing speech–language pathologists in the schools, clinicians frequently group students who stutter with children with other speech and language disorders. This section offers activities that focus on the needs of students who stutter and on the needs of students with receptive, expressive, and pragmatic language difficulties. For example, when making ice cream during Verbal Sequencing–Activity 46, students who stutter practice using speech tools while also being open about their stuttering with nonstuttering peers. At the same time children with language difficulties may work on a vast array of language goals, such as turn-taking skills, sequencing and organizing information, speaking in complete sentences, and learning and using new vocabulary. Children who stutter with concomitant language difficulties will benefit from both the stuttering and language goals of these activities.

Activities Offer Multiple Goals

Although each activity has been placed into one of these five sections to indicate its primary purpose, most activities may be used for multiple purposes. For example, Famous Role Models–Activity 26 has been placed in the Learning the Facts section because it is used to help students learn about famous people who stutter. However, this activity requires open discussions about stuttering and would also fit in the Uncovering Feelings section. Stuttering Quiz–Activity 25 is placed in the Learning the Facts section. Stuttering quizzes also encourage students to identify various aspects of their own stuttering and may be used for identification goals as well. Many stories and poems about stuttering are included in Practicing Speech Tools as a means to help students practice their speech tools while reading. These stories and poems may also be used for discussion purposes and for learning about stuttering and could have easily been placed within other sections.

Using More Than One Activity During a Single Session

After becoming comfortable with the activities in this book, you will be able to use more than one activity, taken from different sections, in a single session. For example, one speech class may consist of the following:

- Review homework.
- Play a game of Stutter Tag–Activity 1, in which you model primary and secondary stuttering behaviors and students compete to be the first to raise their hands and identify how you are stuttering. (Identifying and Exploring Stuttering)
- Discuss one or more stories or poems from You Feel That Way Too?–Activity 31. (Uncovering Feelings)

- Have students practice speaking strategies, such as pausing or stretching, while telling the class about their weekend or other topic. (Practicing Speech Tools)
- Assign new homework.

Where To Start in Speech Therapy

Some speech–language pathologists suggest beginning therapy by targeting the greatest need of the client. Others begin where they believe the client will have the most success. When considering where to start therapy and what activities to use, ask yourself the following ten questions:

1. What are my client's greatest needs at this time?
2. What are the major maintaining factors affecting my client's stuttering?
3. To what level is my client aware of her stuttering?
4. To what level is my client willing or able to discuss stuttering?
5. To what level is my client impaired by her overt stuttering behaviors?
6. To what level is my client impaired by her avoidance behaviors?
7. How much does my client know about stuttering?
8. Is teasing and bullying a major component in my client's stuttering problem?
9. What kinds of tools is my client currently using to manage stuttering?
10. What kinds of "tricks" is my client using to manage or avoid stuttering?

If a student demonstrates very little awareness of her stuttering, you will want to begin with activities in the Identifying and Exploring Stuttering section. If a student has been in speech therapy for several years and is aware of much of her overt stuttering, you may begin therapy by targeting several simultaneous goals that include speech tools, learning about stuttering, and talking about feelings. If a student demonstrates little difficulty identifying stuttering behaviors and little difficulty discussing feelings and stuttering openly, you may wish to concentrate on speech tools and learning about stuttering.

It is important to expose students to the four speech tools (stretching, bouncing, voluntary stuttering, and pausing) as early as possible in the therapy process. Though speech tools are not the most important aspect of therapy, by covering these tools early, the student will be able to practice them during many other activities and assignments, such as Barrier Games–Activity 41, Let's Talk–Activity 42, and Joke Telling–Activity 44.

Occasionally you may focus on an area that does not appear to be the student's primary concern. For example, some students who stutter are teased often, whereas others are teased very little or not at all. You want to focus on teasing issues if this is a concern for an individual student. However, it is worth noting that some children consistently report that they are not teased about stuttering, only to reveal later in therapy that they really are the target of teasers and bullies. Even if students report that they are not teased about stuttering, you may wish to occasionally focus on activities such as Dear Abby–Activity 34 or It's Showtime–Activity 32 that discuss teasing. This way you are giving students the opportunity to talk about an issue that often brings with it feelings of shame and guilt.

Homework

Reproducible homework assignments are presented at the end of many of the activities in this book. These assignments may be used as actual homework or as additional speech class activities. It is suggested that after you make photocopies of each homework handout, you cut apart the individual assignments so that you may hand students a single assignment.

Review each assignment with students before they take them home so that they understand what is expected. Never give homework without reviewing and discussing it—doing so only sends the message that the work was unimportant. Homework assignments may be assigned more than once if you feel they remain productive and fun for students. Use the reproducible Stuttering Homework form in Appendix A to create your own assignments.

Some of the assignments ask students to write down ways in which they stutter. For example, one of the assignments from Stutter Tag–Activity 1 states, "Remember five words that you stuttered on today. Write them below." For assignments such as this one, suggest that students carry the homework and a pencil throughout the day so they are prepared to write down answers.

Assigning too much homework is counterproductive because it takes the fun out of going to speech class. You may wish to give one homework assignment after every session with occasional breaks from homework as a reward. If you work with a child only once a week, you may wish to give two homework assignments at a time; one assignment could reinforce the current speech class activity, whereas the second assignment could review a skill or topic covered in a past activity.

Some students will enjoy "extra" or "bonus" assignments. Try handing out one mandatory and one optional assignment. For completing an optional assignment, you may give students a special reward such as a sticker or points toward an activity of the student's choice.

Each homework assignment has a line for a parent signature. This is one way to encourage parents to participate in their child's speech therapy. Bear in mind that every student brings with them different levels of parental or familial support. Some parents will participate in every homework assignment and sit with students every night to make certain that the homework is completed. Other students have erratic home lives and homework is never completed and is a low priority. You certainly should not reward students who are capable of doing their homework but simply neglect doing so. But on the other hand, do not punish children for incomplete homework when it is beyond their control.

Part 2

50 Great Activities: How-To, Handouts, and Homework

Identifying and Exploring Stuttering

Stutterers do not always know when or how they are stuttering. The activities in this section help students identify, describe, and define overt and covert aspects of stuttering. They also encourage students to begin talking about their stuttering in an open, casual, and honest manner. Donaher (2003a) stated, "The significance of knowing when you are stuttering is extremely important, especially if you want to use techniques [tools] to modify the moments of stuttering" (p. 6). By helping children explore and identify how they stutter, the fears and the mysteries surrounding their stuttering are reduced.

Many school-age children have a low level of stuttering awareness because stuttering is an unpleasant experience (to say the least), and they want to quickly move past a moment of stuttering without analyzing and reflecting upon it. An important aspect of lessening the struggle of stuttering during therapy is for stutterers to allow themselves to stutter and then to stay in the moment and analyze the stuttering (Breitenfeldt & Lorenz, 2000). After all, how can a stutterer change what he is doing if he is unaware of what he is doing? How can a person who stutters react differently if he is unaware of how he is currently reacting to stuttering? By assisting students in identifying and describing their stuttering, you are showing children that they may be objective and rational about a disorder that often evokes emotional and unproductive responses.

At the end of many activities in this section, homework assignments are provided. When appropriate, assignments are discussed so that you understand their purpose and use. Homework assignments are not mandatory. Only assign homework when you feel that the particular assignment meets the specific needs of a student. A reproducible blank Stuttering Homework form is included in Appendix A for writing your own homework assignments.

Note. Reproducible materials, such as homework and handouts, are located at the end of the description of an activity. However, reproducible materials that are used in more than one activity are included in the appendixes.

1

Stutter Tag

Purpose

- To identify moments of stuttering in the clinician, in peers, and in oneself, which will help students talk about and modify their stuttering later in therapy
- To engage stuttering in an open and fun manner

Materials

Scorecard (Appendix A)
Homework

Directions

Explain to students:

> I am going to talk about my weekend (or other recent event). While I am talking, I am going to stutter. When you hear me stutter, raise your hand. The first person to raise his hand gets a point. The person with the most points wins.

Students enjoy this activity and are often amazed that their clinician can also stutter (by doing so on purpose). In describing a similar stuttering identification game called "Catch Me," Dell (2000) wrote, "Children love this, for nothing is more delightful for a child than to be able to correct [catch] the adult" (p. 36). (See Donaher, 2001, for similar activities.) Use the scorecard (photocopy and save the original), because students like to compete during this game. Keep score by putting a check mark in a child's box when he is first to identify a moment of stuttering.

If a child (we will call him "Brian") is not able to earn points, try to help him be successful. A second or 2 before modeling stuttering, direct your eye contact toward Brian. This visual cue alerts him to listen and be ready—thus giving him an advantage and an opportunity for success. If this does not work, try a more direct approach. Say, "I am going to try extra hard to trick Brian; on this turn no one else should raise his hand except Brian." Speak directly to Brian while making an obvious stutter, and when he raises his hand, give him a point and say, "Wow, I wasn't able to trick Brian."

A game of Stutter Tag may last as long as you feel is appropriate. For example, you may decide that the first child to earn 5 points is the winner, or, if you feel that students are enjoying themselves and would benefit from more practice, you could decide that the first child to earn 20 points is the winner.

After you have played one or two games of Stutter Tag, let students take turns stuttering and keeping score. Most students will want to lead the game and will easily begin using voluntary stuttering. Note that at no time do you have to announce or explain that students are using voluntary or fake stuttering. They are simply playing a game in which they have to stutter on purpose. Although there is nothing wrong with explaining these terms to the students, during the early phase of therapy, it is advisable to limit the explanations and to teach by example. You may go into more detail about the purpose of voluntary stuttering during the speech tools activities that are presented later in the book.

When the student leading the game experiences real stuttering during this activity, be sure to include these moments in the game. For example, when a student is talking and stutters for real on the word *ball,* make sure that the leader gives a point to the first person who raises his hand. Keep in mind that it is common for some students to stutter very little when they are expected to stutter. Do not be surprised if a student says, "Hey, it's actually hard to stutter right now." If this occurs, say, "Yes, isn't it interesting that when you do not mind stuttering and when you actually want to stutter, you stutter very little."

Some students may need additional support in identifying moments of stuttering. For example, one student I worked with was able to identify only about half of his own stutters. I realized that in his own mind he was defining stuttering as strictly prolongations and blocks. When he repeated whole words (i.e., "We, we, we, we, we went home"), he did not understand that these whole-word repetitions were also stuttering. To help him understand stuttering, I explained that most children who stutter do so in one of three ways. I then demonstrated repetitions, prolongations, and blocks. I also made a point of using children-friendly language during these demonstrations. I referred to prolongations as *stretchy talk,* blocks as *throaty talk,* and repetitions as *bouncy talk.*

Playing Stutter Tag is a good opportunity to include friends or siblings who do not stutter. This should be done carefully by only including guests who will not tease or laugh at stuttering. As long as the game is fun, students who do not stutter should not care that the game involves stuttering.

More Ideas

Play *Guess That Sound Stutter Tag.* As Stutter Tag progresses, begin to ask students to identify sounds on which they stuttered. For example, if the child stutters on the first sound in the word *dog,* ask, "What sound (or letter) did you just stutter on?" Now students are identifying not only when they stutter but what sounds and letters they are stuttering on.

Play the *Name Game* (Donaher, 2001, 2003b). This game helps students create their own vocabulary to describe stuttering behaviors, which enables them to more easily discuss stuttering. Instead of using standard terminology, such as *blocking* and *repetitions,* students are asked to create their own labels. For example, students may label a block as *sticky speech* and a repetition as *bumpy speech.* A group of students once had a healthy laugh when they recognized that some of them stuttered in a way that looked like a chicken eating. Students began to refer to this "head bobbing" secondary behavior as "the chicken dance."

Begin the Name Game by stuttering on purpose on the word "sssssssseven" in a prolonged fashion. Call on a student and ask, "What can we call the way I stuttered?" Students may respond in ways such as "a snake stutter," "a stretchy stutter," or "a slithery stutter." Then stutter again on "sssseven," but this time add a secondary behavior, such as head bobbing. When called upon, a student may say, "You did another snake stutter, and you also did the chicken dance."

Students will enjoy leading this game. Explain, "Now it is your turn to be the speech teacher, and I will be the student. You speak while stuttering, and I will have to come up with words to describe the way that you stutter." By allowing students to play the role of the clinician, you have the opportunity to demonstrate to students what is expected. For example, if a student stutters by saying "tea-tea-tea-team," you may say, "You just made a bouncy stutter" or "That was a great bumpy stutter."

Incorporate *eye contact.* Slightly increase the difficulty of the task and ask that while students stutter (during a moment of stuttering), they make eye contact with someone else in the speech class (Breitenfeldt & Lorenz, 2000). This way students are still playing a game that is a lot of fun and are also working on eye contact. Of course, you need to model this first by stuttering while making eye contact with each student.

Homework

The following homework assignments are meant to reinforce awareness of stuttering. Assign homework when you feel it is appropriate.

Stuttering 1 Homework

Name ______________________ Date due ____________

List five words that you often stutter on.

1. ____________ 2. ____________ 3. ____________

4. ____________ 5. ____________

Parent signature ______________________ (1)

Stuttering 1 Homework

Name ______________________ Date due ____________

Remember five words that you stuttered on today. Write them below.

1. ____________ 2. ____________ 3. ____________

4. ____________ 5. ____________

Parent signature ______________________ (2)

Stuttering 1 Homework

Name ______________________ Date due ____________

When do you stutter? Think of three times today that you stuttered and write them below. Try to include what you were doing and what word(s) you stuttered on.

Example: This morning during breakfast I stuttered on the word *milk*.

1. ____

2. ____

3. ____

Parent signature ______________________ (3)

2
Stuttering Awards

Purpose

- To desensitize students toward feeling shame about stuttering
- To promote trust, camaraderie, and friendship among students and the clinician
- To introduce the concept of easy stuttering

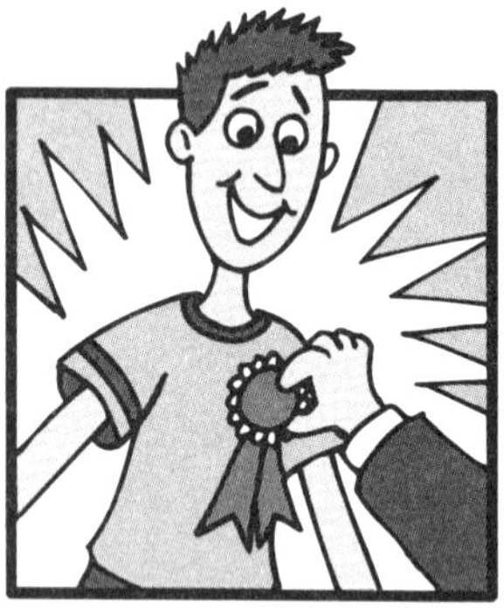

Materials

Stuttering awards (Appendix A)
Homework

Directions

Very few people are willing to discuss stuttering openly and honestly with children. One way to begin these open conversations and to help desensitize children to their fears and shame about stuttering is by giving students awards for stuttering (see Breitenfeldt & Lorenz, 2000; Murphy, 2003). By encouraging children to have fun and manipulate their stuttering for stuttering awards, students begin to understand that stuttering will not be punished or discouraged in any way. When students are asked to compete for stuttering awards, it is common for them to cheer and root for one another. By encouraging students to lengthen, shorten, bounce, increase their volume, and alter their stuttering in other ways, you are showing students that stuttering may be modified and made easier.

For this activity to be successful, you need to demonstrate excitement about stuttering. If you show students that "playing with" their stuttering is fun and normal, then students will easily participate. If you present this activity with apprehension and uncertainty, then students will react the same way.

Begin by holding up a photocopy of the Longest Stuttering Award and asking a student to read what it says. After a student reads the award, ask the class, "Who can give me the longest stutter?" Regardless of the amount of hands that are raised, say, "Wait, I'm the oldest, I'm gonna go first." Then say to one of your students, "Choose a good word for me to stutter on." If she says "dinosaur" then stutter on purpose by saying "ddddddddinosaur." Then energetically ask, "Who can give me a longer stutter on 'dinosaur'?" At this point, students smell competition in the air and are all raising their hands to try to give the longest stutter. After each student has had a turn, give out the Longest Stuttering Award to the child you feel deserves it or would benefit the most from receiving the first award. Students enjoy watching you write their names on the award and presenting the awards to them immediately.

Directly after working on long stuttering, take the chosen word (*dinosaur*) and model a shorter stutter than before by saying "ddddinosaur." Hold up a copy of the Shortest Stuttering Award and ask, "Can anyone make an even shorter stutter?" Now that their competitive juices are flowing, students eagerly modify their stuttering and volunteer to demonstrate a short stutter. This type of modification helps students start to gain control and power over their speech.

Try to move the class through as many stuttering awards as possible. You may want to spend more than one session on these awards and then return to them later in the therapy process. Some of the awards will require students to be creative. For example, once when working on the Coolest Stuttering Award, a third grader asked, "Just wait a minute—how can stuttering be cool?" At this point other students stood up and took rock star and rap star poses and began stuttering on their favorite song lyrics. Students quickly began to realize that stuttering can be cool and that stuttering is okay. It helps to work with a group of children during these awards so that students will want to be creative, imaginative, and competitive. If you do have a group, encourage your client to bring friends, classmates, or siblings.

The Loudest Stuttering Award is useful because so many stutterers lower their voices and try to hide their stuttering. This award encourages students to speak without hiding or minimizing their stuttering. Many times a student will shout out a word such as "ice cream" but will forget to stutter. You may smile and say, "That was great—but you forgot to stutter." Students laugh and realize that you can laugh and bond over stuttering.

The Best Bou-Bou-Bou-Bouncing Award is useful because it helps introduce students to easy stuttering (stuttering modification). Later in therapy when students are introduced to the stretching, bouncing, and pausing speech tools, you may motivate them by giving stuttering awards to help students practice these tools.

Some students are hesitant or ashamed to stutter in their first language. Stuttering awards that feature foreign languages, such as the best Spanish or best Chinese awards, make it clear that stuttering is allowed in any language or culture. Because Spanish is so prevalent, the Best Spanish Stuttering Award is included in Appendix A.

There is also a blank template that you may use to represent any language that your students speak. For example, if you work with children who speak Japanese, you may wish to create "The Best Japanese Stuttering Award" by simply writing in the words "Best Japanese" on the template. Some speech pathologists report that they are uncomfortable treating stutterers who come from culturally diverse backgrounds (Tellis & Tellis, 2003). Clinicians may find that using these "cultural" stuttering awards may open up conversations between the student, the family, and the clinician regarding different cultural issues and sensitivities. For example, one Puerto Rican student I worked with was hesitant to compete for the Best Spanish

Stuttering Award. It turns out that the student did not know the Spanish word for stuttering and felt that she was not supposed to stutter in Spanish. One way I was subsequently able to help this student was by introducing her to Spanish-speaking children and adults who stutter.

Other awards in Appendix A, such as the Strongest Stuttering Award and Weirdest Stuttering Award, are included because they are fun and offer students additional opportunities to play with and modify their stuttering.

Take every opportunity to help your students advertise (be forthcoming and open about) stuttering. After giving out the awards (and, of course, all students earn an award), students decorate the awards and hang them on the speech class walls, in the hallway, or in their classrooms so other students and teachers may see them.

When working individually with a student, create a situation in which you and the student engage in friendly competition. Most students will enjoy having this opportunity to compete with their clinician. Explain: "Today we are going to see who can win more stuttering awards, the teacher or the student. Let's see who can stutter better—me or you."

More Ideas

Design your own awards to meet the specific needs of individual students. You may easily design stuttering awards in any word-processing program or use the blank template available in Appendix A. Other awards might be the Best Rhyming Stuttering Award, the Best Rapping Stutterer, and the Best Rock Music Stuttering Award. During one speech class students began stuttering on the names of their favorite chocolate bars. During this activity one student commented in a joking manner that another student was the "whackest stutterer" (*whackest* is a popular slang term that usually means "uncool" or "the worst"). This was friendly banter that all the students enjoyed. Each student then attempted to demonstrate the whackest stutter. For the next speech class, I prepared the Best Chocolate Bar Stuttering Award and the Whackest Stuttering Award. Students eagerly competed for these awards and seemed pleased that their clinician was able to appreciate their humor and interests.

Homework

Assign the homework you feel will best meet the goals of your students. The first assignment asks students to teach their parents how to produce different types of stuttering. You may wish to contact the parents beforehand and explain that they should participate in a fun and lighthearted way. Or better yet, to prepare parents for this assignment, invite them to speech class to demonstrate how calmly and openly you and your students talk about and work on stuttering.

Stuttering (2) Homework

Name ______________________ Date due ______________

Take home your stuttering award and show it to your parents. If you won the Longest Stuttering Award, teach your parents how to make a long stutter. Teach your parents all of the awards you can remember from class, such as the longest, shortest, loudest, bounciest, and strongest stutters. See who can stutter better, you or your parents!

Parent signature ______________________ (1)

- - - - - - - - - - - - - - - - - - -

Stuttering (2) Homework

Name ______________________ Date due ______________

Think of three ideas that you have for your own stuttering awards. For example, one kind of stuttering award we did not practice in class is the Best Rapping Stutter. Write down your three suggestions for stuttering awards below.

1. ______________________________________
2. ______________________________________
3. ______________________________________

Parent signature ______________________ (2)

3
Stuttering Bingo

Purpose:

- To identify the particular sounds stuttered on in the clinician, in peers, and in oneself
- To identify the manner and place of articulation of stuttered sounds

Materials

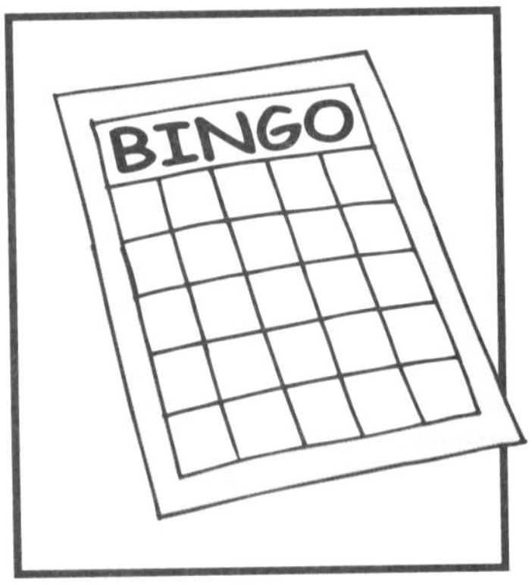

Blank paper (8 ½" x 11")
Pencils
Mirror
Homework

Directions

To make bingo boards, hand out a sheet of paper to each student. Instruct students to fold their papers in half 4 times so that when they unfold their papers, they each have 16 squares. It helps for you to make a bingo board as you give the directions so students may observe you. For some students you may wish to simplify this game by instructing them to fold their papers in half 3 times so that they have 8 squares instead of 16. Then tell the students:

> We are getting ready to play Stuttering Bingo. I am going to name 16 letters or combination of letters. After I say a letter, such as *b* or *o*, or a combination of letters, such as *sh*, write the letter or the letter combination in a box on the board. You may put the letters in any box that you want. Everybody's board should be different.

p	sh	ch	b
m	n	e	y
c	a	h	f
v	th	t	d

Figure 3.1 A completed bingo board

Consonants, blends, and vowels may be used during this activity, but use letters because even though you will be referring to *sounds*, teaching phonetic symbols to students is unnecessary and complicated. As you start to read letters and letter combinations aloud, encourage students to randomly place the letters in boxes on their boards. When using blends you may say, "In one box write the letters *c* and *h*, as in *church*." Figure 3.1 shows an example of a completed bingo board.

Now you are ready to play *Specific Sound Bingo.* Tell students:

> I am going to begin the game by stuttering on a word. When you hear me stutter on that word, you have to figure out what sound I stuttered on. For example, if I say "c-c-c-candy," you have to figure out that I stuttered on the /k/ sound. You will then find the letter *c* on your paper and put a small number 1 in the *c* square. The first student who gets four 1s in a row, either going up and down or across, is the winner.

The fun and practical part about using numbers instead of bingo chips is that for the next game, students are instructed to write a small number 2 in the appropriate boxes. This way you may play the game several times while avoiding the distracting component of having many bingo chips on the table. You may then ask students to turn their boards over so that you can give them a different set of letters and letter combinations. You may repeat some of the letters from the first board.

You may add another element of challenge to Specific Sound Bingo by saying sentences and stuttering on one word within a sentence. For example, you may say, "Today I am going to the pppppark after school. What sound did I stutter on?"

Increase the difficulty of Stuttering Bingo by having students identify how each sound is produced. We can call this game *How Do You Make This Sound? Bingo.* Helping school-age students understand how sounds are produced is a fundamental aspect of therapy and empowering for children who stutter.

Begin by stuttering on /b/ in the word *boy* and asking a student to tell you what letter you stuttered on. Then ask the student to stutter on the word himself and tell you how he made the stuttered sound. Ask, "When you stuttered on the letter *b* in the word boy, did you use your lips, tongue, or throat (vocal cords)?" Begin with simple vocabulary: tongue, back of the tongue, front of the tongue, lips, roof of the mouth, throat, voice box, and vocal cords.

When playing this game students often develop their own vocabulary for sounds. Encourage this self-generated vocabulary because it will be more meaningful to students than clinical terms, such as *plosives* and *fricatives.* For example, several students have classified /s/ and /z/ (fricatives) as "hissing sounds"; other students have called these "snake sounds." When students have correctly identified that /s/ and /z/ are made with air that hisses, take advantage of the situation by asking students to examine these sounds more closely. Using the student-generated terminology, ask "How are the hissing sounds made?" Help students figure out that hissing sounds are produced by directing air through a groove in the tongue and then through the teeth when the tongue is pressed lightly against the roof of the mouth. Try using mirrors and asking students to put their hands in front of their mouths to feel the hissing air. You can say, "Jaclyn, when you make the /s/ sound, where is your tongue? You're right, it is behind your teeth on the roof of your mouth. Now put your hand in front of your mouth and make the /s/ sound; do you feel the air coming out?"

When beginning How Do You Make This Sound? Bingo, it is best to start with sounds such as bilabials (/b/, /p/, /m/, and /w/) and labiodentals (/f/ and /v/) that are made with the lips. These sounds tend to be the easiest to identify because they may be seen readily by students and when using a mirror.

Homework

Review homework assignments before the students leave speech class. Consider writing individualized assignments to specifically target sounds that are most useful for your students (see Appendix A for a blank homework form). If a student has the most difficulty identifying sounds produced with the vocal folds, for example, you may wish to target these sounds during homework.

Stuttering (3) Homework

Name ______________________________ Date due ____________________

We use our vocal cords (also called our "voice box") to help us make many different sounds. Circle four letters below that you say by using your vocal cords. It helps to softly put your hand on your throat and then say each letter.

m p b v s t z

Parent signature ______________________________ (1)

Stuttering (3) Homework

Name ______________________________ Date due ____________________

Circle four letters below that you say *without* using your vocal cords. It helps to softly put your hand on your throat and say each letter.

s b r t d f p

Parent signature ______________________________ (2)

Stuttering (3) Homework

Name ______________________________ Date due ____________________

We use the tongue, lips, and vocal cords to make many of the sounds we use for speaking. They are called our "speech helpers" because they help us say our letters and words. Figure out which speech helpers are used. Circle the correct answer.

Example: The letter "m" is made using your (LIPS) or TONGUE?

1. The letter "b" is made using your LIPS or TONGUE?
2. The letter "s" is made using your TONGUE or VOCAL CORDS?
3. The letter "p" is made using your LIPS or TONGUE?
4. The letter "t" is made using your TONGUE or VOCAL CORDS?

Parent signature ______________________________

(3)

Stuttering (3) Homework

Name ______________________ Date due ______________

Some people who stutter feel that certain letters and words are harder to say than others. How about you? What letters and words do you have trouble saying? Write the letters and words below.

Example: Hard letter: b

Hard words: baseball, big, baby, because, Batman, bike, bus

1. Hard letter: _____

   Hard words: ______________________________

2. Hard letter: _____

   Hard words: ______________________________

3. Hard letter: _____

   Hard words: ______________________________

Parent signature ______________________ (4)

4
Pocket Calendar

Purpose

- To identify and record specific words stuttered on
- To engage stuttering outside of the therapy room

Materials

Rulers
Pencils
Markers
Scissors
Construction paper (12" x 18")
Sample completed pocket calendar

Directions

Constructing a pocket calendar should take anywhere from 15 to 30 minutes. The calendar is then used by the student over 7 consecutive days to record some special homework assignments related to identification. For example, one week's assignment would be for a student to write down 5 words a day that she avoids saying.

Introduce this activity by showing students a completed calendar. Give each student a piece of construction paper, a ruler, a pencil, a marker, and a pair of scissors. It is best to make a calendar yourself while giving directions so that students may follow your lead. The first step is to draw 7 rectangles to represent the 7 days of the week. Show students how to measure 7 squares on the construction paper (make each square approximately 2 ½" x 4").

When finished with the measurements, students cut out their construction paper calendars so that they have one long strip with 7 rectangles, all of an equal size. At the top of each rectangle, students write the day of the week and its number. Refer to Figure 4.1.

2½"

4"

Monday 16	Tuesday 17	Wednesday 18	Thursday 19	Friday 20	Saturday 21	Sunday 22

Figure 4.1 Example of a stuttering calendar with the days of the week

Then show students how to fold the calendar into a stack, like a fan. The first day of the week is on the front cover and on the back cover (which is blank), students write their name and the title "Stuttering Calendar." (See Figure 4.2.)

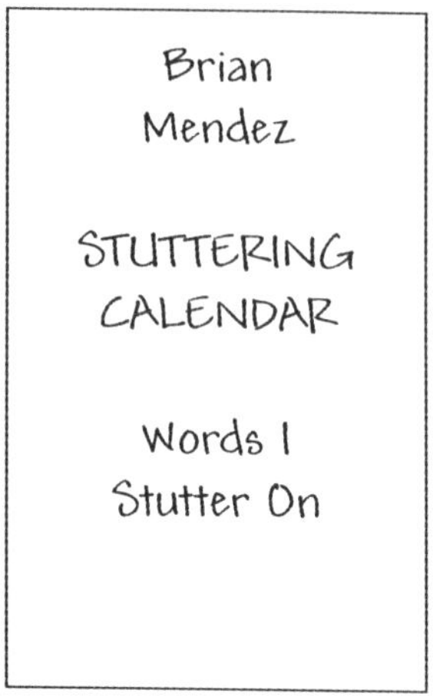

Figure 4.2 Example of back cover

Instruct students to leave a little room at the bottom of the back cover for later use. They will need this space to write down the name of a particular homework assignment, such as "Words I Stutter On." (See Figure 4.2.) This will help students remember what they need to do for homework. Show students how neatly and easily the folded calendar fits into a pocket.

You are now ready to discuss the speech goal for this activity. The first time students use the stuttering calendar, explain that the assignment is to "write down five words you stutter on for each day of the week." For this assignment students number from 1 to 5 under each day of the week. The calendar is now ready to be used for homework. (See Figure 4.3.)

Monday 16	Tuesday 17	Wednesday 18	Thursday 19	Friday 20	Saturday 21	Sunday 22
1.	1.	1.	1.	1.	1.	1.
2.	2.	2.	2.	2.	2.	2.
3.	3.	3.	3.	3.	3.	3.
4.	4.	4.	4.	4.	4.	4.
5.	5.	5.	5.	5.	5.	5.

Figure 4.3 Example of calendar that is ready to be completed as homework

To help students understand their assignment, say, "Think of some words you have stuttered on today." If a student cannot think of a word, refer to a word that the student has stuttered on during the session. You may say, "Sally, I heard you stutter on the word *lunch* today," to which the student may reply, "Oh, yeah." Then ask the student to write the word lunch next to the number 1 on the correct day of the calendar. If the student says, "I stuttered on my name today in class," direct her to "write Sally next to number 2." (Refer to Figure 4.4.)

Monday 16	Tuesday 17	Wednesday 18	Thursday 19	Friday 20	Saturday 21	Sunday 22
1. lunch	1.	1.	1.	1.	1.	1.
2. Sally	2.	2.	2.	2.	2.	2.
3.	3.	3.	3.	3.	3.	3.
4.	4.	4.	4.	4.	4.	4.
5.	5.	5.	5.	5.	5.	5.

Figure 4.4 Example of calendar being used to record words stuttered on

One way to motivate students is to ask them to carry their stuttering calendars and a pencil with them throughout the school day; then when students ask why they need to do this, respond by asking, "Why should you wait to do your homework at home when you can complete it in school?" Students tend to understand this reasoning. It helps if you offer a special treat or reward for completing this assignment. As a school clinician, it is rewarding to pass your students in the hallway and have them wave their calendars in the air and rush over to show you their work.

Once a third grader completed this assignment by writing down several words that started with *b* and *p*, such as *because* and *peanuts.* After showing his completed stuttering calendar to the speech class, the student realized that he often stuttered on words beginning with the letters *b* and *p.* In this example both the clinician and the student were becoming aware of the advent of sound and word fears in this child's stuttering.

More Ideas

When Do I Stutter? Think of three times each day that you were scared of speaking. Write them down on your calendar. We will discuss your answers in class.

How Do I Stutter? You may assign students other stuttering identification goals, such as writing down words to represent how they physically stutter. For example, you may demonstrate a repetition by repeating the first syllable in the word *pizza,* and then write it on your own calendar to read "pi-pi-pi-pizza." Show students this example and then demonstrate other types of stutters. Students may signify a prolongation on a word, such as *lucky,* by writing "llllllllllucky" or a block by writing "........lucky." Refer to Figure 4.5 for a completed calendar that details how a student stuttered on individual words.

Monday 16	Tuesday 17	Wednesday 18	Thursday 19	Friday 20	Saturday 21	Sunday 22
1. llllllunch 2. Bri-Bri-Brian 3. ......pizza	1. to-to-to-today 2. .....class 3. ma-ma-ma-math	1. bbbbbut 2. be-be-be-because 3. mo-mo-mo-mom	1. ni-ni-ni-ni-ni-nine 2. goo-goo-good 3. fffffun	1. ffffirst 2. to-to-to-tomorrow 3. ......test	1. Fri-Fri-Friday 2. stu-stu-stu-stutter 3. aaaaaafter	1. ......Mrs. 2. di-di-di-dinner 3. mmmovie

Figure 4.5 Example of completed calendar from *How Do I Stutter?*

What Makes Talking Easier? Stuttering calendars may also be used to assess or determine a child's self-generated strategies to manage stuttering (i.e., secondary behaviors, such as foot tapping and taking deep breaths). Ask students to write down one thing they do a day that makes talking easier. It is typical for students to list their speech tools, such as stretching and pausing. Students who have had previous speech therapy may list speaking techniques that they have been taught in the past, such as deep breathing or easy onsets. One fourth-grade student listed some unproductive speaking techniques he used, including, "Take a deep breath," "Back up and try saying it again," and "Whisper." In response to such answers, avoid passing judgment and attempt to draw the student into a discussion. You may say, "I hear that you are finding ways to control your stuttering—tell me more." You are then able to address the pros and cons of these student-generated strategies.

5 Candid Camera

Purpose

- To identify moments of stuttering in the clinician, in peers, and in oneself
- To identify the particular sounds stuttered on in the clinician, in peers, and in oneself

Materials

Video camera and TV or tape recorder and tapes
Reading materials
Scorecard (Appendix A)
Homework

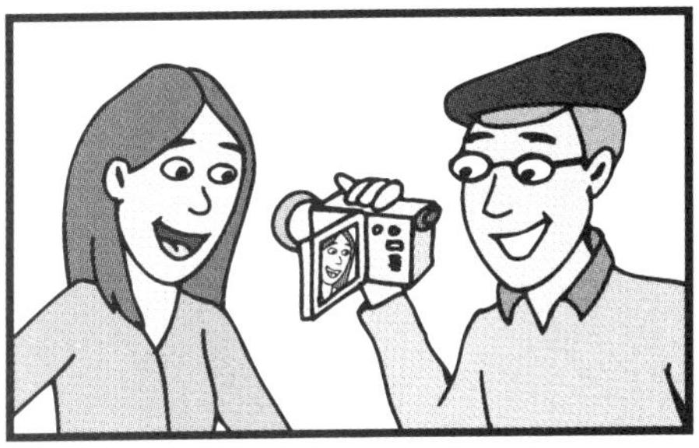

Directions

Another good way to help students identify moments of stuttering is to use a video camera or tape recorder to tape them speaking. Before students arrive, record a few passages or stories in which you stutter on purpose randomly throughout the passages. You may use some of the stories or poems included in this book. See You Feel that Way Too?–Activity 31 or other books or newspaper articles. Or simply talk about a current event or hobby while stuttering on purpose.

Play the videotape or audio recording. Just as in Stutter Tag–Activity 1, begin by asking students to identify moments of stuttering that they hear or see by raising their hands. You may use copies of the scorecard in Appendix A to keep score. After a student has identified a moment of stuttering, ask him, "What sound (or letter) did I get stuck on?" If a student is having difficulty identifying the specific sound stuttered on, ask him to replicate the stutter. Say, "Try stuttering on the word exactly the way I just did." For example, if you stuttered on the word "kkkkickball," ask the student to "stutter on 'kickball' just as I did it." Then ask, "What sound did you stutter on?"

Offer students the opportunity to record their own passages using a video camera or tape recorder. Then play the recording to the group and ask students to identify the moments of stuttering and the sounds stuttered on. Many students are eager to record themselves, but some students find it painful to hear their own voices on tape and to see themselves stutter and will not want to participate. Many adults find this activity particularly challenging. In these situations, use your own best judgment on how fast to proceed.

More Ideas

Many students will demonstrate secondary behaviors. When secondaries occur, ask students to identify them. For example, if a student says "fffffive" while blinking his eyes, you may first ask, "What sound did you get stuck on?" Then ask, "What part of your mouth got stuck on that /f/ sound?" And conclude by asking, "What else did you do when you stuttered on 'five'? " If the student is not aware of the secondary behavior, give a hint such as, "You did something with your eyes when you stuttered." Often times other students waiting for their turn are well aware of the observed secondary behavior and will excitedly offer hints. In the situation above students may blink their eyes to help their friend. You may want to remind students that each child needs his own "think time" and that hints are only welcome when asked for by you.

6
Teach Me How To Stutter

Purpose

- To help students identify how they stutter and then teach others to stutter in the same manner

Materials

None

Directions

Guiding children to teach others how to stutter is one more component in helping children identify, explore, and accept their own stuttering (Guitar & Reville, 2003; Murphy, 2003). Explain to students:

> Everybody stutters in his or her own way. For example, some people repeat their words, some people stretch their sounds, and other people blink their eyes (model examples of these and other stuttering behaviors). It is much easier for me to help you with your speech if you can teach me how *you* stutter. We will go around the room and take turns talking about our favorite movie or TV show. I will go first. When I stutter, be the first to raise your hand, and I will teach you how I stuttered. Then you will have to stutter in the exact same way.

Describe a movie or TV show; be sure to throw in different kinds of obvious voluntary stutters. For example, say, "My favorite movie is Ssssstar Wars." When a student raises her hand, say, "Tami caught my stutter first so I am going to teach my stutter to Tami." Then say:

> Let's see. I stuttered on the /s/ sound in Star Wars. I stuttered like this (duplicate how you stuttered): "Ssssstar Wars." My tongue got caught on the roof of my mouth, and I made a slithering snake sound with the *s*. I also nodded my head a little bit when I stuttered. Tami, let's see if you can stutter just like I did.

Watch Tami try to copy your stuttering. If she does so correctly, congratulate her. If she does so incorrectly, say, "Nice try! You almost got it. Let's try it again." Then again show Tami how you stuttered and let her repeat it. When Tami successfully copies your stuttering, say, "Now you know how to stutter just like me!"

Give each student at least one turn learning how you stutter before allowing her to lead the class. Then ask, "Who wants a turn teaching the class how *you* stutter." Choose a student to speak first and support her in teaching others how to stutter.

You may wish to participate in this part of the activity to add one more player to the game. Students will enjoy playing the game with their speech teacher.

As the student is talking, have her call on the first person to catch her stuttering. Then help her teach the stutter to the student she called upon. You may then say, "Let's see who else can stutter like that (encourage each student to have try and emulate the stutter)." During this game, if one student is slow in identifying moments of stuttering, you may say, "Alex raised his hand second that time, but he hasn't had a turn yet, so let's give him a turn to go first."

At times a student may attempt to emulate a stutter but will do so incorrectly. For example, the leader of the game may stutter on the word *favorite* by saying "ffffavorite," but a student may emulate the stutter incorrectly by saying "fay-fay-fay-favorite." If this occurs, say, "Hey, wait a minute, those were two different stutters. Who can tell me or show me how they were different?"

Often students will not stutter when they are expected to. If this occurs, say, "You really are not stuttering much today. So here is what I want you to do. Just like I stuttered on purpose—I want you to stutter on purpose too. And when you do, call on someone and teach them how you stuttered."

More Ideas

Instead of using conversation, play any game that requires talking. For example, play "Go Fish." While students ask each other questions, ask them to identify each other's stuttering and their own moments of stuttering. Then briefly break away from the game so you and the students may teach one another how to stutter.

Homework

For the first assignment explain that "by teaching your relative or friend how to stutter, you are also showing them that working on stuttering is both fun and hard work." You may wish to explain this assignment to relatives beforehand. Let them know that by completing this first assignment with the child, they are helping her be aware of how she stutters so that she may have an easier time changing how she stutters. The second homework assignment can be used after a speech class guest has attended a session and has begun to learn that stuttering may be talked about openly and casually. You may also have the student call another child who stutters rather than a speech class guest.

Stuttering 6 Homework

Name ______________________ Date due ______________

Choose a partner (any relative or friend) to talk with. Explain to this person that you are working on your stuttering in speech class and that as you talk you need to write down five words that you stutter on. After writing down a word, teach your partner to stutter on the word the same way that you did. For example, if you stutter on the word *video* by saying "vi-vi-vi-video" and blinking your eyes, teach your partner to stutter on it the same way.

1. ______________ 2. ______________ 3. ______________

4. ______________ 5. ______________

Parent signature ______________________

(1)

Stuttering 6 Homework

Name ______________________ Date due ______________

Call ______________ at ______________ . Explain to this person that you will be teaching them to stutter exactly as you do. You may talk about anything you want, such as school, vacation, sports, or hobbies.

When you stutter, stop and teach the other person to stutter in the same way on the same word. Write the five words you used below.

1. ______________ 2. ______________ 3. ______________

4. ______________ 5. ______________

Parent signature ______________________

(2)

7
Stuttering Private Eye

Purpose

- To identify primary and secondary stuttering behaviors in the clinician, in peers, and in oneself, which will help students talk about and modify their stuttering later in therapy
- To label various primary and secondary stuttering behaviors using self-generated terms

Materials

Stuttering Private Eye handout
Pencils
Mirrors (handheld)
Homework

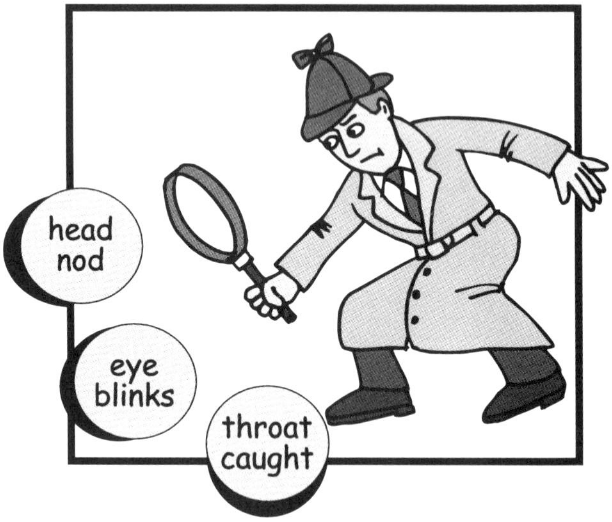

Directions

Begin this activity by initiating a conversation about school, sports, video games, or other topics of interest to the students. Speak using voluntary stuttering and voluntary secondaries. During the conversation ask students to observe and point out your voluntary stuttering behaviors. Just as in Stutter Tag–Activity 1, ask students to raise their hands when someone stutters. Start by saying, "After ssschool I am g-g-going to get pizza." When you voluntarily stuttering, also use some voluntary secondaries, such as nodding your head and blinking your eyes.

Call on students as they raise their hands and say, "Tell me how I stuttered." Students will begin to list behaviors, such as "getting stuck," "rocking while stuttering," "blinking your eyes," "tapping your fingers," "bouncing your head," and "getting caught in the throat." After the group conversation, pass out copies of the Stuttering Private Eye handout and explain:

> Today we are going to break up into pairs (if pairs are not possible, then a group of three is acceptable). You will each have a mirror and a Stuttering Private Eye handout. You are the Private Eye—the detective. Your job is to find out five ways that you stutter and five ways that your partner stutters. You will write your answers on your Stuttering Private Eye handout. You and your partner may talk about anything you want, such as video games, your favorite

toys, sports, or your favorite places to go. As you are talking with your partner, look for the different ways that he stutters. Does he nod his head when he stutters? Does he close his eyes or turn his head? While talking to your partner, use the mirror to look at yourself while you talk to see your own stuttering. The mirror will help you see the different ways that you stutter.

Students begin speaking with one another while looking for stuttering behaviors. Observe each group closely. You may offer advice and suggestions, if necessary, to help students become aware of each other's stuttering patterns. After the pairs have completed the assignment, the group reconvenes for a class discussion.

Although some students are aware of their own stuttering patterns, many others will make comments such as, "I had no idea I did that when I stutter." Once a student mentioned that he was having difficulty observing his own stuttering using a mirror, to which his partner pointed out, "It is hard to see how you are stuttering when you stutter with your eyes closed." Both had a good laugh!

More Ideas

Simplify Stuttering Private Eye by pairing students and giving the following directions: "Fold your handout in half so all you see is the bottom half of the paper on which is written 'Five Ways That My Partner Stutters.' Today you are going to have a conversation with your partner and discover his ways of stuttering. Write down five ways that your partner stutters."

At a later date you can have students complete the top half of the handout. Partners can help each other discover five ways they each stutter.

Homework

Parents may be uncomfortable with Homework Assignment 2, which asks them to describe how their child stutters. Before assigning this homework, you may wish to invite parents to speech class to participate in the Stuttering Private Eye lesson.

Stuttering Private Eye

Name ______________________________ Date ________________

Directions: Describe five things you do when you stutter. Describe five things your partner does when he or she stutters.

Five ways that I stutter

1. ____

____

2. ____

____

3. ____

____

4. ____

____

5. ____

____

Five ways that my partner stutters

1. ____

____

2. ____

____

3. ____

____

4. ____

____

5. ____

____

Stuttering 7 Homework

Name ______________________ Date due ____________

Many children who stutter hide their stuttering from others. Some children do not raise their hands in class when they feel they will stutter. Other children change words, such as asking for chocolate ice cream when they really want vanilla ice cream. How do you hide your stuttering? Write three ways below.

1. ______________________________

2. ______________________________

3. ______________________________

Parent signature ______________________ (1)

Stuttering 7 Homework

Name ______________________ Date due ____________

Tell your parent (or other relative) that in speech class you are learning how you stutter. Sit down with your relative and have a conversation. It is your relative's job to describe five ways he or she sees you stutter. If your relative misses any of your stutters during the conversation, say, "You missed one."

Examples: 1. Stuttered on the letter "b" in ball and closed eyes.

2. Said the word *pizza* six times and moved head up and down.

3. Stretched the letter "s" in the word *sister* for a few seconds like this: "sssssssister."

Below, your relative (not you) writes down the five ways that you stuttered.

1. ______________________________

2. ______________________________

3. ______________________________

4. ______________________________

5. ______________________________

Parent signature ______________________ (2)

Practicing Speech Tools

Speaking is both effortful and frustrating for stutterers. School-age children need tools and strategies that will help them reduce the struggle of stuttering and make talking easier. As mentioned earlier, the speech tools used in this section integrate stuttering modification techniques with pausing, a progressive fluency-shaping tool.

It is important to present speech tools as early in therapy as possible. Once students are able to use their speech tools, they may practice them while participating in many other activities offered throughout the book, such as Out in the World–Activity 19, Stuttering Interviews–Activity 30, You Feel That Way Too?–Activity 31, and It's Showtime–Activity 32.

Using speech tools to manage stuttering is not an option if the school-age child is unable to openly discuss and analyze his stuttering. Students need to understand that although they speak differently from other children, their stuttering is not something that needs be hidden or avoided—doing so only exacerbates the problem. With your guidance students learn that stuttering is not shameful or bad. By dealing openly and compassionately with feelings and attitudes, you lay the groundwork that enables children to practice and use speech tools.

The speech tools offered in this section are viewed as a vital part of a comprehensive therapy approach that gives an equal emphasis on dealing with the feelings and emotions that accompany stuttering. Learning and using speech tools will help stutterers manage one component of a complex and multidimensional disorder. Although using appropriate eye contact is not considered a speech tool, it is an important and closely related speaking strategy that is also discussed in this section.

There are many homework assignments in this section that provide students with opportunities to practice their speech tools. After teaching a speech tool (stretching, bouncing, pausing, or voluntary stuttering), it is best to assign homework that reinforces the use of that tool. Then, later in therapy, periodically assign homework from previous speech tool activities so that students continue to practice and use speech tools.

Note. Reproducible materials, such as homework and handouts, are located at the end of the description of how to facilitate an activity. However, reproducible materials that are used in more than one activity are included in the appendixes.

8
Tools of the Trade

Purpose

- To introduce students to items in the Stuttering Kit
- To introduce and explain the concept of controlling stuttering by using speech tools

Materials

Chalkboard with chalk (or large writing tablet or poster board with magic marker)
Stuttering Kit(s)—see Assembling a Stuttering Kit, page 33
Speech Tools handout

Directions

This lesson is relatively short and should be planned as an introduction to using speech tools. Spend approximately 10 minutes completing this lesson and then go directly into the stretching activity that follows (Stretching–Activity 9).

Introduce the concept of speech tools to students by writing "Professions" at the top of a chalkboard. Underneath list several professions, such as "construction worker," "baseball player," "police officer," and "firefighter." Then go around the room and ask each student to think of tools that one of these people uses. For example, ask, "Who can tell me one tool that a police officer uses?" For a police officer students may list gun, baton, and handcuffs; for a baseball player students may list hat, ball, and glove; for a construction worker students may list hammer, nails, and hard hat; and for a firefighter students may list hose, axe, and protective glasses.

After discussing several professions, say, "Tell me one tool that a stutterer can use." If a student does not yet understand the term *stutter,* you may ask, "What is one tool we can use to help us with our speech?" New students usually look at each other for the answer. Veteran or returning students may respond, "We can use our stretching, bouncing, pausing, and stuttering on purpose." Students who have worked with other clinicians might say, "We can use our easy speech," "We can use our deep breathing," or "We can relax." Then explain:

> It is helpful for you to have a set of tools that you can use to manage and control your stuttering. Just as a firefighter needs to be taught how to use an axe and an air mask, stutterers need to be shown how to use speech tools. To help you learn speech tools, I have a special Stuttering Kit just for you.

Then pass out the Stuttering Kits (one per student or one per speech group) and allow students to explore all of the toys and items contained in the kit. You may say, "We will be using all of the items in your Stuttering Kit to help us with our speech and with our stuttering. Take a minute now to look at them." I often say, "You may each blow one set of bubbles, no more." This way students do not become overly distracted by the bubbles.

After students have had the chance to briefly explore the items, ask them to put everything back in the Stuttering Kits except for the Silly Putty. You will want to collect the Silly Putty and hold it for them until you are ready to use it in the stretching activity that follows. Collect the kits and put them away. Then announce to students:

> You will be learning four speech tools in speech class to help you control your stuttering. These four speech tools are called *stretching, bouncing, pausing,* and *voluntary stuttering.* In this handout (give each student a copy of the Speech Tools handout) each speech tool is briefly explained. I am giving you each a copy so that you may study your speech tools whenever you want. Also, we will be having a few fun quizzes and many guests during speech class. We will need to review this handout before the quizzes and when explaining our speech tools to friends and guests.

Then explain, "The first speech tool we will be focusing on is called stretcing. Look at your Speech Tools handout and follow along as I read to you about stretching." Next read, "Stretch the first sound of a word, lllllllllike this. This will help you start sentences and will help you to stretch-out of a stutter."

You are now prepared to move directly into the Stretching Activity. It is recommended that you have students put their handouts away in their speech folders so that they may focus on the stretching lesson.

Speech Tools

Stretching

Stretch the first sound of a word, lllllllllike this. This will help you start sentences and stretch-out of a stutter.

Bouncing

Bou-bou-bou-bounce the first sound of a word li-li-li-like this. This will help you start sentences and bounce-out of a stutter.

Pausing

Take short pauses between words. This will help you stutter less often. Commas indicate places to pause.

> **Example:** I, practice pausing, so that, I may stutter, less often. A, good time, to practice pausing, is when, I have, to read, aloud. I, also practice pausing, when, I am stuttering, a lot, or when I am, feeling, scared of talking. I, may still stutter, when, I use, my pausing, and that is, okay.

Voluntary Stuttering

Stutter on purpose to reduce the fear of talking and to practice stuttering easily.

9
Stretching

Purpose

- To help students initiate and move forward through sounds, syllables, and words
- To help students smooth-out or stretch-out of moments of stuttering

Materials

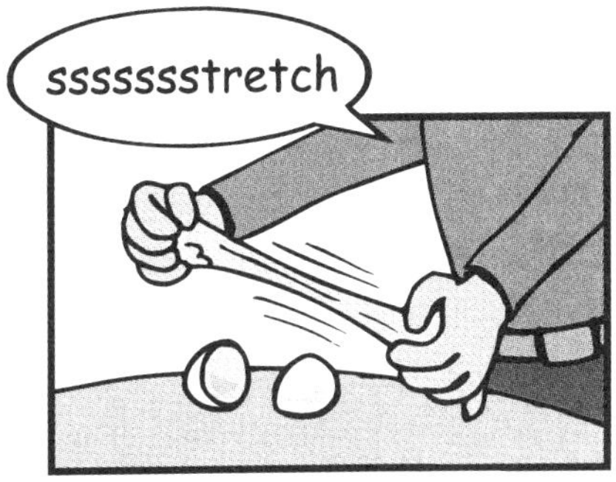

Silly Putty
Stretching Practice handouts
Homework

Directions

Explain to students that stretching is used for two reasons:

1. As a way to begin smooth and forward-moving speech
2. As a way to stretch-out of and repair stuttering moments

Silly Putty Stretch. When describing prolongations (what I call stretching), Breitenfeldt & Lorenz (2000) suggest:

1. Keep all [articulator] contacts light.
2. Prolong on the first sound of a word.
3. Say the rest of the word crisply at a normal rate of speed. (p. 88)

Begin by teaching stretching at the single-word level. At first, focus on stretching words that begin with continuants because these sounds are the easiest to stretch. Start by gently and slowly stretching the Silly Putty (from the Stuttering Kit) while simultaneously stretching the initial sound of words such as "sssssssssssoda" or "mmmmmmmountain." Stretch only the first sound. *Do not prolong or stretch the rest of the word.*

The ultimate outcome is for students to be able to reliably use stretching to move forward through sounds. It is helpful for students to learn they are able to make their stuttering as long or short as they would like—this provides them a strong sense of control over their speech. Stuttering is struggled, so stretching should be demonstrated and practiced without struggle, in a gentle and easy manner. Show your students long, smooth stretching (5–7 seconds); medium, smooth stretching (2–4 seconds); and, finally, short, smooth stretching (1 second or less).

After demonstrating long, medium, and short stretching variations, pass the Silly Putty around the group and ask each student to practice stretching the first sound of a word. Engage students by providing them with fun words. For example, choose favorite foods that start with continuant sounds, such as *fries, hamburgers,* and *ice cream.* If you have a student who is a big baseball fan, give him the names of famous baseball players, such as Mickey Mantle or Sammy Sosa.

You need to stress that stretching is typically used on the first sound of words. Students will often want to stretch the vowel sound after the first phoneme (i.e., saying "ruuuuning" instead of "rrrruning"). Explain that *it is best to stretch on the first sounds of words because this is where stuttering usually occurs.* If a student stretches a word on the second sound, such as in "maaaaaybe," you may say, "That was really good, but I want you to try it again and stretch on the first sound—like this: "mmmmmaybe." If a student continues to stretch the wrong sound, write out the word and underline the first sound (letter or blend) to make it clear where the stretching should occur.

Because of each student's individualized sound and word fears, different students may have difficulty stretching different sounds. For example, a student who has grown to fear /d/ and /f/ may have more difficulty stretching these sounds than others. When a student uses stretching to productively move forward through his feared sounds, he will come to understand the tool's usefulness.

As mentioned earlier, continuants are viewed as the easiest sounds to stretch. For many, stop sounds are more difficult to stretch than vowels, diphthongs, fricatives, affricates, nasals, liquids, and glides because stops are not continuants. When stretching stops (/p/, /d/, /t/, /d/, /k/, /g/), you need to treat them as continuant sounds (see Breitenfeldt & Lorenz, 2000). You may need to guide your students as to how to do this. For example, here is how you can help them stretch the /p/ in *panda.* First, take out the mirrors from the Stuttering Kits and explain:

> Let's say the /p/ sound together while watching our lips in our mirrors. We are not going to say a whole word, just the /p/ sound. First, put your lips together gently—so softly that if you put an egg between your lips, it wouldn't break. Now stretch on the /p/ sound—gently let the /p/ sound out. You will feel air smoothly leaving your lips. Now put down your mirror and let's try it again. This time, put your hand in front of your mouth and feel the air gently leave as you say /p/.

After students are able to stretch on the /p/ sound, continue by saying: "Now let's try stretching on the /p/ sound while saying panda. Remember, be sure to put your lips together lightly, not hard. Gently let the /p/ come out and say the word panda."

Student/Clinician Switch. Next ask students to stretch their Silly Putty to control your speech. Explain in this manner:

> Now everybody will get the chance to be the speech teacher, and I will be the student. You will use your Silly Putty to control my stretching. I will start

> saying a word, and you will slowly stretch your Silly Putty. As you start gently pulling apart the Silly Putty, I will stretch that sound and hold it until you stop stretching the Silly Putty. Then I will complete the word.

For example, let's say the student chooses the word *Spiderman* for you to stretch. Begin to say Spiderman by stretching the initial /s/. The student stretches the Silly Putty as you stretch the /s/ sound. When the student stops stretching the Silly Putty, you smoothly stretch free of the /s/ sound and *complete the rest of the word at a normal rate.*

Students enjoy being able to modify their clinician's speech, and by doing so it shows them that control is possible. Do not be surprised if students stretch their Silly Putty slowly—they may want to have fun and make you produce a very long stretch. Be a good sport and do so!

Finger Stretching. Another way to teach and practice stretching is to hold two fingers about a foot or two apart and ask a student to stretch "this far." The student then tries to stretch a word until his Silly Putty is as wide as your two fingers. Then move your fingers closer together and repeat the activity. Continue this activity until you are starting from a position in which your fingers are so close that they are almost touching. Then ask students to put away their Silly Putty and practice this activity without the prop. This demonstrates to children that they can control and modify moments of stuttering themselves, without external aids.

Allow students to play the role of the teacher again. Students take turns controlling your modeled stuttering by slowing moving their fingers together as you stutter. At this point you will not be using Silly Putty to help you stretch. Explain, "I will keep stretching as you move your fingers together. When your fingers touch, I will smoothly stretch free of the stutter."

Once you feel that students understand how to use stretching, *the Silly Putty prop should be phased out.* This is done so that hand movements do not become part of the child's stuttering pattern. I often compare using Silly Putty to using training wheels:

> Stretching our speech with Silly Putty is a lot like riding a bike with training wheels. Once we learn how to ride a bike, we no longer need the training wheels. And once we learn how to stretch with our mouths, we no longer need the Silly Putty to help us. Stretching is done with our mouths, not our hands.

As therapy progresses, students may want occasionally to use the Silly Putty because it is fun—and that is acceptable. Teaching stretching to guests is an ideal time to revisit Silly Putty. You just need to be clear that the purpose of using such props is only for learning the tool and teaching it to others.

Stutter Punch—Using Stretch-Outs. Stretching and stretch-outs are basically the same tool (both may be referred to as stretching). The distinction is that stretching is used to initiate speech, and stretch-outs are used to smooth-out of (or modify) a stutter. The goal of teaching stretch-outs is to show students that they may move forward through and repair moments of stuttering in a smooth and easy way. Although stuttering most frequently occurs at the beginning of sentences and words, stuttering also occurs in the middle of words (i.e., "toddday"). It is appropriate for students to use and practice stretch-outs at different locations within a word where they typically stutter. As a reminder, stuttering rarely occurs at the end of words, so there is no reason to practice stretching or stretch-outs at the end of words. Begin by explaining the game:

> Today we are going to play a game called Stutter Punch. While talking, I am going to stutter. When you hear me stutter, grab my stutter with a stutter punch (as a demonstration, extend your hand and tightly close your fist). I will hold the stutter until you begin to slowly unclench your fist. When you unclench your fist, I will gently stretch-out of the stutter.[4]

Give each student the opportunity to control your stuttering. After each student has had a chance to catch your voluntary stuttering, explain:

> Now you will each take turns speaking about any topic that you want, such as a favorite sport or hobby. As you are speaking, I will listen closely for moments of stuttering. When I hear you stutter, I will throw out a stutter punch and hold the stutter for a few seconds before gently unclenching my fist. You need to hold the stutter until I begin unclenching my fist. As I let go of the stutter punch, gently stretch-out of the stutter.

At first you, the clinician, may hold each stutter for 2 seconds or more. As therapy progresses, you will want to vary the duration of each stretch-out. Eventually, you will reduce the duration of the stretch-outs to a second and then less. This procedure is very similar to working on the longest and shortest stuttering awards. Students are shown that they may stutter in different ways with a certain level of control and management. Even if a student immediately demonstrates the ability to stretch-out of a stutter in less than a second in a smooth and nonstruggled fashion, you and the student should not expect this at all times. If a student demonstrates difficulty with shorter stretch-outs, move back to practicing longer ones before returning to shorter stretch-outs.

Stuttering Stories. Use the four stories contained in the Stretching Practice handouts ("The Wrong Answer," "Special Talking Time," "Reading Out Loud," and "Pizza and Stuttering") to practice stretching. You will need to make photocopies of the stories so that students may read along. Begin with the first story "The Wrong Ans-

---

[4] This is a commonly used therapy technique and is demonstrated by Guitar (2005) in the Stuttering Foundation of America's video "Therapy in Action: The School-Age Child Who Stutters."

wer" and read through the directions with students. Watch students closely to make sure they underline the correct words (the first word in every sentence). Then demonstrate the assignment by reading a few sentences from "The Wrong Answer" while stretching the initial sound of each underlined word. Stretch initial sounds for about a second before completing the word. Then ask students to take turns reading aloud. Be sure that the stories you choose are at your students' reading levels. If students are struggling to read, they will not be able to focus on using stretching or any other assigned tool.

After reading through a story in class, I often assign it for homework that same day or later during the course of therapy so that students may have a second opportunity to consider the content. Do not feel obligated to read through all four of the stretching practice stories at one time. You may use them later in therapy as you continually review speech tools.

You can also use stories from Appendix C to practice stretching. In this case you will need to assign the words the students will stretch on. For example, ask students to underline the first word in each sentence. Or ask them to underline two words or more in every sentence.

Take a break from practicing stretching to discuss the content of the stories, especially if students initiate the conversation. If students do not comment on the content of these stories, ask questions. For example, after reading "Reading Out Loud" by Leslie Furmansky, you may ask, "What do you think about the way that Leslie avoided stuttering?" or "How do you deal with stuttering in the classroom?"

More Ideas

Assign stretching during many of the activities in this book, such as Stuttering Interviews–Activity 30, It's Showtime–Activity 32, and Questions and Answers–Activity 33.

Homework

Assign homework you feel will best meet the needs of your students. These assignments provide students with the opportunity to practice stretching and to share this speech tool with family and friends.

After moving on to the other speech tools and activities in this book, you will want to revisit the stretching activities so that students continue to practice and use this tool. Also consider assigning stretching homework for several consecutive sessions for reinforcement.

Homework Assignments 7 through 10 ask students to read the stories contained in the Stretching Practice handouts and to answer questions about them. There is no harm in reading through the stories first in class and then assigning them for homework as well. Sometimes students reconsider their answers and have a new viewpoint to express.

The directions for the stories ask students to underline the first word in each sentence to show which words will be stretched. Some students demonstrate specific sound and letter fears. For these students you may give the additional assignment of underlining words in the stories that begin with their feared sounds. If a student fears saying /b/ and /p/, ask him to underline all words in the stories that begin with these letters. This way students practice stretching on the first words in sentences and on words that begin with feared sounds.

Stretching Practice

Name: ______________________________

Directions: Read the following story and underline the first word in every sentence to show which words you will stretch on. The first sentence is completed for you. Then practice reading the story aloud using stretching.

The Wrong Answer

by Peter Reitzes

When I was 8 years old, I had to take a geography test. Our teacher went around the classroom and asked students to name the capitals of all 50 states. I was very upset because it was suppose to be a written test, but at the last minute the teacher changed his mind and thought it would be fun to give an oral test. I studied for days and knew the answer to every question. When the teacher called on me, I felt my mouth and throat get tight. It felt like I was choking. The teacher asked, "What is the capital of New York state?" I tried to say "Albany," but I got really stuck on the letter "A." So instead of stuttering I said, "I don't know" and failed the test. I felt really bad afterward but did not know what else to do.

— — — — — — — — — — — — — — — — — —

Stretching Practice

Name: ______________________________

Directions: Read the following story and underline the first word in every sentence to show which words you will stretch on. The first sentence is completed for you. Then practice reading the story aloud using stretching.

Special Talking Time

by Lee Goodman

My name is Lee and I am 10 years old. I go to speech class because I stutter. My mom is very busy—she works at a hospital and sometimes has to work very late. My speech teacher said that every night my mom and I should have "special talking time" together. Sometimes when my mom gets home late, she kisses my brother goodnight and then sits next to me in bed and we talk. This is our special time. Mom rubs my head, and I get to tell her about my day. Mom doesn't tell me to slow down any more or to think before I talk. Now we just talk. I like this time. Maybe if more kids stuttered, they would get special talking time with their moms too.

Stretching Practice

Name: ______________________________

Directions: Read the following story and underline the first word in every sentence to show which words you will stretch on. The first sentence is completed for you. Then practice reading the stories aloud using stretching.

Reading Out Loud

by Leslie Furmansky

In elementary school the thought of reading out loud in class was horrible. Some days my speech was good, and some days my speech was bad. But I was not always able to know when my speech would be good and when it would be bad. Even worse than reading out loud was reading or singing out loud in a foreign language. I remember being in school and having the teacher pick a leader to read a paragraph. Fortunately, I had a plan, and, boy, did I think I was clever. I was usually able to figure out when my turn would be, and I would escape to the bathroom just in time!

Stretching Practice

Name: ______________________________

Directions: Read the following story and underline the first word in every sentence to show which words you will stretch on. The first sentence is completed for you. Then practice reading the stories aloud using stretching.

Pizza and Stuttering

by Matthew Hall

I am 32 years old now. When I was younger, in elementary school, I went once a week to speech therapy. Every week my mother and my grandmother had to drive me 45 minutes in the car to get to the special doctor who tried to help me with my stuttering. The speech doctor was very cool—he had a real video game in his office, and it was free to play. I liked it when the doctor was busy because I got to play with all of his toys. Sometimes the doctor helped me talk, and other times he would stop by the speech room while someone else was helping me. I don't really remember what we worked on, but I had fun. On the way home my mom and grandma would take me for pizza. That was the best part of the trip.

Stuttering 9 Homework

Name ______________________ Date due______________

Show your parents how you have learned to stretch your words. Explain that stretching will help you to stretch-out or smooth-out of moments of stuttering. Write down five words that you stretched on. Also ask your parents to try stretching. You might have to teach them!

1.______________ 2. ______________ 3. ______________

4.______________ 5. ______________

Parent signature ______________________ (1)

Stuttering 9 Homework

Name ______________________ Date due ______________

Call ______________ at ______________ and practice using stretching on the first word of every sentence. Talk for at least 5 minutes with this person.

Parent signature ______________________ (2)

Stuttering 9 Homework

Name ______________________ Date due ______________

Telephone or visit a relative and explain that you are using stretching to help you stretch-out or smooth-out of moments of stuttering. Show them how you use stretching. Ask them to try stretching too.

What did your relative say about your speech? ______________________

____

____

How did they feel about trying stretching? ______________________

____

____

Parent signature ______________________ (3)

Stuttering 9 Homework

Name ______________________ Date due ______________

List five words that you have a hard time saying.

1.______________ 2. ______________ 3. ______________

4.______________ 5. ______________

Teach your parents how to make a "long" stutter and a "short" stutter using stretching. Teach them how to stutter on at least five different words. See who can make the longest and shortest stutters, you or your parents!

Parent signature ______________________

(4)

Stuttering 9 Homework

Name ______________________ Date due ______________

Write down five words that you want to stretch.

1.______________ 2. ______________ 3. ______________

4.______________ 5. ______________

Call a relative or a friend and explain that you are using stretching to help you with your stuttering. Tell them that your speech teacher thinks it is helpful for you to show other people your speech tools. Then show them how you use your stretching on the five words you wrote above. You could say, "I am now going to show you my stretching by stretching on five words."

Parent signature ______________________

(5)

Stuttering 9 Homework

Name ______________________ Date due ______________

On a separate sheet of paper, write a story about your own stuttering. Then underline the first word in each sentence. You will read the story aloud during the next speech class while stretching on the underlined words.

Parent signature ______________________

(6)

Stuttering 9 Homework

Name ______________________ Date due ______________

Read "The Wrong Answer" by Peter Reitzes. In school, is it better to stutter and say the correct answer or to speak without stuttering and say the wrong answer? Explain below.

What do you feel about stuttering in school? Are certain teachers harder to talk to than others? Explain below.

Parent signature ______________________ (7)

Stuttering 9 Homework

Name ______________________ Date due ______________

Read "Special Talking Time" by Lee Goodman. What is special and good about your stuttering? ______________________

Who do you like talking to the most? Explain why. ______________________

Parent signature ______________________ (8)

Stuttering (9) Homework

Name ______________________ Date due ____________

Read "Pizza and Stuttering" by Matthew Hall. Matthew liked playing the video game before speech therapy and liked getting pizza after speech therapy. What do you like about going to speech class?

____

____

____

____

Matthew could not remember what he did in speech class. Can you? List two things you do in speech class that help you with your stuttering.

1. ____

2. ____

Parent signature ______________________ (9)

Stuttering (9) Homework

Name ______________________ Date due ____________

Read "Reading Out Loud" by Leslie Furmansky. Leslie said that she would run to the bathroom every time it was her time to read out loud in class. What do you do to get out of talking?

1. ____

2. ____

3. ____

Parent signature ______________________ (10)

10
Bouncing

Purpose

- To help students initiate and move forward through sounds, syllables, and words
- To help students bounce-out of moments of stuttering

Materials

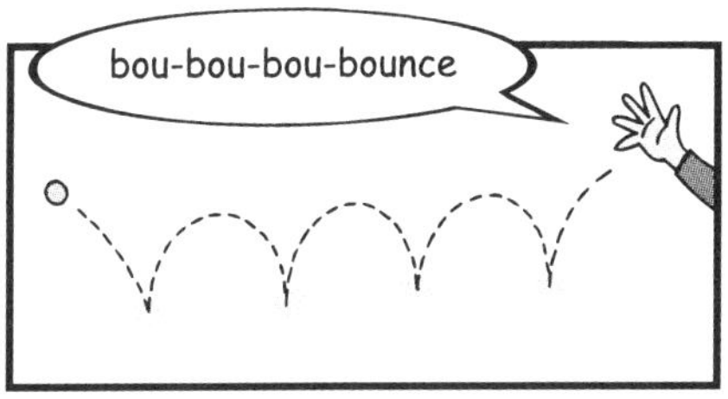

Bouncy balls (the small, hard rubber type that bounce high and are sold in gumball machines)
Homework

Directions

Explain to students that bouncing is used for two reasons:

1. As a way to start smooth and forward-moving speech
2. As a way to bounce-out of stuttering moments

Bouncy-Ball Bouncing. Be sure to demonstrate bouncing on the first syllable or sounds of words. Begin by taking a bouncy ball out of a Stuttering Kit and saying to a student, "Choose a good word for me to bounce on." Then drop the ball and each time the ball hits the ground, repeat the first consonant/vowel or vowel/consonant combination of the word. For example, drop the ball and say, "so-so-so-soda." For a word such as *team* that is only one syllable, say "tea-tea-tea-team." Initially, bounce a syllable or sound three times before continuing the word (i.e., "po-po-po-potato"). If a student chooses the word *Barbie,* drop the bouncy ball and say, "Bar-Bar-Bar-Barbie" in time with the ball. Each time the ball hits the ground, say, "Bar." The fourth time the ball hits the ground, say the entire word. Bouncy balls will bounce at a slower rate than stuttered dysfluencies, and this encourages the child to slow her repetitions, thus approximating normal disfluencies.

During bouncing activities you need to be careful to offer students clear and accurate models. Unlike typical speakers, people who stutter often use the schwa vowel in place of the correct vowel (Ainsworth & Fraser, 2002; Shapiro, 1999; Starkweather, 1987; Van Riper, 1982). A stutterer may say "gu-gu-gu-going" instead of "go-go-go-going." When clinicians and students bounce on a word such as *baseball,* it is incorrect to say "bu-bu-bu-baseball. There is no short *u* or schwa vowel sound in baseball. The correct way to teach bouncing on the word baseball is to model "bay-bay-bay-baseball." By encouraging students to stutter using the correct vowel sound and by slowing down their repetitions, you help students change their stuttering pattern to approximate normal, nonstuttered disfluencies.

After demonstrating bouncing give students the opportunity to practice bouncing. Assign each student a word. For example, say, "Briana, I know you love animals, so your word is *penguin.*" Begin by asking students to bounce on the first syllable three times (i.e., "pen-pen-pen-penguin"). The student drops the ball on the floor or table. Each time the ball hits the ground, the student says a syllable or the beginning of a syllable. After three bounces the student completes the word.

Mouth Bouncing. Using bouncy balls is fun, but students learn the concept quickly and may become silly when using the balls. For these reasons the balls are promptly phased out. Props can always be brought back into therapy if the student needs to be reminded how to bounce. Explain:

> Now we are going to practice our bouncing without using bouncy balls. We are going to bounce only with the help of our mouths. We are each going to take a turn bouncing on the name of our favorite television show. My favorite TV show is "Sta-Sta-Sta-Star Trek" (at this point each sound or syllable is still being bounced three times). Notice how I bounced only with my mouth. Now everyone will get a turn to try it.

After students are given turns to bounce three times on the name of their favorite TV shows, focus on varying the number of bounces in much the same way you taught various lengths and durations of stretching. Explain, "Let's try to practice bouncing with two instead of three bounces. Let's see who can bounce the word *video* two times." Then demonstrate this by saying "vi-vi-video." (Remember to say the correct vowel.) Now ask each student to try. If a student demonstrates any difficulty, increase the bounces to three or more. Then when the student is successful, try to reduce the bounces again. At this point ask, "Who has a word that you want to bounce two times?"

After two bounces, encourage students to attempt bouncing only once, (i.e., "tay-table"). And, of course, if the student is having difficulty bouncing at any time, encourage the child's attempt. For example, say, "Bouncing only once can be difficult, but I can see that you are trying really hard to do it—good job!" If a student is having difficulty reducing the number of bounces, ask her to bounce more times (i.e., 3–6 times) before reducing the number of bounces again. You may even ask the student to bounce as many times as she can before completing the word. This takes much of the speaking pressure off the child. Because students are often competitive, you may suggest, "Let's see who can bounce the greatest number of times."

Stutter Punch and Bounce-Outs. Just as with stretch-outs, you may play a game of Stutter Punch to teach students bounce-outs. Because moments of stuttering occur not only at the beginning of words but within words as well, students may use bounce-outs at the beginning of words and in the medial position. As a reminder, stuttering rarely occurs on the last sound or syllable of words, so there is no need to practice bouncing at the end of words. Say:

> Just as we have learned how to stretch-out of a stutter, today we will learn how to bounce-out of a stutter. We are going to have a conversation. When you stutter you will be expected to gently bounce-out of the stutter.

Lead the game by speaking first while using voluntary stuttering. Assign a student the task of grabbing your stutter with a stutter punch (closing her fist tightly and holding it closed when you stutter). It is your job to keep bouncing on a sound or syllable until the student releases you from a stutter punch (opens fist). For example, say, "This weekend I spent most of the day in the park riding my bike. Everything was fine until my chain broke. Then I had to walk all the way to the bu-bu-bu-bu-bu-bus." Keep bouncing on the word *bus* until the student releases you from the stutter.

Students may want to hold your stutter a long time so that you have to bounce many times. Again, be a good sport and do so. Remember, you can return the favor when it is the student's turn to speak! After demonstrating several bounce-outs, students then take turns speaking and holding each other's stutters. It is best if you also take a turn holding each child's stutter.

Different groups of students will play Stutter Punch in different ways. Some students find that when it is their turn to speak they do not stutter at all. It is normal for people who stutter to become fluent when they are expected to stutter. These students will often start using voluntary stuttering without being asked to do so. When this occurs be pleased that students are so willing to stutter on purpose. If a student is not stuttering at all, suggest, "Try throwing in some fake stutters so that your friends can catch you."

Stuttering Stories. Use the four stories contained in the Bouncing Practice handouts ("I Know How You Feel"; "The First Day of School"; "Thumbs Up, Thumbs Down"; and "The Soda Man") as one way to practice bouncing. You will need to make photocopies of the stories so that students may read along. Read through the directions with students, and then watch as they underline the assigned words. As a demonstration read several sentences aloud from the first story "I Know How You Feel" while bouncing on the assigned words. Then have students take turns reading aloud while practicing bouncing.

These stories will often elicit emotional responses from children because they relate to the experiences expressed in them. Take a break from practicing bouncing and spend some time talking about the content of the stories. Students will appreciate that you are not fixated on the singular goal of practicing bouncing. For example, after reading the story by Sam Hatahet, you may ask, "Sam says that he doesn't like to speak in class because other students laugh at him. How do you feel about speaking in class?" You may read all four stories at one time or go over some of them later in therapy.

More Ideas

Invite guests to speech class and teach them bouncing. The bouncy ball may be used in this situation. Students enjoy teaching their speech tools to guests, and it offers them an opportunity to truly own their speech tools.

Homework

After teaching bouncing consider assigning bouncing homework for several consecutive sessions to reinforce this tool. Also, spend some time reviewing and practicing bouncing during your next several sessions.

Homework Assignments 5 through 8 ask students to read the stories contained in the Bouncing Practice handouts and to answer questions about them. These stories are a good way to encourage students to talk openly about stuttering. You will need to make photocopies of the stories so that students may take them home to review them for the homework.

The directions for the stories ask students to underline the first word in every sentence to show which words will be bounced on. You may give students the additional assignment of underlining words in stories that begin with their feared letters or sounds. Then students practice bouncing on challenging letters and sounds.

Homework Assignment 7 is a good way for you to assess which speaking situations are the hardest for your students as well as the ways in which your students avoid speaking. You may then discuss these avoidances and help come up with ways to face these difficult situations.

Bouncing Practice

Name: ______________________________

Directions: Read the following story and underline the first word in every sentence to show which words you will bounce on. The first sentence is completed for you. Then practice reading the story aloud using bouncing.

I Know How You Feel

by Sam Hatahet

My name is Sam Hatahet, and I am going to St. Andrew School. I am in the fifth grade, and I am 12 years old. I know how you feel because I stutter too. When I moved to America, I was 6 years old. I am from Syria. My sister is coming to America in April. Her name is Majaleen. I haven't seen her for 6 years. I can't wait to see her again. When I go to the airport, she probably won't recognize me.

When I stutter I feel lower than all the other kids. Sometimes when I want to ask the teacher something, I feel that I can't ask her because if I stutter all the other kids will laugh at me. I feel that I'm not as capable as I really am. It kind of makes me mad because I was born this way. Sometimes I feel that I'm glad because I don't have another problem. I'm also glad that I'm seeing a speech teacher. She understands how I feel. I feel I could trust her with everything.

Sometimes when my teacher calls on me I freeze. Then my teacher tries to help me. And she doesn't go on to another person. She stays until I get the answer. Then I can remember all my speech helpers that I learned in speech.

— — — — — — — — — — — — — — — — — —

Bouncing Practice

Name: ______________________________

Directions: Read the following story and underline the first word in every sentence to show which words you will bounce on. The first sentence is completed for you. Then practice reading the story aloud using bouncing.

Thumbs Up, Thumbs Down

by Leslie Furmansky

Passover, a Jewish holiday, is usually shared with family members while at a special dinner called a seder. During Passover dinner, family members take turns reading the history of the Jews, like in a play. Since my dad usually assigned the speaking parts, I made a special code that only the two of us understood. When it was my turn to speak, my dad would look at me for the code. If I gave him a thumbs up, I was okay to read, but a thumbs down meant don't even think of calling on me!

Bouncing Practice

Name: ______________________

Directions: Read the following story and underline the first word in every sentence to show which words you will bounce on. The first sentence is completed for you. Then practice reading the story aloud using bouncing.

The First Day of School

by Peter Reitzes

My first day of school is still clearly in my memory. I was 5 years old. Our mothers sat with us on mats on the floor. The mats had our names on them. The teacher, Ms. Mahoney, went around the room and asked each student to say his or her name. I was very scared. I didn't know what the word *stuttering* meant at that time, but I knew that my mouth was going to get stuck when I had to say my name. When it was my turn to say my name, my mouth froze. I quickly gave up and didn't even try. My mom looked at me like I was crazy and said, "Peter, you know your name." I didn't want to say my name and stutter, so I just sat there and pretended to be shy. Ben, my first friend at school, stood up and pointed at me and yelled, "His name is Peter Cottontail." Everyone laughed in a nice way, including me, but I also felt bad at the same time.

Bouncing Practice

Name: ______________________

Directions: Read the following story and underline the first word in every sentence to show which words you will bounce on. The first sentence is completed for you. Then practice reading the story aloud using bouncing.

The Soda Man

by Joseph Williams

On Sundays, my father and I watch football together. Before the games begin, we go to the sub shop and buy several subs. Some people call subs "hoagies;" other people just call them sandwiches. When my dad was paying for the subs, a man came in delivering sodas. He was talking to the guys making the subs in a loud voice and he was stuttering a lot. I never heard anyone stutter like that before. Every time he stuttered, his eyes closed really tight, but he just battled right through it. My father looked at me, but we both chose not to talk about it. I wanted to ask my dad if I also stuttered with my eyes closed, like the soda guy, but I never did.

Stuttering 10 Homework

Name ______________________ Date due ______________

Show your parents how you have learned to bounce your words by showing them five bounces. Write the five words below that you bounced on.

1. ______________ 2. ______________ 3. ______________

4. ______________ 5. ______________

Explain that bouncing will help you to start sentences, say words, and bounce-out of moments of stuttering. Also, ask your parents to try bouncing on the five words. You might have to teach them!

How did your parents do? ______________________________

____

Parent signature ______________________ (1)

Stuttering 10 Homework

Name ______________________ Date due ______________

Teach a friend or relative how to use bouncing and how to bounce-out of a stutter. Ask them to try bouncing.

Who did you speak to about bouncing? ______________________

How did they do? ______________________________________

____

Parent signature ______________________ (2)

Stuttering 10 Homework

Name ______________________ Date due ______________

Call ______________ at ______________ and practice using bouncing on the first word of every sentence. Talk for at least 5 minutes.

Parent signature ______________________ (3)

Stuttering 10 Homework

Name ______________________ Date due ______________

Make a list of 10 words—any words that you want. Write the words on the back of this homework. Call or visit a relative, and tell them that you are practicing your speech tools and need them to listen to you. Explain that you are going to read them 10 words using bouncing and stretching. Bounce on the first five words and stretch on the last five words.

Then, ask your relative to try bouncing three times and stretching three times using any words they want. How did they do?

____

____

Parent signature ______________________ (4)

Stuttering 10 Homework

Name ______________________ Date due ______________

Read "The First Day of School" by Peter Reitzes. Peter said that he would rather pretend to be shy than stutter in front of his class.

What do you do to get out of and avoid stuttering? Write your answer below.

____

____

____

Parent signature ______________________ (5)

Stuttering 10 Homework

Name ______________________ Date due ______________

Read "I Know How You Feel" by Sam Hatahet. Sam said that when he stutters, he feels "lower than all the other kids" in his class. How do you feel when you stutter in class? Write your answer on a separate sheet of paper.

Sam says that when he stutters, other children laugh at him. What do you want your teacher to do if students laugh at your stuttering? Write your answer on the same sheet of paper you used above.

Parent signature ______________________ (6)

Stuttering 10 Homework

Name ______________________ Date due ____________

Read "Thumbs Up, Thumbs Down" by Leslie Furmansky. Leslie had a secret code she gave her father when she didn't want to speak at the dinner table. What are some things you do to tell or show others that you do not want to speak? ______________________________

____

____

____

Parent signature ______________________ *(7)*

Stuttering 10 Homework

Name ______________________ Date due ____________

Read "The Soda Man" by Joseph Williams. Joseph wanted to talk to his father about stuttering but never did. Do you talk to your father or other relatives about your stuttering? What do you say or what would you like to say?

____

____

____

____

Parent signature ______________________ *(8)*

11
Pausing

Purpose

- To provide students with a strategy to stutter less often by pausing (briefly stopping) between words
- To provide students with a way to reduce the domino effect of stuttering

Materials

Pausing Practice handouts
Abacus
Picture cards (i.e., verb or "action word" pictures)
Photocopies of reading materials (i.e., story handouts from this activity and books)
Homework

Directions

Pausing is taught as a means to help students reduce the frequency of their stuttering by reducing muscle tension and time pressure considerations felt by the speaker. It is typical for stutterers to increase their rate of speech when they stutter, thus increasing their frequency of stuttering. This is often referred to as a "domino effect" or "clustering." By teaching pausing, you are offering students a valuable skill that will help prevent the domino effect.

Use an abacus to demonstrate to students the concept of pausing. Simply move a bead from one side of a bar to the other side while you say a word. Moving one bead per word will reduce the rate of speech of the speaker and will significantly reduce the frequency of stuttering. Be sure to pause *between* words, not within words. Try to keep your pauses from a fraction of a second to a full second in duration.

Initially, students practice pausing after every word by using the abacus. Once the abacus is phased out, students practice pausing after the first word in every sentence and then after every two, three, four, or five words. Many students use pausing after the first word of every sentence and then at linguistically appropriate boundaries, such as the beginning of phrases or in other comfortable or individualized ways. One fifth-grade student would pause after every three, four, or five words. He would say, "I like going, to visit my mother, at her job, after I get home from, Boy Scouts."

Pausing Using an Abacus. Students are intrigued by the abacus and will all want a turn using it. The following is an example of what you can say when demonstrating the use of the abacus. (Commas indicate when to pause.)

> Stuttering, is, all, about, struggle. When, people, stutter, their, muscles, get, tight, and, stiff, like, when, you, pick, up, something, very, heavy. It, is, really, hard, to, speak, when, your, muscles, are, tight, and, stiff. Pausing, between, words, lets, your, muscles, relax, and, will, help, you, to, stutter, less, often. Pausing, is, useful, because, it, helps, people, who, stutter, to, immediately, gain, control, of, their, speech, during, tough, talking, times.

Although pausing after every word might seem excessive, this exaggerated demonstration of pausing helps students learn the tool. Each pause need only be a fraction of a second and all pauses occur between words. *When using pausing, students should not prolong sounds within words.*

Give each student a turn speaking while using the abacus. You may say, "While, using, the, abacus, tell, us, about, your, favorite, vacation" or "favorite, place, to, go, during, the, summer." Watch students as they speak with the abacus. Occasionally a student may move one bead per syllable. Instead, make sure that students move *one bead per word.* If students move one bead per syllable, stop them and show them how to move one bead per word. Also, you may need to explain, "When we first use pausing, speech may sound unnatural, robotic, or weird. To learn a new skill, it often helps to overdo it. Over time, with some practice, pausing will sound more natural and more normal."

Another way to practice pausing with the abacus is to take out simple picture cards, such as those found in verb or "action word" decks. You go first by choosing a card and making up a short story about the picture while using pausing with the abacus. Then give each student a turn. You may also show students a picture and explain that everyone will work together to create a group story while using pausing. Begin by telling a story while using the abacus. Then, after a few sentences, pass the abacus to a student and ask, "What, happens, next?"

Pausing Without the Abacus. After students become comfortable with slowing their rate by using the abacus, remove it and announce, "Now, let's, practice, speaking, the, same, way, with, pausing, between, words, like, I, am, doing, now, only, without, using, the, abacus." A 5-year-old student has referred to this as using his "mental abacus." Use any topic of conversation that interests your students.

By this time everyone should understand that pausing occurs between words, not within words. Students should have also experienced reduced struggle and far fewer moments of stuttering as a result of pausing after every word. Now it is time to demonstrate pausing after the first word in every sentence, for a fraction of a second, and then after every two or three words. By pausing in this manner, you begin to demonstrate to students how this speech tool may be used in more natural sounding ways. Explain:

> My, name is, Ms./Mr. ________, and I am, a teacher at________. I, was born in ___________, and my, favorite hobby, is __________. I, love eating pizza,

after school. Now, each of you, will get a chance, to introduce yourself, while practicing, your pausing.

Ask students to practice pausing by introducing themselves (much as you did). You may also ask students to choose a popular topic of conversation to pursue, such as a local sports team, music, or favorite activities. I often introduce topics such as video games or trading cards that students can speak about at length. I even keep a pile of the most popular trading cards in my office so that I can quickly take them out to stimulate conversation. If students demonstrate difficulty remembering to pause between words, bring out the abacus and try again. When reviewing pausing during subsequent sessions, you may wish to have students briefly use the abacus to set a strong model for reducing their rate. Then remove it and practice pausing after the first words in sentences and after every two, three, four, or five words.

Pausing While Reading. Children are frequently called upon to read aloud in class. Learning to use pausing while reading aloud is a skill that children may use frequently. Begin by choosing reading materials that are within or slightly below the student's reading level. Place commas after the first word in every sentence and then after every two or three words to signify when to pause. You may wish to make a photocopy of the text ahead of time so as not to mark up reading materials. Begin reading while pausing noticeably at each comma. After this demonstration ask the student to read aloud and remind him to pause briefly at each comma.

You may use the four stories contained in the Pausing Practice handouts ("My Frozen Mouth," "Stutter Ball," "Climbing to the Top," and "About Stuttering") as one way to practice pausing or use stories from Appendix C. You may also use stories from You Feel that Way Too?–Activity 31. You or your students need to add commas to any reading materials to signify when to pause. As always, take the time to engage students in discussing the content of the stories.

Once students are comfortable reading while using pausing, explain that you want to see if they are able to use pausing when reading without the commas. Provide students with reading materials that do not have commas added. Students often view this as a challenge and try hard to use their pausing without reminders from you. If a child is reading and forgets to pause, you might whisper "pausing" as a reminder, which often helps refocus the student.

More Ideas

To continue to practice pausing, use 20 Questions–Activity 40. Many other activities may be used to practice pausing as well, including Barrier Games–Activity 41 and Joke Telling–Activity 44.

Revisit Pocket Calendar–Activity 4 and give the following assignment for homework: "Use pausing once a day while talking in class. Write down on your calendar when you used pausing and if it helped you. We will talk about your answers in class."

Homework

After teaching pausing, assign pausing homework for several consecutive sessions to reinforce this tool. Also, spend some time reviewing and practicing pausing during your next several sessions.

Homework Assignments 1 through 5 allow students to practice pausing and to share this speech tool with their family and friends. Homework Assignments 6 through 9 ask students to read the stories contained in the Pausing Practice handouts and then answer questions that relate to them. Make photocopies of the stories so that students may take them home. If you like you may practice reading the stories first in speech class and then assign them for homework. This allows students to reconsider the content of the stories.

Pausing Practice

Name: ______________________________

Directions: Read the following story and put commas **after the first word** in every sentence. The first two sentences are done for you. Then we will practice reading the story aloud using pausing.

My Turn

by Jeff Shames

I, was very quiet in my school days. It, was hard for me to say my name. But worse than that was having to read out loud in class. Many times the teacher would go around the room in order having each of us take turns reading a paragraph. I counted the paragraphs to figure out which one I would have to read. I would get more and more nervous as my turn drew closer. I hoped that my reading would be short and not have too many sounds that I would stutter on. I became so worried that I didn't hear anything that was said by the other kids.

Now that I have grown up, I am more open and more comfortable about being a person who stutters. In business meetings I sometimes have to say my name or even read out loud. At these times I might or I might not stutter. Either way it's okay; I get the job done. I no longer fear my turn.

— — — — — — — — — — — — — — — — — — —

Pausing Practice

Name: ______________________________

Directions: Pausing marks (commas) have been added to this story. We will practice reading the story aloud using pausing.

Stutter Ball

by Angel Soto

My, brother, Eric, and I, play baseball, in our basement. We, make, a soft ball, out of socks. And, take turns, hitting the ball, and running, the bases. One day, Eric, did not pitch, the ball to me. I, tried to say, "Pitch it to me," but I had a big stutter. It came out "pppppppitch it." I, was mad, that it was, so hard to say, but then Eric laughed in a nice way. He said, "Let's, call, this game, Stutter Ball." I laughed too. Now, we play, Stutter Ball.

Pausing Practice

Name: ______________________

Directions: Read the following story and put commas **after the first word** in every sentence and then **after every two or three words.** The first two sentences are done for you. Then we will practice reading the story aloud using pausing.

Climbing to the Top

by Amy

My, name is, Amy and, my speech, gets bumpy, and stuck, sometimes. My, speech teacher, and I, talk about, climbing the mountain, of stuttering. Sometimes the mountain looks small and sometimes it looks big. It all depends on how I see it.

It's neat that I have all the tools I need to climb. I have a tool belt like the mountain climbers do, and it has lots of different tools. In case one doesn't work, I can try another.

My speech teacher is my trainer. He gives me the tools and shows me how to use them and tells me I can do anything. My mom and dad are my coaches. When I fall off the mountain, they say it's okay and help me back on. But I am the mountain climber.

Only I can learn and practice. If I don't practice, my tools get rusty and won't work. Sometimes I climb easy. Sometimes I can't climb at all. But that's all okay.

My speech teacher says all I need to know is that I can get to the top of the stuttering mountain.

And I know I can.

Pausing Practice

Name: ______________________

Directions: Pausing marks (commas) have been added to this story. We will practice reading the story aloud using pausing.

My Frozen Mouth

by Sarah Kaplan

My, mouth, does not always work, the way, I want it to. Sometimes, I can't, say my own name. My mouth, won't even open. My, tongue, feels like it is glued, to my lips. I, just sit, there, like, I am frozen. I, push, and push, but my name, does not come out. When, this happens, I get, very mad. Once, I even cried. I, want, to be like, other kids, who don't have this problem.

Stuttering 11 Homework

Name ______________________ Date due ____________

Explain to your parents that you use pausing in speech class because it helps you stutter less often. Choose a book at home to read to your parents. Pause briefly after the first word in every sentence and then after every two, three, or four words. Read with your parents for 5 minutes. Remember, it's okay if you stutter.

Parent signature ______________________

1

Stuttering 11 Homework

Name ______________________ Date due ____________

Telephone or visit a relative of yours and explain that you are using pausing because it may help you stutter less often. Talk for 5 minutes while pausing between every couple of words.

What did your relative say about your speech? ______________________

____

____

Parent signature ______________________

2

Stuttering 11 Homework

Name ______________________ Date due ____________

Call ______________ at ______________ and practice pausing after every couple of words. Talk for at least 5 minutes with this person.

Parent signature ______________________

3

Stuttering 11 Homework

Name ______________________ Date due ____________

Think of three speaking situations in which it may help you to use pausing. Write them below.

1. ____
2. ____
3. ____

Parent signature ______________________

4

Stuttering 11 Homework

Name ______________________ Date due ______________

Think about something that happened to you recently that includes your stuttering. Maybe a friend asked you a question about stuttering, or maybe you had an easy or a difficult stuttering day in school. Using a separate sheet of paper, write a few sentences describing what happened and put pausing marks (commas) after the first word in every sentence. Then read your homework to your parents. Be sure to stop briefly at each comma.

Parent signature ______________________ (5)

Stuttering 11 Homework

Name ______________________ Date due ______________

Read "My Turn" by Jeff Shames to a relative while using your pausing. Jeff dreaded having to sit in class and wait to be called on to speak. What are two ways that your teacher could make speaking easier for you in your classroom?

1. ______________________

2. ______________________

Parent signature ______________________ (6)

Stuttering 11 Homework

Name ______________________ Date due ______________

Read "Stutter Ball" by Angel Soto to a relative while using pausing. Angel's brother Eric helped Angel laugh about stuttering. He called the game they were playing "Stutter Ball." This was a nice way to tease about stuttering. What are some other nice or funny ways to talk about stuttering?

____

____

____

Parent signature ______________________ (7)

Stuttering 11 Homework

Name ______________________ Date due ______________

Read "My Frozen Mouth" by Sarah Kaplan to your parents while using pausing. Sarah described her mouth as feeling "frozen" when she stuttered. How does your mouth or body feel when you stutter? ______________________

____

Parent signature ______________________ (8)

Stuttering (11) Homework

Name ______________________ Date due ______________

Read "Climbing to the Top" by Amy to a relative while using pausing.

Amy talked about "the mountain of stuttering." She wrote, "Sometimes the mountain looks small and sometimes it looks big. It all depends on how I see it." What did Amy mean by this? ______________________

____

What is your stuttering like? Is your stuttering like a mountain or something else? ______________________

____

Parent signature ______________________ (9)

Stuttering (11) Homework

Name ______________________ Date due ______________

Read "Shaky Speech" by Kayla Hernandez (below).

My, words get stuck, when I talk.
This, is called, shaky speech.
This, is called, stucky speech.
This, is called, stopping speech.
This, is called, sticky speech.
This, is called, hard speech.
This, is called, stuttering.

In her poem Kayla used the word *shaky* to describe her speech. What are two other words that Kayla used to describe her speech?

1.______________ 2.______________

What are two words that you can use to describe your speech?

1.______________ 2.______________

Parent signature ______________________ (10)

12 Voluntary Stuttering

Purpose

- To help students reduce their fear of talking (desensitization)
- To help students practice altering their stuttering (modification)

Materials

Scorecard (Appendix A)
The Best Stuttering on Purpose Award (Appendix A)
Stuttering on Purpose Plays handout
Speech Class Permission Form (Appendix A)
Letter to Parents: Stuttering on Purpose
Homework

Directions

Note: This activity may require two or three sessions.

There are many names for voluntary stuttering, including *pseudo stuttering, purposeful stuttering,* and *negative practice.* When working with elementary school children, you can use the terms *stuttering on purpose, fake stuttering,* and *pretend stuttering.*

Voluntary Stuttering at the Word Level. Tell the students the reasons for using voluntary stuttering:

> Sometimes people who stutter are very scared to speak in public places, such as restaurants or stores, because they often worry about other people hearing them stutter. We are going to practice stuttering on purpose on the very first words we say so that other people know that you stutter. The goal of this activity is to use stuttering in a clearly noticeable way. Later, when we are ready, we will go out and try our pretend stuttering in public.

Begin by teaching voluntary stuttering at the single-word level. Model smooth and easy voluntary stutters *that are clearly recognizable as stutters.* Try using easy repetitions (bouncing) and easy prolongations (stretching). Students may say, "Stuttering on purpose is just like using stretching and bouncing." Let students know, "Yes, you are correct—stuttering on purpose is very similar to using those other speech tools."

Begin by choosing any game to facilitate stuttering on purpose at the single-word level. Here is just one idea: Play *How Many Can You Name?* While modeling easy voluntary stuttering, explain to students:

> WWWWWe are going to play How Many Can You Name? The first topic is sports. We will take tu-tu-turns mentioning the name of a sport. You must stutter on pppurpose on the name of the sport. I will call on sssstudents by going aaaround the room in a circle. For each sport you name, you get a point. The students with the mmmmost points iiis the winner. If you forget to stutter on the nay-nay-name of the sport, you lose a point. The first sport that I will name is bay-bay-baseball.

The game ends when students are unable to think of the name of a sport that has not been mentioned already. Consider using the scorecard (Appendix A) to keep score. Doing so often raises the level of excitement and interest in the game. Also, occasionally forget to stutter on purpose so that students can "catch" you forgetting to use the assigned tool. This will helps students monitor their own speech more effectively.

After naming sports, introduce other topics, such as names of television shows, movies, junk food, video games, books, and athletes. Make sure the topics will hold the group's attention.

Although you want to encourage easy stuttering during this activity, you also want the stuttering to be noticeable. Sometimes a student will "cheat the stutter" by speaking so smoothly that it does not sound like a stutter. If a student is stuttering in a subtle or barely noticeable manner, say, "You can stutter better than that!"

Voluntary Stuttering at the Sentence Level. Continue playing How Many Can You Name? but students are now expected to speak using complete sentences while stuttering on purpose. Explain:

> The new topic is "favorite foods." But now you have to speak in complete sentences. I will go first. "My favorite thing to eat at Burger King is ffffffrench fries." If you forget to stutter at least one time, or if you forget to say a complete sentence, you lose a point.

Role-Playing Voluntary Stuttering. Students should have plenty of opportunities to role-play stuttering on purpose in speech class before using this technique in public. Begin by holding up your hand and announcing, "I have five fingers on my hand; we need to come up with five places where speaking is difficult. Ordering food at restaurants is often hard. What are some other difficult speaking situations?" You may write down student answers on a chalkboard or on poster board for the group to see. Then ask students to choose a difficult speaking situation to use when role-playing. Next, role-play the situation while using voluntary stuttering. You may use the Stuttering on Purpose Plays handout to get you started. Inform students that it is completely acceptable for any character in the play to stutter. Students should not feel ashamed or concerned about stuttering when playing the role of the cashier. You might say, "When playing roles other than the stutterer, I still expect that you might stutter. Don't worry if you do!"

Appropriate eye contact should be stressed throughout role-playing activities (see Eye-to-Eye–Activity 13). Tell students that they do not have to hold solid, unbreaking eye contact but should maintain eye contact during moments of stuttering (Sheehan, 1968). Model the assignment by speaking first. For example, if students wish to practice ordering ice cream in a store, you will order first (assign a student the role of working at the ice-cream counter). You may say, "Eeeexcuse me, cccould I plea-plea-please have a vvvanilla ice-cream cone?" Be sure to make eye contact while stuttering. After you model the assignment, give each student a turn to order.

In the real world, students will often forget to stutter on purpose because they are not sure when they should be stuttering. To avoid this, assist by providing specific words for students to stutter on. Say, "Stutter on the first word that you say" or "Be sure to stutter on the flavor of ice cream that you want." Then role-play the situation so that students may practice stuttering on their assigned words. If a student forgets to stutter, make a humorous comment, such as, "How can a stutterer forget to stutter?" Repeat the activity until all students remember to stutter.

Voluntary Stuttering in Public. When students feel comfortable in their ability to stutter on purpose during role-playing situations, practice voluntary stuttering outside of the therapy room. Be sure to secure the necessary permission to take students off site. Use the Speech Class Permission Form in Appendix A. Read through the form and print your name on the appropriate line. Then have the form approved by your site's administrator. Your site may ask you to add specific language, or they may offer you a preexisting form to use in its place. It is best to include your site's official letterhead on any permission form you use so that parents understand you have the support of your administration.

Plan the activity around your student's interests. Ask them, "Where do you want to go today to work on your stuttering?" Answers may include a corner store, a bakery, or a local fast food establishment. If students choose to go to a local bakery and buy a treat, you may wish to briefly have them role-play this situation.

Then go out to the bakery and encourage students to watch you closely *as you order first* while using fake stuttering. Say, "I am going to make eye contact with the counter person when I stutter on purpose so be sure to look at my eyes." This will show that you are not ashamed of stuttering, and it provides a strong model for your students. Then give each student the opportunity to order a treat while stuttering on purpose and maintaining eye contact. Remember to give students very specific directions. There are some employees who will look to the adult (you) when a child is ordering. To circumvent this, it is best that you look at the student while he is talking so that the employee also knows to focus on the student.

After all of your students order, reward them for their attempts. Do not wait to get back to speech class. Congratulate the students in the store or as soon as you leave the store. If a student uses voluntary stuttering but forgets to make eye contact, be sure to reward him for trying. You may say, "You are so strong and brave to come out here and stutter on purpose. I can tell you are really working hard on your stuttering." When you get back to speech class or while heading back to speech class, discuss the experience with students.

Students will report a wide variety of feelings and thoughts after this assignment. Some students return from a voluntary stuttering assignment and cannot believe how helpful it was to get their stuttering quickly out in the open. Some students are fearful of using voluntary stuttering and choose not to participate the first time. Some do not have strong feelings one way or the other but feel it is just another way to practice talking.

When using voluntary stuttering, it is common for students to report different levels of real stuttering. Some may say, "By trying to stutter on purpose, I wasn't able to stutter at all," whereas others will state, "Stuttering on purpose only made me stutter more." All responses need to be validated and discussed. Whether a student reports stuttering less or stuttering more, you are correct to say that both are typical responses to stuttering on purpose. Over time, stuttering on purpose reduces the fear of stuttering and that in turn reduces the frequency and severity of stuttering.

You need to show much patience and compassion when working on voluntary stuttering. Do not push students too fast. At first a student may be too fearful to attempt stuttering on purpose in public. Just "tagging along" and observing is success and needs to be respected and rewarded. If a student chooses not to order his own treat, buy him a treat anyway and be sure to tell him, "You are so courageous to join us today."

There is no limit to how many times students may use and practice voluntary stuttering. Revisit this activity as much as you deem necessary and useful. I often use voluntary stuttering in public as a reward for completing other assignments and activities. For example, I may say, "When we complete our stuttering newsletter (see Big News–Activity 36), I will take everyone out for an ice-cream cone, and we will order it by stuttering on purpose." Although this may sound like work to an adult, to many children it is seen as a special reward.

More Ideas

Voluntary stuttering activities are a great time to have guests and visitors attend therapy. Students will learn much by explaining the purpose of voluntary stuttering. Guests are also expected to use voluntary stuttering; this often provides guests with a greater appreciation for the difficulties that stutterers face. Teach guests voluntary stuttering using a hierarchy (i.e., single words, sentences, and role-playing). You may even have guests participate in voluntary stuttering activities in public.

When playing the game How Many Can You Name? change the point system and give students points for forgetting to use voluntary stuttering. Played this way, the student with the most points loses and the student with the fewest points is the winner. Although this may seem like a minor change, children often find it exciting to play a game in this manner. This is a "trick" I use during many games to keep them fun and fresh.

Homework

Voluntary stuttering is a speech tool that should be explained to parents before they are expected to assist their children with related homework. Although many parents will easily understand the importance of voluntary stuttering, some will not. It is not uncommon or unreasonable for a parent to say, "I thought my child was going to speech therapy to stop stuttering, not to stutter more." Take the necessary time to explain the importance of voluntary stuttering. Speaking to parents in person and including them in therapy is the best way to proceed; but if this is not possible, send home the Letter to Parents: Stuttering on Purpose located at the end of this activity. Homework Assignment 4 asks parents to stutter on purpose in public. Just as you do not want to push your students too hard, it is important not to push parents either. Before using this assignment, you want to make sure that the parents are willing and ready. Invite them to one or more sessions and include them in voluntary stuttering activities.

Stuttering on Purpose Plays

Fast Food

CASHIER: How can I help you today?

STUDENT: May-may-may-may-may I please have a large order of french fries?

CASHIER: Okay, would you like anything to drink with that?

STUDENT: Yyyyyyyes, a large chocolate milkshake.

CASHIER: I'm sorry, we are out of milkshakes. Would you like something else?

STUDENT: I-I-I-I will have a large cola instead, please.

The Corner Store

STUDENT: Eeeexcuse me, sir. Hhhhow much are your chocolate bars?

CASHIER: Some are 75 cents and others are a dollar or more.

STUDENT: Ccccccould I please have a Rrrrreese's Peanut Butter Cup?

CASHIER: No problem. Anything else?

STUDENT: Nnno, thank you.

Letter to Parents: Stuttering on Purpose

Dear ______________________________ ,

In speech class we work on talking about stuttering, and we also work on using "speech tools" to help students stutter more easily and less often. Speech tools is a term used with children that means speaking strategies. For example, one speech tool we use is called "stretching." Your child ssssstretches the first sound of a word in an easy and gentle manner to help him or her move through moments of stuttering.

Many children have a difficult time using speech tools because they have built up a lot of fear and shame around talking. One way to reduce this fear of speaking is by using a speech tool called "voluntary stuttering." Voluntary stuttering is the same as stuttering on purpose. Students learn that when facing a difficult speaking situation, they may use this pretend stuttering to help them be less afraid of talking. As they get their stuttering out in the open, they are also able to concentrate on what they want to say.

Students will occasionally bring home assignments that ask them to practice stuttering on purpose with a family member. Some assignments may ask a family member to try stuttering on purpose. If you have any questions about voluntary stuttering, please contact me at ______________________________ . I am happy to talk with you about this important speaking strategy.

Sincerely,

Stuttering (12) Homework

Name ______________________________ Date due ______________

Think of three speaking situations in which it may help you to use voluntary stuttering. Write them below. We will discuss them in class.

1. ____

2. ____

3. ____

Parent signature ______________________________

(1)

Stuttering (12) Homework

Name ______________________________ Date due ______________

Explain to your parents that you are using voluntary stuttering to help reduce your fear of talking. Then call up a relative, such as a grandparent or aunt, and talk to him or her for 5 minutes. Stutter on purpose at least three times. How did this feel? ______________________________

____

____

____

____

____

Parent signature ______________________________

(2)

Stuttering 12 Homework

Name ______________________ Date due ______________

Teach your parents how to stutter on purpose. Ask your mother or father to try stuttering on purpose on at least three words. Make sure that their stuttering is hard enough so that it sounds like real stuttering. Ask them how it felt to stutter and write their answers below.

____

____

____

____

____

Parent signature ______________________ (3)

Stuttering 12 Homework

Name ______________________ Date due ______________

Go out with a parent for ice cream. Explain that you are working on stuttering on purpose to help reduce your fear of stuttering. Your parent's homework is to order ice cream while stuttering on the kind that he or she wants. For example, if your mother wants chocolate ice cream, then she needs to say, "Could I please have ch-ch-ch-chocolate ice cream." You may have to teach your parent how to stutter! Then ask your parent how it felt to stutter in public and write the answer below.

____

____

____

____

____

____

Parent signature ______________________ (4)

13
Eye-to-Eye

Purpose

- To learn that making eye contact while stuttering leads to increased confidence and self-respect

Materials

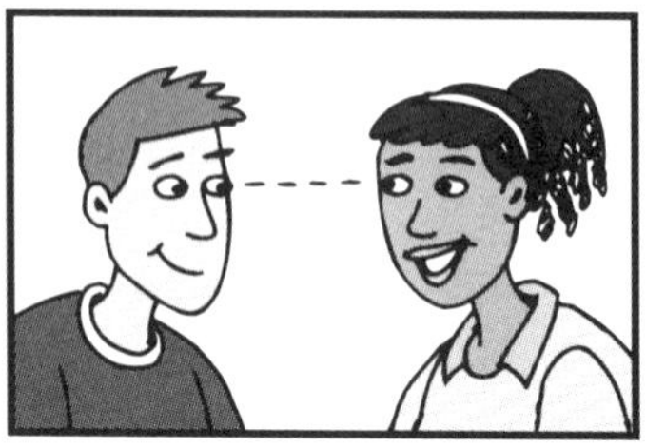

Toy glasses
The Best Eye Contact Stuttering Award (Appendix A)
The Worst Eye Contact Stuttering Award (Appendix A)
Homework

Directions

Introductions. One way to stress the importance of eye contact during moments of stuttering is by showing students a demonstration. Explain, "Let's pretend that I am introducing myself to someone at a party. Watch the two ways that I introduce myself and tell me what you think."

Then walk out of the room and reenter by walking up to one of the students, shaking her hand, and introducing yourself while stuttering on purpose. Make a point to look away from the listener by looking at your feet; this demonstrates a clear example of poor eye contact. Then leave the room again and reenter. This time shake the student's hand and introduce yourself using voluntarily stuttering while maintaining eye contact; this demonstrates a clear example of good eye contact. After these two brief demonstrations, ask, "Which was a better way to introduce myself?" Most students will easily recognize that stuttering while looking away indicates shame and fear. Students learn that good eye contact shows confidence and self-respect. Continue by explaining the following:

> You tell other people a lot about yourself by the way that you stutter. If you stutter while looking at the floor and avoiding eye contact, you are showing others that you are ashamed and scared of the way that you talk. If you stutter while making eye contact, you show others that you are not ashamed of stuttering and they need not be either.

Ask students, "Who wants to show the class one good and one bad example of eye contact while stuttering just like I did?" Then give students the opportunity to introduce themselves to each other using voluntary stuttering—first with poor eye contact and then with good eye contact. Most students will have little difficulty stuttering on purpose if you present it casually. If a student forgets to stutter, say, "Hey, you forgot to stutter during your introduction. Try it again and throw in a few fake stutters like I did." You may even revisit Stuttering Awards–Activity 21 and award the Best Eye Contact Stuttering Award and the Worst Eye Contact Stuttering Award.

Conversation. Continue by asking the students to talk about a topic, such as rollerblading, trading cards, music, basketball, or a hit television show. Say, "When you stutter, make eye contact with someone in the room." If students are not stuttering during this activity, ask them to use fake stuttering while practicing eye contact.

Pass out the toy glasses from the Stuttering Kits for students to use while practicing eye contact. Ask students to wear or hold their toy glasses during conversations. The glasses are used because they are symbolic and fun.

Homework

Be sure to review assigned homework in class before sending it home so that students fully understand what they are expected to do. Parents may be uncomfortable holding eye contact with their children during stuttering moments. Thus, before assigning homework from this activity, consider inviting parents to join a therapy session in which eye contact is discussed and practiced.

Stuttering 13 Homework

Name ______________________ Date due ______________

Explain to your parents or other adult relative that you are practicing making eye contact when you stutter. Tell them that by looking at people when you stutter, you are showing them that stuttering is nothing to be scared of or ashamed of.

Next, introduce yourself to your relative, just like we did in speech class, with "bad" eye contact while stuttering and then with "good" eye contact while stuttering. Then ask them which one they liked better.

What did he or she say and why? ______________________

____

____

Then ask your relative to try stuttering with good eye contact and bad eye contact. How did he or she do? ______________________

____

Parent signature ______________________ (1)

Stuttering 13 Homework

Name ______________________ Date due ______________

Sit down with a sibling, neighbor, or friend and explain that you are practicing making eye contact when you stutter. Explain that by making eye contact, you are showing everyone that you are not scared of how you talk. Then demonstrate "good" eye contact and "bad" eye contact and ask this person to try both. How did he or she do? ______________________

____

____

____

____

____

____

Parent signature ______________________ (2)

14
Stuttering Grab Bag

Purpose

- To practice stuttering easily tools (stretching, bouncing, and voluntary stuttering)
- To provide students with the opportunity to identify correct and incorrect use of speech tools

Materials

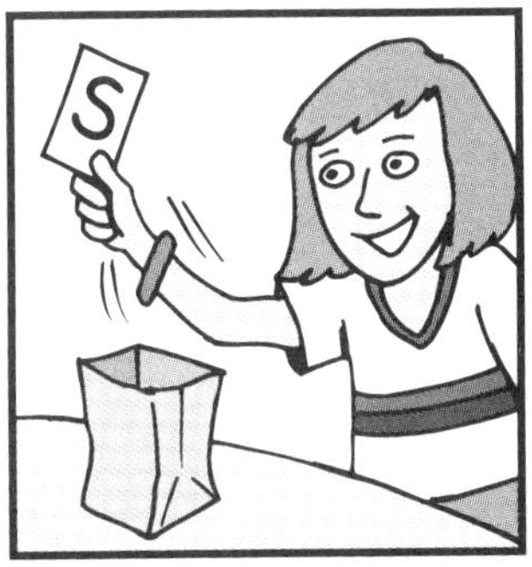

Flashcards with letters of the alphabet and blends (i.e., *s* and *th*)—purchased at educational or office supply stores, or you can make them
Cloth, plastic, or paper bag
Scorecard (Appendix A)
Bingo chips or other tokens

Directions

Stuttering Grab Bag requires that students possess basic phonemic awareness abilities (see More Ideas for working with students without these skills). Begin playing by putting the flashcards with the sounds you wish to target in a bag. Explain:

> Today we are going to practice stretching. You will each take a turn picking a card with a letter or blend out of the bag. Then you will think of a word that starts with that letter or letters and say it by stretching the first sound. If you remember to stretch the first sound of the word, you get a point (use the scorecard or tokens to award points). If you forget to stretch the first sound or if you accidentally stretch the wrong sound, then I get the point. The first person to get 10 points is the winner.

Demonstrate a few correct stretches to students using letters and blends. As the game progresses and as students are able to stretch single words, increase the difficulty by asking students to stretch words within sentences. For example, if a student picks the letter *z* out of the bag, then she would say, "After school I am going to the zzzzzzoo with my sister."

As the game progresses, encourage students to pay close attention to the assigned speech tool. For example, you may say,

> Anyone who identifies someone using a speech tool in the wrong way will receive an extra point. For example, if the assigned tool is stretching and I say the word "tuuuuurtle," I would be stretching on the second sound of the word,

which we all know is not correct. The first person to raise his hand and catch this mistake gets the extra point.

Remember that in general, stops may be more difficult to stretch than vowels, diphthongs, fricatives, nasals, affricates, liquids, and glides. (See Stretching–Activity 9 to understand how to stretch stops.) After practicing stretching use this game to practice bouncing and voluntary stuttering as well.

You will need to be flexible during this game because different students have different letter/sound correspondence abilities. For example, if the letter being discussed is *s* and a student suggests *city,* tell the class, "*City* does not start with the letter *s,* but it does start with the /s/ sound, so it is worth a point."

More Ideas

Bonus Points. Offer students a bonus point for using stretching, bouncing, or voluntary stuttering on two words in a sentence. Give an example by explaining, "I am going to use two bounces in the following sentence: A-a-a-after school I am go-go-go-going to play basketball."

Board Games. Incorporate a common board game such as Chutes and Ladders or checkers. A student picks a letter or blend from the bag and is asked to bounce, stretch, or voluntarily stutter on a word beginning with the assigned sound. Every time a student successfully completes a turn, she gets to take a turn on the board game.

Working with Children with Limited Phonemic Awareness Abilities. When using this activity with children with limited phonemic awareness abilities, try using letter–alphabet cards that contain both a letter and a corresponding picture. This way, when a student picks up the card with the letter *s,* she is able to see the picture of a sun or a snake and is thus able to successfully say at least one word that starts with the letter *s.* Then say, "Let's practice stretching more words that begin with the letter *s.* At this point suggest a few words such as *sister, Saturday,* and *Santa.* Then, if you feel it is appropriate, ask the child if she can think of her own words that begin with the letter *s* or the /s/ sound. Often times, I will find an object in the room that begins with the chosen letter or blend. For example, if a student picks up a *b* card and cannot figure out a word that begins with *b,* I might point to a child and say, "William is not a girl; William is a __________." This hint enables the student to then stretch the word *boy* and earn a point.

15
Stuttering Potluck

Purpose

- To demonstrate that stretching and bouncing (stuttering easily tools) and pausing (stutter less often tool) may be used in conjunction with one another

Materials

None

Directions

Pausing can reduce the frequency of stuttering at any one time but will not eradicate stuttering entirely. Although not all children feel this way, one fourth-grade student explained that he viewed using stretch-outs and bounce-outs as emergency tools to be used when pausing did not completely diminish his moments of stuttering. Here is a way to practice this integrated therapy approach. Explain (while using pausing after the first word of each sentence and then after every two, three, four, or five words):

> Today we are going to practice our speech tools while playing Stutter Punch. Everyone will get a turn to speak while using pausing. You can talk about your favorite hobbies, such as TV shows or playing basketball or anything else you want to talk about. When you start to stutter, I will grab your stutter with my fist and hold it in my "stutter punch." As I start to slowly unclench my fist, you have to stretch-out (or bounce-out) of the stutter.

Have the students take turns talking while you "grab their stutters" and hold them as they stretch-out or bounce-out of the stutters. Then reverse roles by letting a student play the role of the clinician, reaching out and holding your stutters in his fist. You might say:

> Now I am going to explain to you how I cook my favorite meal. I will use pausing, as I am doing now, and when I stutter, the assigned student needs to grab my stutter with a stutter punch and slowly let it go. As the student lets my stutter go, I will bounce-out (or stretch-out) of the stutter.

Then, in great detail, explain how you cook or prepare something that is somewhat complicated. If you choose something simple like making a bowl of cereal, your turn will be over very quickly. Also, by choosing something complicated, you are demonstrating to students that speech is fun and that they are allowed to take their time and enjoy speaking. When your turn is over, ask each student to think of something they are good at making such as homemade pizza, sandwiches, or pancakes. If a student says that he is not allowed to cook at home, ask him to describe something he has seen a relative prepare. Explain:

> Now it is your turn to tell us how to cook something while using your pausing. When I hear you stutter, I will catch your stutter and hold it until I am ready to let go. You will hold the stutter and then release it with a bounce-out (or a stretch-out).

Next, give students the opportunity to catch each other's stutters. You may move on from cooking to other topics and say, "Tell us all the rules of baseball" or "How do you play checkers? Tell us all the rules."

At times students will not stutter at all because of the combined effect of using pausing and being expected to stutter. In such situations, ask students to use their pausing while also using some voluntary stuttering. When an assigned student uses voluntary stuttering, catch the stutter and gently release your fist. As your fist unclenches, the student stretches or bounces out of the voluntary stutter.

16
Speech Tool Bingo

Purpose

- To practice stuttering easily tools (stretching, bouncing, and voluntary stuttering)

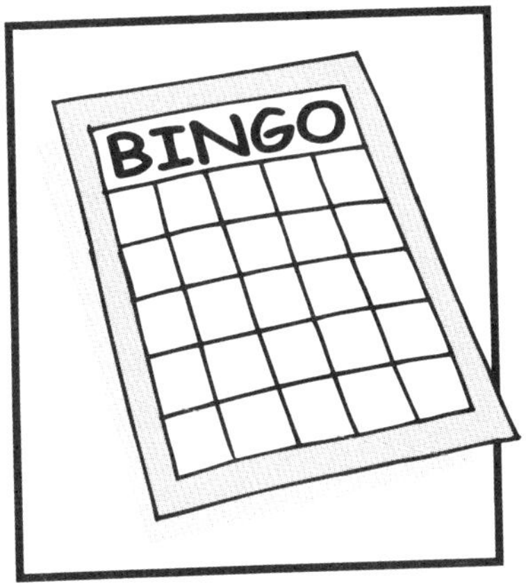

Materials

Blank paper (8 ½" x 11")
Pencils
Mirror
Bingo chips
Homework

Directions

Have each student construct a Stuttering Bingo board (as described in Stuttering Bingo–Activity 3). Students create a bingo board by folding a piece of paper into 16 squares. Assign 16 letters and blends that students randomly write in bingo squares. For example, if you say *r*, students write the letter *r* in any bingo square. If you say *s* and then *n*, students write the *sn* blend in a bingo square. The purpose of random placement is so that all students use the same letters and blends but have a differently configured board. Then explain:

> Each student is going to get a chance to be the teacher. The chosen student will look at her bingo board and choose a letter or a blend. But she shouldn't tell anyone what she has chosen. Then she will say a word that begins with the chosen letter or blend by stretching (or bouncing or using voluntary stuttering) on it. Everyone will have to find the letter or blend that the word begins with on their bingo boards. For example, if the student says "ssssoda," put a bingo chip on the square with the letter *s*. The first person to complete a line of chips across the board shouts "bingo" and is the winner.

After students have success playing this game at the word level, you may increase the difficulty of the task by saying to students, "Use your voluntary stuttering (or stretching or bouncing) on a word within a sentence." Give an example by saying, "Today I am going to eat ppppizza after school." Now find the letter *p* on your boards."

More Ideas

It is helpful to work on identifying how sounds are made so that students think about how they can use their speech tools on these sounds. For example, if a student is practicing stretching on the /b/ sound in *Batman,* he might ask, "How do you stretch the letter *b?* (Children and adults often find stops to be the hardest sounds to stretch.) You may respond by asking, "Well, tell me how you make the /b/ sound in Batman." At that point the student may say, "By putting my lips together." You may then say, "Now try saying Batman by putting your lips together very softly so that there is just a little space between them. Your words should now have a little room to come out." During Speech Tool Bingo, occasionally stop students and ask, "What sound did you stretch on?" Then, "How did you stretch on it?"

By knowing how sounds are made, students have a better understanding of how to initiate them and work through them with reduced struggle. I recall working with a fifth-grade student who was having difficulty moving from the /h/ to the /o/ in the word *home.* He just kept blocking on the /h/ with his lips pressed together tightly. This student gave up and said, "I can't say it." I then asked him to explain how the /o/ sound is made. He said, "You make the /o/ by using your voice box and opening your mouth." The student then realized that he would not be able to complete the word home until he opened his mouth to make the /o/. The student tried saying the word home again, became stuck on the /h/, and then opened his mouth and completed the word. Taking the time to consider how sounds are made helped this student move forward through moments of stuttering.

Homework

Use the following homework assignments or assign homework from previous activities.

Stuttering 16 Homework

Name ______________________ Date due ______________

Take home a completed bingo board from speech class. Teach a family member how to stretch or bounce a word that begins with each letter or blend on the bingo board. Ask your relative to stretch or bounce after you do. Make sure they do it correctly!

Parent signature ______________________ (1)

Stuttering 16 Homework

Name ______________________ Date due ______________

Think about letters and sounds that are easy and hard for you to say. Some children find the letter "s" in *snake* easy to stretch, and others find the "ch" blend in *church* difficult to stretch.

List three letters or blends that are easy for you to stretch and bounce on.

1. ______________ 2. ______________ 3. ______________

List three letters or blends that are difficult for you to stretch and bounce on.

1. ______________ 2. ______________ 3. ______________

Also, write down one way that you would like to practice stretching and bouncing during our next speech class.

____

____

____

____

____

____

Parent signature ______________________ (2)

17
Stutter Bubbles

Purpose

- To help students understand the concept that speaking gently is often more helpful when trying to speak easily than pushing hard
- To help students understand that taking deep breaths will not help speech improve

Materials

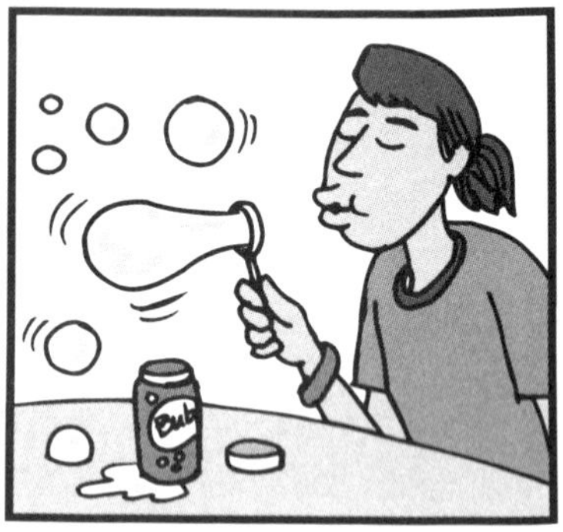

Bottle(s) of bubbles
Homework

Directions

This activity may take as little as 10 minutes. Thus, be prepared to move into a second activity, preferably one that asks students to practice stretching or bouncing. Begin the activity by taking out bottles of bubbles from each Stuttering Kit and passing them out. After allowing students to play with the bubbles for a minute, collect them all. Allowing students to play with the bubbles first makes it easier for them to concentrate on your lesson.

Dip the wand from a bottle of bubbles into the liquid and blow extremely hard into it so that the bubbles cannot form. Ask, "What happened?" to which students respond, "You blew too hard!"

Dip again and blow very softly into the bubble wand; blow so softly that the bubbles cannot form. Ask, "What happened?" to which students respond, "You blew too softly." Then dip and blow using the appropriate amount of air. Students will watch as you create a wave of bubbles.

Then ask, "How is blowing bubbles like stuttering?" There is usually a student or two who will respond, "When you try too hard to speak, the words don't come out." Sometimes a student will say, "When you use too much air, you stutter." Explain:

> You never need to take a deep breath to speak, and when you do take a deep breath, speaking will often become harder. When you whisper and use too little air (as stutterers often do), you cannot be heard. Part of speaking is using the right amount of air and the right amount of force. If you push too hard or breathe in deep breaths, you will probably stutter a lot more.

The visceral and visual experience of using bubbles is one that students not only enjoy but it helps them understand stuttering and speech tools better. When students are having a difficult stuttering day and are speaking with a lot of effort, remind them of the bubble activity. For example, say, "I see you pushing very hard today. Do you remember what happened when we blew too hard with the bubbles?"

More Ideas

Continue this session by practicing stretching and bouncing using any appropriate activity, such as 20 Questions–Activity 40 or Barrier Games–Activity 41. When students stutter remind them of the bubbles and ask, "How is your stuttering like blowing bubbles?" You may follow with, "Speaking and using speech tools is a lot like blowing bubbles; if you push too hard they don't work."

Homework

Homework Assignment 1 requires students to take bubbles home with them. If you choose to assign this homework, expect that some of the bubbles will spill at home, and some students will forget to bring them back to school. You may want to let students keep the bubbles as a treat.

Stuttering 17 Homework

Name ______________________ Date due ______________

Take home a bottle of bubbles from speech class and sit down with an adult family member. Show this person that stuttering is a lot like blowing bubbles. Explain and show them that

- when you blow too hard, the bubbles break;
- when you blow too soft, the bubbles won't come out; and
- when you blow with just the right amount of air, the bubbles come out nicely.

Tell them that just like with bubbles, when you push too hard with your speech, you stutter, and when you do not use enough air, your speech cannot be heard. Write down any comments from your family. ______________

____

____

____

____

____

Parent signature ______________________ (1)

Stuttering 17 Homework

Name ______________________ Date due ______________

When you blow bubbles too hard, the bubbles break. When you speak too hard, you sometimes stutter. What else does not work when you push too hard? For example, sometimes when you try to open a door that is stuck, pushing hard only makes it become more stuck. Think of two things that do not work right when you push too hard and write them below.

1. ____

____

2. ____

____

Parent signature ______________________ (2)

18
Pick-Up Sticks

Purpose

- To help students consider the amount of struggle they put into speaking
- To reward students for hard work

Materials

Pick-Up Sticks (available from toy stores and the Internet)

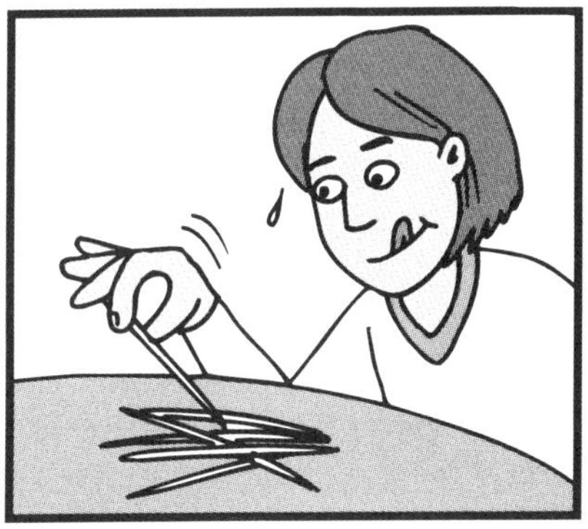

Directions

Pick-Up Sticks is a fun game to play occasionally as a reward or as a way to start or end a session. The game comes in a tube and has approximately 30 different colored sticks—each stick being approximately 10" long and very narrow (like long toothpicks).

After dropping the sticks on a steady table, students take turns trying to pick up one stick at a time, without moving any other sticks. At first the game is simple because several sticks are usually lying on the table without touching other sticks. But as the game continues, students have to try to pick up sticks that are lying under, on top of, or between other sticks *without moving any other sticks.*

While playing this game, you will have several opportunities to discuss stuttering concepts. For example, some students end up quickly losing their turns because they move so quickly and work so fast that they accidentally move several sticks before successfully picking up a single stick, thus losing a turn. When appropriate, suggest to students that just as with speaking, "When you work too fast, you may not get what you want." One student has stated, "When you move too fast, you lose control over your game."

Typically you can play this game by allowing a player to continue picking up sticks until he loses a turn. However, in speech class you may want to adapt the rules and allow only one stick to be picked up per turn. This means that even when a player successfully picks up a stick, his turn is over. This allows students with poorer hand coordination to have equal playing time. Sometimes when I am playing Pick-Up Sticks with a student who is capable of taking his time but always rushes, I revert to the original rules so that the student begins to understand that other children who are moving deliberately and carefully are amassing many more sticks and are winning.

Some students will unsuccessfully attempt to pick up the same stick many times in the same way. Students who have never played the game will not know strategies for picking up sticks. For example, students may attempt to pick up sticks with only one hand rather than two. Other students will not think to roll up their shirt-sleeves and will repeatedly lose their turns when a sleeve moves a stick. You may suggest that just as with stuttering, there are several strategies (tools) to use to achieve success. Show students several strategies that may be used to pick up sticks, such as the following:

- Move slowly, without excessive force.
- Using two hands, gently touch both ends of a stick with one finger on each point, squeeze the fingers together, and lift.
- Push down on one side of the stick so that it lifts up like a seesaw—then use the free hand to safely pick up the stick.
- Use a stick you have already picked up as a tool to gently push a desired stick out of the larger pile. Most Pick-Up Stick sets have one black stick that is the only stick that may be used for this purpose. Sometimes I adapt the rules and say that any stick—or any blue stick—may be used for assistance. In the latter case, if there are five or six blue sticks in a set, then each student has a pretty good chance of obtaining one during the game.

After playing a game of Pick-Up Sticks, have students explain different strategies they have for picking up sticks. Then you can relate this to the different uses of speech tools. Ask students questions such as, "When playing Pick-Up Sticks, you have several ways of easily picking up sticks. What ways do you have to help make talking easier?" Students often list speech tools, such as stretching and pausing. Sometimes students will share their own self-generated strategies. As a reminder, it is important to note that some student self-generated strategies are functioning as secondary behaviors. For instance, students may say that "taking deep breaths" or "snapping my fingers" makes talking easier.

More Ideas

Toy Trains. Other toys, such as trains, are a fun way to help students understand the concept that *struggle often leads to more struggle.* There are several different brands of toy trains that come with tracks that are put together with interlocking pieces. Students often find that when putting away these train tracks, they are not always easy to separate. Some students will struggle with the tracks and pull harder and harder to separate them. Sometimes the tracks will separate, but at other times they will remain stuck or even break. This is a good time for you to demonstrate that by pulling gently on the train tracks, they come apart easier. Discuss this concept with students and compare it to stuttering. For example, you may say,

> Just like with our stuttering, sometimes when we push hard we only get more stuck. By pulling and pushing hard on the train tracks, the tracks may remain

> stuck and may even break. By gently stretching and bouncing our words, we often find that they just come out. Try gently pulling apart the train tracks.

Keep in mind that toy trains may seem babyish to some students, especially those in the fourth and fifth grades. This activity is typically suitable for students from kindergarten through the second and third grades.

Chinese Finger Traps. Try using Chinese finger toys or finger traps. Finger traps are short tubes, as long as a finger, that are available through the Internet, the Oriental Trading Company catalogs, and some party stores. Students are given one finger trap and asked to insert a finger on each side. The two fingers immediately get stuck in the toys and students respond by pulling hard and struggling. Demonstrate that by pulling and pushing gently, the fingers are released. These finger toys also fit nicely into Stuttering Kits. When guests come to speech class, students often enjoy explaining how finger traps relate to stuttering.

19
Out in the World

Purpose

- To practice using stretching, bouncing, and pausing in public
- To reduce the fear of speaking in public

Materials

Prop-making materials (i.e., paper, pencils, magic markers, and tape)
Out in the World Stretching Play

Directions

By now the students are probably familiar with using voluntary stuttering in public. This activity will focus on practicing the specific techniques of stretching, bouncing, and pausing in the real world. Using stretching and bouncing is a great way to practice modifying speech during stressful speaking situations, and students will benefit from the desensitization aspect of this activity.

Role-Playing. Ask students to decide upon a local shop or store they would like to visit to practice their speech tools out in the world. Make sure that the final choice is appropriate and practical. You may want to make suggestions, such as a local fast food establishment or a neighborhood deli. If students decide they would like to use their speech tools while asking for a candy bar or other treat at a local deli, role-play this situation first. You and your students may create a makeshift deli in the therapy room with a deli sign and other appropriate props.

Some students may play the role of deli employees, and the others can be stutterers. Remind students, "When playing roles other than a stutterer, it is completely acceptable if you stutter. Don't feel you need to speak without stuttering." The first assignment for the students playing stutterers is to stretch (or bounce) on the first syllable they say. Demonstrate the assignment by taking the role of a stutterer and asking the student playing the cashier, "Eeeeexcuse me, could I please have a Milky Way bar?" Continue by having the students act out their parts while stretching the first sound of the first word that they say.

It is important to stress the importance of initiating and maintaining eye contact when using speech tools. Remind students that using eye contact shows confidence. Just as during Voluntary Stuttering–Activity 12, students will enjoy constructing a role-playing scene, such as a restaurant, in the speech room.

Using Speech Tools in the Real World. It is best if you take the group out in public directly after practicing role-playing. If possible, consider extending speech class to a double period so that there is continuity between the role-playing exercise and using speech tools in the real word. If this is not possible, simply take your students out in public during their next speech class.

For the first assignment, take the situation your students role-played into the real world. To continue with the earlier example, take students to a local deli and ask them to stretch the first sound of the first word that they say. You need to order an item first, using the assigned tool in a noticeable way.

Try other public-speaking assignments, practicing by role-playing first. Be sure to give very specific directions so that students do not forget to use their speech tools. Some assignments follow:

- Use frequent pausing after every one, two, or three words. For example, "May, I please have, a hot chocolate, with, whipped cream?"
- Ask students to bounce on the first word of a sentence. For example, "Wh-wh-wh-where are the comic books?"
- Ask a librarian where to find a certain book while stretching (or bouncing) on the name of the book. For example, "Sir, do you have any Ssssspiderman books?"
- Ask a store clerk several questions about products at the store while pausing after every couple of words. "Excuse me, do you carry, baseball cards? I, am looking, for one, to buy, my brother for, his birthday. How, much is it?"

More Ideas

Use the Out in the World Stretching Play at the end of this activity. This is a play that helps students role-play stretching at an ice-cream parlor. You may also write your own plays and underline words to signify stretching or bouncing or put in commas to indicate where to pause.

Out in the World Stretching Play

The scene is an ice-cream parlor.

COUNTER PERSON: How can I help you today?

CHILD 1: Ccccould I please have a chocolate ice-cream cone with sprinkles?

COUNTER PERSON: No problem. Do you want one scoop or two?

CHILD 1: Ooooone scoop please.

COUNTER PERSON: Here you go.

CHILD 1: Thanks a lot.

CHILD 2: Dddddo you have vanilla fudge?

COUNTER PERSON: Yes we do.

CHILD 2: Llllet me have vanilla fudge in a bowl with whipped cream and a cherry.

COUNTER PERSON: Do you want one scoop or two?

CHILD 2: Tttttwo scoops please.

COUNTER PERSON: Here you go.

CHILD 2: Thanks for your hhhhelp.

20
Phone Fun

Purpose

- To reduce the fear of speaking on the telephone
- To practice speech tools during stressful situations

Materials

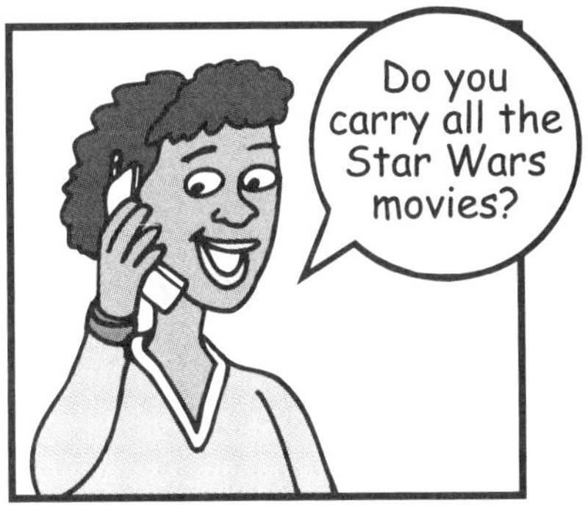

Telephone
Local phonebook
Index cards
Pencil
Questions: Telephone Assignment handout
Create-Your-Own Telephone Assignment handout
Homework

Directions

Many stutterers report that talking on the telephone is one of the most terrifying, frustrating, and difficult times for them to talk. In one questionnaire study, 63% of 223 participants indicated that speaking on the telephone is more difficult than speaking to someone in person (James, Brumfitt, & Cudd, 1999). Using the telephone during therapy is an ideal time for students to face this feared situation and to practice speech tools.

Prepare for this activity by writing the names and phone numbers of local stores on index cards with corresponding questions for students to ask. Leave space on each card so that students may write down their answers. Try to create the phone cards to reflect student interests. For example, many students will be more excited to call a video game store with a question than to call a clothing store. If you are unable to create phone cards from scratch, see the Questions: Telephone Assignment handout. This handout includes prepared questions for the caller to ask; all you need to do is add the names and phone numbers of local stores and assign speech tools. It is always good to have a large stack of completed phone cards so that you do not run out of assignments.

When working on speech tools, use an underline to signify where stretching, bouncing, or voluntary stuttering should occur and use commas to signify where pausing should occur. Be well prepared during phone activities—students need to know the name and phone number of who they are calling, how they should begin their phone conversation, and what questions they should ask (in writing). See Figure 20.1 for an example of a prepared index card for pausing practice. Figure 20.2 shows a prepared index card to practice stretching, bouncing, or voluntary stuttering.

Call Peter's Pets at 888-8888 and ask them—

Could, you please, tell me, what kind, of animals, your store, carries?

Answer ______________________________

____

____

____

____

Figure 20.1 Example of a prepared index card for pausing practice

Call Michelle's Music at 999-9999 and ask them—

What time do you close today?

Answer ______________________________

____

____

____

____

Figure 20.2 Example of a prepared index card for stretching, bouncing, or voluntary stuttering practice

Begin by asking students to explain their experiences and feelings about talking on the phone. Some students will have great fear of using the phone; others will have little fear or be indifferent. Some students will say that they rarely or never use the phone at home. Discuss each child's phone experiences. Then explain:

> Many people who stutter do not like talking on the telephone because they often find it frustrating and embarrassing to stutter on the phone. Talking on the telephone is a great time to practice using speech tools. Using speech tools will help you work through words and deal with the fear of talking

on the phone. Today we will role-play making phone calls while practicing speech tools. Then we will make real phone calls.

Role-Playing. Give each student an index card assignment and ask him to review it. Break students into pairs to practice role-playing as you have in other activities. Make sure that students remember to use their assigned speech tool.

Making Real Phone Calls. You need to complete the first phone call or first few phone calls to demonstrate this activity and to create a safe working environment. Ask students to listen closely to make sure that you use the assigned speech tool. For example, say, "I'm going to make a phone call while pausing after every few words. Watch me closely to make sure I do it right."

Students can use an assignment they were given during role-playing to complete their first real telephone call. As the first student completes his assignment, the rest of the class quietly observes. You may use a speaker phone so that those observing may hear both sides of the phone conversation (Guitar & Reville, 2003). When a student completes an assignment, be sure to reward him for having the courage to use a speech tool on the phone. If a student forgets to use the speech tool, reward him for his attempt.

After students have completed their assignments, discuss how it feels to use speech tools on the telephone. Were they scared or nervous beforehand? How do they feel now having completed the phone calls? What would they change? Would they like to choose their own speech tools for making calls? Many students feel strong and confident after participating in phone activities. After the discussion, continue having them make phone calls by giving each one an additional card.

More Ideas

Students Create Their Own Phone Assignments. Pass out local phone books and copies of the Create-Your-Own Telephone Assignment handout (page 151), so that students may go through the phone books and write down their own telephone assignments. You or the student may decide which speech tool or tools to use. Each student should be expected to prepare for several phone calls (in case any of the phone numbers are out of service). When ready, students takes turns making their phone calls and writing down their answers.

Calling Parents. After students make several phone calls, ask them to call a parent or a close relative to explain the Phone Fun activity. For example, give the following assignment, "Using pausing, call your mother and talk to her about the phone calls you just made. Be sure to tell her about the speech tools you used and how you feel now that we are finished."

Calling Stuttering Organizations. There are many fine nonprofit organizations dedicated to helping people who stutter (see Resources in Appendix E). Have students call these groups and request catalogs and membership information. Tell students that they should not give out their own names or addresses and that all requests for information should be mailed to your office or the school. Write down the appropriate mailing address for students to have in front of them. The following is an example of what the student could say if calling the Stuttering Foundation of America.

> My name is ________________, and I am a calling you during my speech class. My speech teacher is ________________. Could you please mail us a catalog of your stuttering books and videos? Please address the catalog to my teacher, Mr./Ms. ________________. My school's address is________________. Thank you.

Homework

Assign homework from this activity that you feel best meets the needs of your students. If you noticed that a student was having particular difficulty using one of the speech tools, you may assign homework that includes practice on that speech tool.

Questions: Telephone Assignment

Name ______________________

Call ______________________ at ______________ and ask them—
(name of store) (phone number)

What time does your store close today?

answer ____

Questions: Telephone Assignment

Name ______________________

Call ______________________ at ______________ and ask them—
(name of store) (phone number)

Could you please tell me what bus lines run closest to your store?

answer ____

Questions: Telephone Assignment

Name ______________________

Call ______________________ at ______________ and ask them—
(name of store) (phone number)

How much does a large pepperoni pizza cost? Do you deliver?

answers ____

Questions: Telephone Assignment

Name ______________________

Call ______________________ at ______________ and ask them—
(name of store) (phone number)

Does your store carry video games? What time do you open on weekends?

answers ____

Questions: Telephone Assignment

Name ____________________

Call ____________________ at ______________ and ask them—
(name of store) (phone number)

Does your store sell board games? I am looking for games for children.

answer ____

____

Questions: Telephone Assignment

Name ____________________

Call ____________________ at ______________ and ask them—
(name of store) (phone number)

I collect comic books. What type of comic books do you carry?

answer ____

____

Questions: Telephone Assignment

Name ____________________

Call ____________________ at ______________ and ask them—
(name of store) (phone number)

Does your store carry children's sneakers? What brands do you carry?

answers ____

____

Questions: Telephone Assignment

Name ____________________

Call ____________________ at ______________ and ask them—
(name of store) (phone number)

I collect baseball trading cards. What kind of selection do you have?

answer ____

____

Create-Your-Own Telephone Assignment

Name ______________________

Call ______________________ at ______________ and ask them—
(name of store) (phone number)

question ____

____

____

answer ____

____

____

Create-Your-Own Telephone Assignment

Name ______________________

Call ______________________ at ______________ and ask them—
(name of store) (phone number)

question ____

____

____

answer ____

____

____

Create-Your-Own Telephone Assignment

Name ______________________

Call ______________________ at ______________ and ask them—
(name of store) (phone number)

question ____

____

____

answer ____

____

____

Stuttering 20 Homework

Name ______________________ Date due ______________

Take home a Create-Your-Own Telephone Assignment handout. Use your family's phone book to find some stores that you would like to call. Fill out the handout. Make sure you include the name of the stores, the phone numbers, and questions that you want to ask. We will make the phone calls in speech class using a speech tool.

Parent signature ______________________

(1)

- - - - - - - - - - - - - - - - - - - -

Stuttering 20 Homework

Name ______________________ Date due ______________

Take home two telephone note cards that your speech teacher has created for you. With your parents watching, call the stores while using the assigned speech tool. Remember, commas show you when to pause and underline marks show you when to stretch or bounce.

Parent signature ______________________

(2)

- - - - - - - - - - - - - - - - - - - -

Stuttering 20 Homework

Name ______________________ Date due ______________

Next time you come to speech class, we will practice using speech tools while calling stores.

Which speech tool do you think would help you the most on the telephone? ______________ Why do you think using this speech tool would help you?

____

____

Which speech tool do you think would help you the least when talking on the telephone? ______________ Why is it your least favorite speech tool to use on the telephone? ______________________________

____

____

Parent signature ______________________

(3)

21
All Together Now

Purpose

- To demonstrate to students who stutter frequently and with little control that they are physically capable of producing forward-moving speech. This is done through choral reading in unison.
- To begin speech class with easy, forward-moving speech.

Materials

Books or reading handouts (preferably one copy per person).

Directions

For most stutterers, stuttering is greatly reduced or even temporarily eliminated while talking in chorus (also known as speaking in unison). Van Riper referred to this fact as "one of the curious features about the disorder" (1982, p. 422).

When children are asked to read a passage aloud in chorus, these children are often amazed to see that they rarely stutter. Speaking in chorus promotes forward-moving speech. Although a child should never be made to feel that he is expected to speak without stuttering, this activity helps restore confidence in those who are experiencing a period of great difficulty speaking.

You may read in chorus with a single student or include additional students and have the group read together. Begin the activity by obtaining enough copies of a book or reading passage so all present may read aloud at the same time. Choose a book that is below every student's reading level. This way students are not challenged by the reading level of the activity. It is fun to try counting down to the reading, such as, "On the count of 3, let's all start reading."

Choral reading is a great way to begin speech class for students who are having a particularly difficult day controlling their stuttering. The first time I used choral reading was when working with a second grader who was unable to say two consecutive words without stuttering, showed great struggle, and had several pronounced secondaries. His parents and teachers could rarely understand him. This child began to withdraw from speaking, and after seeing a commercial on television about deaf education, he decided he wanted to learn sign language. I began to engage this student in choral reading activities simply to remind him that he was capable of producing forward-moving speech. Twice a week for several weeks, this student came to speech class and read for 5 or 10 minutes in chorus before being engaged in play. This student often brought a friend who also participated in the choral reading and the playing. My student seemed surprised that he was able to talk with much less stuttering during the reading assignments. The forward-moving speech he experienced during choral reading began to carry over to playtime and to his classroom and home. His speech began to flow more smoothly. After several weeks this student was saying 11- and 12-word sentences with much less struggle. Although I cannot be certain, I felt that by allowing him to experience forward-moving speech in this manner, this student was able to regain his speaking confidence.

Homework

Homework Assignment 2 requires that students read a story about stuttering along with a relative. Choose any story from this book that you feel is appropriate and send it home (see stories in You Feel That Way Too?–Activity 31 and in Appendix C).

Homework Assignment 3 asks students to bring one or more books to speech class. Make sure students understand that the book or books they choose should not be academically challenging. They may want to impress you by choosing high-level reading books. Be clear that you want them to bring "easy" books.

Stuttering 21 Homework

Name ______________________ Date due ______________

Choose a book from home that you and a parent can read together. Make sure the book you choose is easy for you to read. Read the book in chorus (at the same time) with your parent. If the book is short, then choose a second book and read that as well. Let your parents know that reading together helps you get the feeling of speaking easily.

What book or books did you read? ______________________

How did it feel to read together? ______________________

____

Parent signature ______________________ (1)

Stuttering 21 Homework

Name ______________________ Date due ______________

Your speech teacher will provide you with a story or poem about stuttering. Read it in chorus with a relative. Explain that reading in chorus helps you practice talking easily.

What story or poem did you read? ______________________

How did it feel to read in chorus with your relative? ______________________

____

Parent signature ______________________ (2)

Stuttering 21 Homework

Name ______________________ Date due ______________

Bring to speech class one or two books from home or from your classroom that you would like to read with your speech teacher. Make sure that the books you choose are easy for you to read; do not choose hard books.

What book or books did you choose? ______________________

____

Parent signature ______________________ (3)

22
The King of Pausing

Purpose

- To challenge students to maintain their focus on using pausing while the clinician uses stuttering-inducing "triggers" to distract them
- To prepare students for real-world interaction

Materials

None

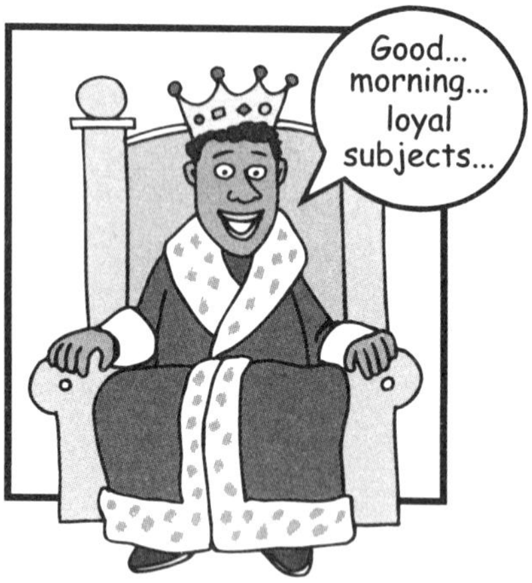

Directions

This activity involves challenging students by assigning pausing and then attempting to trigger stuttering. The King of Pausing is intended for students who are very comfortable with using pausing. (This activity should not be used to teach pausing or as practice for students who are still learning pausing.) There are many ways to trigger moments of stuttering. These triggers or "barbs" include interrupting students, speaking at a fast rate, and asking students to repeat themselves. Do not introduce this activity when students are having a "bad" day or with children who are extremely sensitive about stuttering or who do not yet fully trust the clinician.

This activity arose during a therapy session in which a student was bragging to his friends that he was "the king of pausing." The other students good-naturedly disagreed and started to tease each other about who was the best at using pausing. I decided that we would play a game in which the class would all engage in a conversation while using pausing, and I would do my best to cause the students to stutter. This group did not include any students who I felt would be caused pain or embarrassment by playing this game. I explained (as you might):

> We are going to find out who really is the king (or queen) of pausing. We are going to have a class conversation about anything you want, such as video games, sports, cars, or our favorite music. Your job is to speak politely while using pausing. My job is to be rude. I will interrupt you, ask you to repeat yourselves, act like I am not interested, cut you off, rush you to speak faster, ask you to explain complicated tasks, and do just about anything I can to make you forget to use pausing. Let's see who can remember to use their pausing.

As the group begins to have a conversation, use the stuttering triggers just mentioned while students are talking. For example, a student may say, "I was playing my new video game and got to Level 5. I have never gotten so high in the . . ." Quickly cut the student off by saying, "Come on, speak faster—you are taking too long—speed it up." Wave your hands in a motion to signal, "Hurry up." While a student is describing the video game, you can also interrupt him frequently by using a fast rate of speech and asking a quick series of questions such as, "Where did you buy the game? Who bought it for you? Why do you like it? How do you play?" As a student tries to answer, interrupt again and ask more questions.

You need to visibly have fun for students to do the same. If you show apprehension about acting the part of a rude person, then your students may feel that they should not be participating or that you are doing something wrong. Students will find it funny when you pretend to be rude; just remember to keep it light.

Try to exaggerate your behaviors. For example, when you interrupt a student, do not be subtle. When a student responds to your barbs by forgetting to pause, energetically exclaim with a smile, "You forgot your pausing—I got you that time!" This will not be taken as punishment if it is said in a light and friendly way. Also, when students respond to your barbs by staying on target, congratulate them by saying, "Wow, I can't catch you forgetting to pause."

The King of Pausing is not being played to stop students from stuttering; it is being played to challenge students to use pausing during difficult situations. This distinction is not minor. If a student stutters but is using pausing, reward him for remembering to use the speech tool.

23

Stuttering Private Eye–Revisited

Purpose

- To help students identify their own stuttering patterns
- To help students modify stuttering behaviors
- To review self-generated terminology

Materials

Mirrors
Homework

Directions

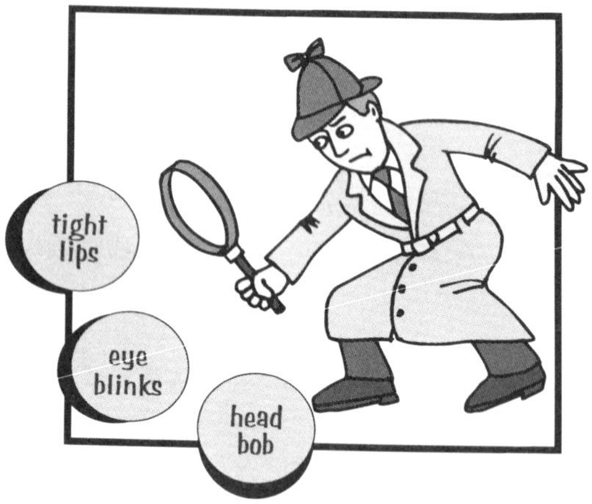

This visual awareness activity helps students identify and modify their own stuttering. Begin by passing out the mirrors from the Stuttering Kits. Explain, "You are using mirrors today to help you learn about your stuttering." Ask all students to voluntarily stutter on the /m/ sound in the word *moon* while looking in their mirrors, and then ask, "Where did you feel the stutter?" or "Where did you see the stutter?" Most students will say that they felt or saw their stuttering on their lips, but a stutterer might report feeling the stutter in her voice box. For those who need it, review the names of the speech helpers (i.e., tongue, lips, voice box, and teeth). Some students may demonstrate secondary behaviors and say that they saw head bobbing or eyes twitching.

Continue this activity by asking students to stutter on the name of an occupation they want to have when they grow up or the name of their favorite teacher or their favorite food. You may go first by giving the following example while using your mirror: "When I was a child I wanted to be a professional bay-bay-bay-baseball player. Let's see. I got stuck on the /b/ sound in baseball. My lips got stuck. I think I will call that my 'tight-lip stutter.' "

Encourage students to stutter on purpose on their chosen words while using their mirrors. Ask each student to explain how and where she stuttered. Then ask the student if she has a name (self-generated terminology) for how she stuttered (i.e., tight-lip stutter).

After students get accustomed to watching and describing their stuttering, introduce a topic of conversation that is sure to get their attention. Talk about music, sports, a recent field trip, or any other topic that your students are excited about.

While students are talking encourage them to alternate between speaking to the group and looking in the mirror. Remind them that it is most important to look into the mirrors when they are stuttering so they can see it. When students stutter, let them work through the sentence or thought and then stop and ask them to explain how and where they were stuttering.

More Ideas

When a student stutters, ask her to teach her stuttering pattern to the class. For example, if a student stutters on the /k/ sound in the word *kitten* and uses a secondary behavior such as head rocking, have her teach the class to stutter in the exact same way. Students better understand and modify their stuttering when they have to teach their stuttering pattern to others.

Another idea is to ask each student to say five words that she usually stutters on. After she says each word, ask her to explain how she stuttered on that word. Because it is common for stutterers not to stutter when they are expected to do so, if this occurs, ask them to use voluntary stuttering while saying the words.

See Breitenfeldt and Lorenz (2000) and Bryngelson, Chapman, and Hanson (1950). Both offer activities called "Mirror Work" in which stutterers look at themselves while stuttering openly (without avoidance) to learn their stuttering patterns.

Homework

Homework Assignment 2 asks students to list three situations in which they would like to see themselves stutter. If you have access to a video camera, you may want to follow up by using it to help students observe their stuttering behaviors. If a student lists that she would like to see how she stutters in class, arrange a time when you can videotape the student while speaking in class. Then view the videotape with the student and discuss it.

Stuttering (23) Homework

Name ____________________ Date due ______________

Explain to an adult relative that you are using mirrors in speech class to practice watching how you stutter. Then have a conversation with this relative about anything that you want. During the conversation, use a mirror to see your stutters.

During your conversation, write down three ways you saw yourself stutter in the mirror:

1. ______________________________________

2. ______________________________________

3. ______________________________________

Ask your relative to remember three ways that he or she saw you stutter. Write them down.

1. ______________________________________

2. ______________________________________

3. ______________________________________

Parent signature ____________________ (1)

Stuttering (23) Homework

Name ____________________ Date due ______________

Think of three situations in which you would like to be able to watch yourself stutter. List these three times below.

1. ______________________________________

2. ______________________________________

3. ______________________________________

Parent signature ____________________ (2)

Learning the Facts

Children who stutter are generally curious about how they talk and often view stuttering as a mystery and a puzzle. They have many questions and want to know why they stutter and why they are different from other children. The advice and information that children often receive about stuttering tends to be "confusing and misleading" (Williams, 2003, p. 5). Children want to feel "normal" and want to know that they are not alone. By providing students with facts and information about stuttering and about people who stutter, clinicians are helping to normalize, de-awfulize, and demystify stuttering. Manning (2000) writes, "The clinician who is able to help the client decrease the mystery and understand the lawfulness of the stuttering syndrome provides a valuable service to the client" (p. 227). This book was written with the belief that understanding stuttering is an essential component of managing and controlling stuttering for the school-age child.

Some students will ask questions about stuttering at the beginning of therapy, whereas others will wait until they are comfortable enough with their clinician and comfortable enough with talking about stuttering. Some students may resist or avoid talking about stuttering for the first several months of therapy, and then all of a sudden, in the middle of a speech class, ask several questions in quick succession. Students will want to know the answers to questions such as, "Why do I stutter?" "Is there a cure for stuttering?" and "Will I always stutter?"

The activities contained in this section will help students learn about stuttering and will also provide opportunities for students to talk openly about stuttering.

Note. Reproducible materials, such as homework and handouts, are located at the end of the description of how to facilitate an activity. However, reproducible materials that are used in more than one activity are included in the appendixes.

24
Facts

Purpose

- To help take the mystery and shame out of the way students speak by exposing them to basic facts about stuttering
- To prepare students to take stuttering quizzes (see Activity 25) and to teach peers about stuttering (see Activity 28)

Materials

Stuttering Facts handout
Homework

Directions

Pass out the Stuttering Facts handout and discuss it with students. Have students take turns reading the facts aloud with or without speech tools. If using a speech tool, you may instruct by saying, "Read the first fact about stuttering while stretching on the first word of each sentence," or ask, "Choose a speech tool—stretching, bouncing, or pausing. Which one would you like to use while reading the first fact?"

Students often have questions about the facts presented and will want to discuss certain issues. For example, one year I worked with a group of students from Grade 3 through Grade 5. From the Stuttering Facts handout they read, "You cannot 'catch' stuttering. When a child who stutters plays with other children, stuttering will not be passed along like a common cold." One of the students had been told that he had caught his stuttering from a neighborhood child who stutters. Another student was informed that his younger brother had caught his stuttering. I explained:

> Many people believe that stuttering can be caught by spending time with people who stutter. This is just not true. But sometimes stuttering does run in families. Many parts of us such as eye color, hair color, and height are passed down from our relatives. In many cases stuttering also is passed down or *inherited.*

During one speech class, a fourth grader read the fact that says, "There is no cure for stuttering." He was concerned about this fact and asked, "Then why am I coming to speech class?" It was important for this student to know that he was coming to speech class to learn how to manage his stuttering—not to be cured. It turns out that his mother was telling him that speech class would cure him of stuttering. As is often the case, I realized that I needed to sit down and work closely with both the student and his family.

The Stuttering Facts handout helps to clarify incorrect or negative information about stuttering that children often come to believe. Students also begin to feel safe asking questions about stuttering. When students take home their Stuttering Facts handout for homework assignments, parents also benefit from reading it because it helps demystify stuttering for them as well. And parents see that stuttering is discussed openly and honestly in speech class.

More Ideas

Engage students in Do You Read Me?–Activity 35 by writing teachers and parents letters that include facts about stuttering.

Arrange a time to meet with a student's teacher to discuss facts about stuttering. This may be a good time to discuss therapy activities and goals as well.

Homework

Several of the homework assignments ask students to collect questions about stuttering from family members or friends. Discuss these questions in speech class. You may wish to have a stuttering text handy (i.e., Guitar, 1998) to help students research answers. Students then write down responses to the questions. For example, during homework a student may write down several questions about stuttering that his grandmother wants answered. The student brings the questions to speech class for discussion and writes down the answers. The next time homework is given, the student is assigned the task of taking the answers home and sharing them with his grandmother. If the student brings a question to speech class such as, "When will my son's stuttering go away?" you will want to answer this important question by directly speaking to the parent.

Stuttering Facts

- Over 3 million Americans stutter (about 1 in every 100 Americans stutter).
- Approximately 4 times as many males stutter as females.
- Most stutterers begin stuttering between the ages of 2 and 8.
- After many years of research, experts still do not know why people stutter.
- You cannot "catch" stuttering. When a child who stutters plays with other children, stuttering will not be passed along like a common cold.
- It is normal for people who stutter to speak without stuttering for hours, days, weeks, and even months, and then the stuttering comes back.
- There is no cure for stuttering.
- Research shows that people who stutter are as smart as people who do not stutter.
- People of every religion, culture, color, and from every country stutter. People all over the world stutter.
- Most stutterers do not stutter when singing, speaking to little children or animals, speaking when alone, swearing, speaking with an accent, or speaking in chorus with other people.
- Stuttering is often hereditary (stuttering often "runs in families"). Many stutterers have family members, such as parents, brothers and sisters, and grandparents, who stutter.
- Many very successful people stutter, including doctors, lawyers, police officers, and teachers.
- Many famous people stutter, including James Earl Jones (Darth Vader) and Marilyn Monroe.

Stuttering 24 Homework

Name ________________________ Date due ____________

Take home the Stuttering Facts handout and look it over. Write down two facts that you find interesting. Then explain why you found each fact interesting.

Example: Stuttering Fact: **There is no cure for stuttering.**

Why did you find this interesting? **I found this fact interesting because I just always thought that there was a cure out there somewhere to take my stuttering away.**

Stuttering Fact: ____

____

Why did you find this interesting? ____

____

Stuttering Fact: ____

____

Why did you find this interesting? ____

____

Parent signature ________________________ (1)

Stuttering 24 Homework

Name ________________________ Date due ____________

Look over your Stuttering Facts handout. Is there anything about stuttering you want to know that is not on the handout? Write down two things you would like to ask your speech teacher about stuttering.

1. ____

____

2. ____

____

Parent signature ________________________ (2)

Stuttering 24 Homework

Name ______________________ Date due ______________

Sit down with a parent or other relative and read him or her the Stuttering Facts handout while bouncing the first word of each sentence. Then ask this person to think of two questions to ask your speech teacher about stuttering. Write the two questions below.

1. ______________________________

2. ______________________________

We will talk about these questions in speech class, and then you can give your relative the answers.

Parent signature ______________________ (3)

Stuttering 24 Homework

Name ______________________ Date due ______________

Call or visit a relative or family friend and tell him or her what you are learning about stuttering in speech class. Read this person your Stuttering Facts handout using pausing. Then ask the relative or friend to think of two questions to ask your speech teacher about stuttering. Write the two questions below.

1. ______________________________

2. ______________________________

We will talk about these questions in speech class, and then you may give your relative the answers.

Parent signature ______________________ (4)

Stuttering 24 Homework

Name ______________________ Date due ______________

Sit down with your teacher and read him or her the Stuttering Facts handout while stretching the first word of each sentence. Then ask your teacher to think of two questions to ask your speech teacher about stuttering. Write the two questions below.

1. ______________________________

2. ______________________________

We will talk about these questions in speech class, and then you can give your teacher the answers.

Parent signature ______________________ (5)

25 Quizzes

Purpose

- To help students express what they feel, think, and know about stuttering
- To assess the student's beliefs about stuttering

Materials

Stuttering Quiz 1
Stuttering Quiz 2
Homework

Directions

Stuttering Quizzes allow you to measure and assess your student's reactions to stuttering. Each quiz may be given several times over the course of therapy—first as a baseline assessment and then as ongoing assessment. Before reading further, it will be helpful to go to the end of this activity and read through Stuttering Quiz 1 and Stuttering Quiz 2 to familiarize yourself with them.

Stuttering Quiz 1

Begin by handing out Stuttering Quiz 1 as if it were any other quiz or test. Give verbal instructions such as, "Today we are taking a quiz on stuttering. There are no right or wrong answers; I just want to see what you know about stuttering." While students are taking the quiz, it is best to occupy yourself with work so that students feel that they are not being watched. This often allows them to feel more comfortable about their answers. After the quiz is completed, begin a discussion by having students take turns reading their answers to the quiz questions. After each student reads her answer to a question, engage the class in a discussion. Then move on to the next question. The most valuable aspect of these quizzes is the discussion afterward in which you help students express and evaluate how they feel about stuttering.

Following are the questions from Stuttering Quiz 1, a sampling of typical student answers, and suggestions for discussing the questions with students:

1. *Why do you stutter?* Children as well as adults who stutter often believe that they became stutterers for a variety of inaccurate reasons. Students may report that they stutter because they "learned to stutter from a friend," "fell down," or are "being punished by God." Students may write, "I don't know" or respond with an insightful view such as, "Maybe I learned to talk wrong as a kid." This question helps you to identify why students believe that they stutter. Talk to students about their answers and the etiology of stuttering. For

example, when a student writes that he "caught stuttering from a neighbor," you could mention that if stuttering were truly "catchable," then most children in his neighborhood would be stuttering because all of the children play together. If a student suggests that she began stuttering when her uncle dropped her during a game, you can mention that almost every child has fallen or been dropped numerous times and say, "If stuttering were caused by falling, then everyone would stutter." Students tend to relate to this type of straight talk. You might say, "We really do not know what causes a person to start stuttering, but we know what makes many people stutter more and stutter harder." Then discuss some of the things that make stuttering grow and become more struggled.

2. *When will you stop stuttering?* Students respond to this question with a wide range of answers that have included "in about 2 years," "when my speech teacher is done teaching me," "by eighth grade," and "soon." A student taking the quiz for a second time may respond, "I won't stop stuttering completely because there is no cure for stuttering" or "I am learning to control my stuttering." Sometimes students turn the question around and ask their speech teacher, "When will I stop stuttering?" You may respond in a straightforward and honest way, "I do not know if you will stop stuttering, but I do know that you are working very hard at controlling your stuttering." This gives you the opportunity to discuss the variability of the disorder. For example, you may say, "Some days you stutter a lot, and some days you stutter very little. It is normal for you to go days, weeks, or even months without much stuttering, only to have the stuttering come back." Explain:

> Some people who stutter simply stop stuttering, while many others do not. I can't cure you, and I don't know if you will stop stuttering, but I do have some really good ways to help you face and manage your stuttering. What are some ways that we work on facing and controlling stuttering in speech class?

3. *Why do you come to speech class?* Student responses to this question have included "to stop stuttering," "so I don't have to stutter any more," and "so I can talk right." Sometimes students will write "to have fun." After spending a few months in speech class and taking the quiz a second time, some students have responded, "to learn my speech tools" and "to learn about stuttering." The discussion following this question allows you the opportunity to explore the main objectives of coming to speech class.

4. *List two jobs that a person who stutters **cannot** do.* When taking the quiz for the first time, some students will list jobs that they feel a stutterer cannot do. Students may write that they cannot be doctors or lawyers because they stutter. When taking the quiz a second time, students may leave this item

blank or cross it out. On one occasion a student wrote, "I can do anything." A strong sign of progress and growth is when a student initially lists several jobs that she cannot do because she stutters and then during subsequent quizzes or discussions, states that a stutterer can hold any job or position. It is your duty to demonstrate to students that *children who stutter can do anything they want to do in life, and they can do so while stuttering.*

5. *List two jobs that a person who stutters **can** do.* Student responses to this request vary greatly. Many children who stutter enter therapy believing that there are a whole host of jobs and careers that they cannot hold. One former student responded that he could sell candy in a candy store or be a janitor. He explained that he could hold these jobs because they do not involve a lot of talking. This question allows you to identify students' self-perceptions about their potential and abilities.

6. *List five words that you stutter on.* Students have listed words that start with specific letters, words they frequently have to say in class, or words associated with specific speaking situations. This item allows you and the student to identify sound and word fears, situational fears, and strategies to approach these situations. For example, if a student lists five words that begin with plosives, you may then help the student face this difficulty in a number of ways, such as by practicing stretching-out or bouncing-out of words that begin with plosives.

7. *List one person you **like** to talk to.* This item helps you identify a person in the student's life with whom he feels comfortable and trusts. During the discussion after the quiz, ask each student why he likes talking to the person he identified. Students have responded "because they listen," "because they don't cut me off," or "because they don't tease me when I talk."

8. *List one person you do **not like** to talk to.* Students easily identify at least one person that they do not like to talk to (sometimes students list several people). During the discussion ask, "Why don't you like talking to this person?" Many students report that the person may speak for them, interrupt them, tease them, give them frustrating speaking advice, skip over them, or generally create a difficult speaking environment. This request helps you to determine people in the student's life who would benefit by learning ways to respond to stuttering.

9. *List two things that you are **good** at doing.* This item gives students an opportunity to list their strengths and interests. This is important for building confidence and self-esteem. It will also help you plan future lessons. For example, one student informed me that he is very good at playing basketball and being the captain during pick-up games at the park. Soon after, the class wrote a play about playing basketball in the park in which the student who stutters

practices dealing with being teased.

10. *List two things that you are **not good** at doing.* Some students will write that they are not good at "talking," whereas other students will write that they are not good at "rollerblading," "standing on my hands," or "doing math." This helps you assess how students view not only their speech but themselves.

Stuttering Quiz 2

Stuttering Quiz 2 should be given after you have presented all four speech tools (stretching, bouncing, pausing, and voluntary stuttering) and after students have participated in Facts–Activity 24. This quiz helps you assess how well students have digested and understood this information. Stuttering Quiz 2 should then be repeated at varying intervals during therapy as ongoing assessment. An explanation will follow each question from Stuttering Quiz 2. Correct answers are in bold.

1. *How many people in the United States stutter?—300, 3,000, or **3 million.*** Students are often surprised to learn that approximately 3 million Americans stutter. When teaching this fact to students, explain that 1 out of every 100 people stutters. Attempt to personalize this fact for students. For example, if the child's school has 500 students, you may ask, "Out of the 500 people who go to your school, how many children should stutter?" I worked in a school with a population of 1,400 students. My students figured out that there were only 5 children who stutter in speech class. They determined that there should be, statistically speaking, 9 more stutterers in speech class. One of the students then made an insightful comment, "Maybe the other stutterers are hiding." In this situation I informed the student, "Many children who stutter *do* hide their stuttering so well that others are not aware of it." Also, discuss overall averages to let them know that one school is a small sampling of a much larger population. For example, you could say, "A school with 2,000 children may only have 4 stutterers, whereas a school with 500 children could have 6 children who stutter."

2. *Most stutterers begin stuttering between the ages of—**2 and 8**, 8 and 14, or 15 and 20.* Most students will report that they remember stuttering between the ages of 3 and 8. During the discussion, students are often surprised to discover that they all began stuttering at approximately the same age. This fact helps explain stuttering to children and helps to normalize stuttering. If a student says, "I didn't start stuttering until I was 9," you may respond, "That is normal too" or "Sometimes children stutter when they are very young and then the stuttering comes back."

3. *People who stutter are as smart as people who do not stutter—**True** or False.* Most students will understand that they are supposed to answer True (students are very adept at knowing what their clinician expects). Explore this

statement during the discussion and ask students questions such as, "Do you really think stutterers are as smart as everyone else?" This type of questioning may uncover doubts or misperceptions that students may hold. If students ask how you know that stutterers are as smart as everyone else, you would be correct to tell them that many studies have been conducted that found stutterers to be as smart as people who do not stutter.

4. *By, using, pausing, when you speak, you, will, stutter—Never, All the time, or* ***Less often.*** Even though clinicians spend much time explaining why speech tools such as pausing are used, some students may continue to believe that they are coming to speech class to be cured. This item helps to determine if students understand the reasoning behind pausing.

5. *Choose two answers. Stretching and bouncing are used to—Avoid hard work,* ***Smooth-out of a stutter, Start a sentence smoothly,*** *or Never stutter again.* This question helps to determine if students understand why they use stretching and bouncing. During the discussion following the quiz, you may review these tools and ask students to suggest several situations in which it would be helpful to use stretching and bouncing.

6. *Name two famous people who stutter.* This request may be used to determine if students are internalizing information learned in class or to interest students in learning about famous people who stutter. If this is the first time you are giving the quiz and you have not covered famous people who stutter yet (see Famous Role Models–Activity 26), this is a good time to discuss some famous stutterers, such as James Earl Jones and Marilyn Monroe.

7. *More girls stutter than boys—True or* ***False.*** This is another statement that allows you to assess whether students are internalizing information learned in speech class.

8. *Write five things that you can do when someone teases you about stuttering.* The answers to this item help you understand what options students feel are at their disposal to deal with teasing situations. Student answers include "Tell the teacher," "Tell my parents," "Tease back," and "Hit the bully." Remember to validate how a child feels. For the student who says that fighting and hitting are the answer to being teased, it is best not to say that these are the wrong feelings to have. Instead, help this child consider the consequences of her actions and other choices she has. For example, you may suggest that students notify their teachers and parents. You may even offer students the option of inviting teasers to speech class to learn about stuttering.

9. *List the names of four tools used in speech class.* This item offers you the opportunity to review speech tools with students and to assess how well students are learning their speech tools.

10. a. *In the story "Teasing on the Way to School," put commas (pausing marks) after the first word of every sentence. We will practice reading it, using pausing, when we discuss the quiz.* During the discussion you may want to ask students to go back and add extra commas where they feel it would help. Then ask a student to read the story with his additional commas. Many children will relate to this story and want to discuss it.

b. *What could Peter have done to help the child who was being teased?* Discuss student answers. Talking about this story may also lead into other story discussions, such as in You Feel That Way Too?–Activity 31. Ask questions such as, "What would you do in this situation?" and "Does anyone have a teasing story that they would like to tell?"

More Ideas

It is often helpful to teach speech class guests about stuttering and quiz them as well (Murphy, 2003). You and your students who stutter can teach the guests about stuttering and speech tools. Use Facts–Activity 24 or similar activities to educate the guests. Then have everyone complete a stuttering quiz and follow it with an open discussion about stuttering.

Homework

Some of the homework assignments that follow this activity require you to consider creating follow-up activities and assignments. For example, one assignment asks students to think of three people in their lives who they think would benefit from knowing more about stuttering. Students are then asked, "What are some things you would like to tell them about stuttering?" When discussing this assignment, consider ways to help students talk about stuttering with the people they listed. One student returned the homework and stated that he wanted his grandmother to understand how hard it was for him to speak. This homework was followed up by inviting the grandmother to speech class so that she could learn about stuttering.

Stuttering Quiz 1

Name ______________________________ Date ____________________

1. Why do you stutter? ____

2. When will you stop stuttering? ______________________________

3. Why do you come to speech class? ____________________________

4. List two jobs that a person who stutters **cannot** do.

   a. ____

   b. ____

5. List two jobs that a person who stutters **can** do.

   a. ____

   b. ____

6. List five words that you often stutter on.

   a. ____________________

   b. ____________________

   c. ____________________

   d. ____________________

   e. ____________________

7. List one person you **like** to talk to. ___________________________

8. List one person you do **not like** to talk to. _____________________

9. List two things that you are **good** at doing.

   a. ____

   b. ____

10. List two things that you are **not good** at doing.

   a. ____

   b. ____

Stuttering Quiz 2

Name ______________________________ Date ____________________

Circle the correct answers.

1. How many people in the United States stutter?

   a. 300

   b. 3,000

   c. 3 million

2. Most stutterers begin stuttering between the ages of—

   a. 2 and 8

   b. 8 and 14

   c. 15 and 20

3. People who stutter are as smart as people who do not stutter.

   True or False

4. By, using, pausing, when, you speak, you, will stutter—

   a. Never

   b. All the time

   c. Less often

5. Choose two answers. Stretching and bouncing are used to—

   a. Avoid hard work

   b. Smooth out of stutter

   c. Start a sentence smoothly

   d. Never stutter again

6. Name two famous people who stutter.

   a. ____

   b. ____

7. More girls stutter than boys.

True or False

8. Write five things you can do when someone teases you about stuttering.

a. ______________________________

b. ______________________________

c. ______________________________

d. ______________________________

e. ______________________________

9. List the names of four tools used in speech class.

a. ______________

b. ______________

c. ______________

d. ______________

10a. In the story "Teasing On The Way to School," put commas (pausing marks) after the first word of every sentence. We will practice reading it, using pausing, when we discuss the quiz.

Teasing on the Way to School

by Peter Reitzes

When I was in the seventh grade, I was walking to school, and there were several boys and a girl teasing a kid because he was adopted. They were saying mean things to him like, "You don't have real parents." They even called him "Little Orphan Annie." The kid was crying and the teasers kept calling him "baby." I didn't know him well, but I felt bad for him. I know what it is like to get teased because I stutter, and other children have teased me about my speech. I don't tease anyone else because I know how bad it feels to get teased.

10b. What could Peter have done to help the child who was being teased?

____

____

____

____

____

Stuttering 25 Homework

Name ______________________________ Date due ________________

Should people who stutter be allowed to hold any job, such as a lawyer or a police officer? What do you think? Write at least three sentences below explaining how you feel.

____

____

____

____

____

____

Parent signature ______________________________ (1)

Stuttering 25 Homework

Name ______________________________ Date due ________________

Create your own stuttering quiz with new questions. Think of four questions about stuttering that you would like to ask other people. Write your questions below.

1. ____

____

2. ____

____

3. ____

____

4. ____

____

Parent signature ______________________________ (2)

Stuttering 25 Homework

Name ______________________ Date due ____________

Ask a relative or a teacher the four questions you came up with about stuttering. On a separate piece of paper, write down their answers.

Parent signature ______________________ (3)

Stuttering 25 Homework

Name ______________________ Date due ____________

We have learned a lot about stuttering in speech class. Who do you think needs to know more about stuttering? Think of three people and write their names below.

1. ______________________
2. ______________________
3. ______________________

What are some things you would like to tell them about stuttering? Write three sentences below.

1. ____

____

2. ____

____

3. ____

____

Parent signature ______________________ (4)

26
Famous Role Models

Purpose

- To help children internalize the belief that they may be successful in life as people who stutter
- To give students the opportunity to advertise (share) their stuttering with others

Materials

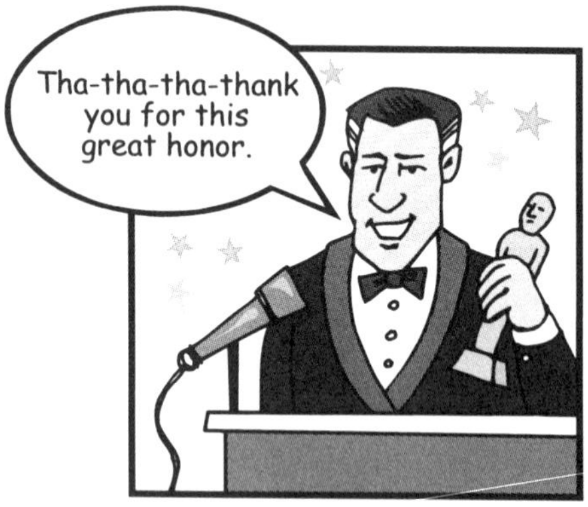

One photograph of each student
Poster board (27" *x* 34" or larger)
Magic markers
Scissors
Internet accessible computers and printers
16 Famous People Who Stutter brochure (free Internet download, www.stutteringhelp.com/download/004416fp.pdf)
Famous People Who Stutter: Essay handout
Famous People Who Stutter: Sample Essay handout
Homework

Directions

Note. Completing this activity will take several sessions.

Many famous and talented people stutter. Some of these people are actors James Earl Jones, Marilyn Monroe, and Nicholas Brendan; athletes Bob Love, Bill Walton, and Bo Jackson; singers Carly Simon, Mel Tillis, and "Scatman" John Larkin; politician Joseph Biden; and television reporter John Stossel. During this activity students will make a poster that consists of photographs of famous people who stutter with short biographies of their lives. Alongside these biographies of famous people, each student will put a photograph of himself and a short biography of his own life.

There are many resources available to learn about famous people who stutter. The Stuttering Foundation of America (SFA), FRIENDS, and the National Stuttering Association all publish posters of famous people who stutter (see Appendix E for contact information). Consider purchasing one or more of these posters for the therapy room. The posters often fascinate students and teachers and encourage open conversations about stuttering. Several of these posters hang in the lunchroom in my school. Often I see students and teachers looking at the posters and talking openly about stuttering. When I walk by, students and teachers have felt free to approach me to talk about stuttering. These posters not only remind children who stutter that they may be successful but also serve to educate teachers and classmates about stuttering and stutterers.

The SFA publishes a brochure of famous people who stutter titled *16 Famous People Who Stutter* (Stuttering Foundation of America, 2005). This brochure is available free on the SFA Web site and also may be inexpensively purchased from the organization (see Appendix E for contact information).

Students will be working together to make one large poster of talented and famous people who stutter. This will require several sessions and may be broken down into the following steps. Each student

1. brings in a photograph of himself for the poster,
2. chooses a famous person who stutters to research,
3. conducts Internet research and prints out articles and pictures on his chosen stutterer,
4. writes a summary paragraph about his famous stutterer,
5. pastes a photograph of his famous stutterer onto the poster board and then copies his summary paragraph next to the photograph, and
6. pastes his own photograph on the poster board and adds a paragraph describing his own talents and interests.

Begin by handing out copies of the *16 Famous People Who Stutter* brochure. After discussing several people featured on the brochure, explain:

> You will be making a poster of talented and successful people who stutter. We will learn about famous people who stutter on the Internet and will put a picture of each one on the poster with a paragraph that describes their lives. Then you will each put your own photograph on the poster with a paragraph describing your talents. Next time you come to speech class, bring in a picture of yourselves.

Internet Research. Typically, set aside one to two sessions for internet research. An excellent place to start learning about famous people who stutter is at www.stutteringhomepage.com; go to this site and then click on "Famous PWS."

Another way students may use the Internet to learn about famous people who stutter is by using popular search engines, such as www.Google.com or www.Yahoo.com. If a student is researching Bob Love, in the search box help him type the words "Bob Love Stuttering." You will find a number of Web pages that have information about Bob Love and his history of stuttering. I usually tell students, "There is a lot of information on the Internet—only print out the information you feel will be helpful for making our poster."

Students should search the Web with your guidance until they find several app priate Web pages or articles that discuss famous people who stutter. Each stu should print out articles about and a picture of their chosen person for this

Make sure the information is appropriate; some will be too advanced for students to read or understand. And, of course, there are Web pages that may be accidentally accessed that are inappropriate for children to visit. For example, some of the Web sites devoted to Marilyn Monroe are not appropriate for children. Thus you will need to work closely with children as they search the Internet.

If your setting does not have Internet access, create your own library of articles about famous people who stutter by using a home computer. Students may then search through your library. Depending on the student and his resources, you may assign some of this Internet research as homework.

Essay Writing. After completing the Internet research, set aside one or two sessions for students to write their summary paragraphs or assign the essays for homework. Pass out copies of the handout titled Famous People Who Stutter: Essay. Explain: "On your handouts I want you to use your research and write a summary paragraph about your famous stutterer."

Students may need some help putting their Internet research into essay form. You may need to review the components of a single topic essay (i.e., a topic sentence, body and details of the paragraph, and a closing sentence). It is often best to assign a specific length. For example, when working with a group of fourth-grade students, you may say, "I want each essay to be at least six sentences long." Be sure to teach students not to copy but to put the information they have gathered in their own words.

You may pass out the handout titled Famous People Who Stutter: Sample Essay about Bob Love and discuss it with students. If a second example would helpful, you may read aloud the following paragraph about actor Nicholas Brendan.

> Nicholas Brendon is a famous actor who stutters. Brendon was born in 1971. After years of working in the food industry, Brendon decided to try acting and went on to star as Xander Harris on the television show *Buffy the Vampire Slayer.* Because of stuttering, Brendon grew up being scared to talk in public and to talk to strangers. Even though many people think he is handsome, Brendon was scared to date because he stutters. Brendon now speaks often about stuttering and gives other stutterers this advice: "Challenge yourself to speak in front of people and make mistakes."

Presenting Completed Essays to Speech Class. After writing their essays, students take turns presenting their famous person who stutters. When working individually with a child, both you and the student can research several famous stutterers. This way the poster will include several stutterers.

Making the Poster and Writing Personal Essays. After completing their essays, at the top of a piece of poster board, students write the title "Talented People Who Stutter." Each student pastes a photograph of his chosen stutterer onto the poster board. Next to each photograph students paste their essays (or copy them by hand onto the poster).

Next, engage students in writing essays for the poster about their own talents and skills by explaining: "We have studied several talented people who stutter. But I know a few more talented people who stutter, and they are sitting right here. Everyone think of one thing that you are really good at doing."

Ask the students to tell the class what they are talented at. Students often take pride in their athletic abilities. When athletics is the topic, ask questions such as, "Why is baseball your best sport?" "What position do you play?" "Why are you so good at soccer?" or "Who is your favorite team?" Assist students while writing their summary paragraphs about themselves. The following is an example:

> My name is Jonathan and I am 9 years old. I am a talented athlete and I stutter. I attend Public School 29. My favorite sport is football. I like football because I am very fast and tackle the best. My brother and sometimes my father take me to the park to play football. It is fun. I can throw the ball far and never drop it. I play on the Sunset Tigers and my favorite team is the Giants. I am the best at football.

After students write their summary paragraphs, they paste photographs of themselves to the poster and copy (or paste) their essays onto the poster.

More Ideas

Instead of having students write their own paragraphs, you may act like a reporter and interview students about their chosen talents. After interviewing students, write summary paragraphs for each one. By writing these summary paragraphs yourself, you can significantly shorten the amount of time this activity will take to complete. This is also helpful for students who have difficulty writing.

Encourage students to bring a guest to speech class for this project. One year a student brought his best friend to speech class for this entire project. This guest participated in all aspects of making the poster. The group created a poster that included information about several famous people who stutter, several students who stutter, an adult woman who stutters who spoke to them as a guest, and the speech class friend.

Homework

Assign homework that you feel best meets the needs of your students.

Famous People Who Stutter Essay

Name ______________________________ Date ____________________

Directions: Use your research about a famous person who stutters to write a summary paragraph about this person.

Famous People Who Stutter
Sample Essay

Name Steven Date 3/24

Bob Love was born in 1942 and was nicknamed "Ole' Butterbean." He grew up very poor with 13 brothers and sisters. Bob Love had a big stuttering problem. He dreamed about becoming a basketball player. He played on the Chicago Bulls NBA basketball team. He was an All-Star three times and was the Bulls' second leading scorer of all time. Even though people thought he was the best player on the Bulls at the time, Bob Love was never interviewed after a game and never got to do commercials because of his stuttering.

Bob Love had to stop playing basketball because he hurt his back. After leaving the Bulls Bob Love was not able to get a good job because of his stuttering. After looking for a steady job for 7 years, he finally took a job washing dishes. He then got a speech teacher and started feeling good about himself. So with the help of his speech teacher, he went back to the Chicago Bulls. Then he ran the Chicago Bulls' Community Affairs Office. Now Bob Love is a professional speaker.

Stuttering 26 Homework

Name ______________________ Date due ______________

Take home your brochure of *16 Famous People Who Stutter.* Talk to a relative or a family friend about the people featured in it. What did your relative or family friend think? Were they surprised to find out that so many famous people stutter?

____

____

Parent signature ______________________ (1)

Stuttering 26 Homework

Name ______________________ Date due ______________

Take home your brochure of *16 Famous People Who Stutter.* Who is your favorite famous person who stutters? Why?

____

____

Parent signature ______________________ (2)

Stuttering 26 Homework

Name ______________________ Date due ______________

With the help of a relative, search the Internet for famous people who stutter who do not appear on your *16 Famous People Who Stutter* brochure. Choose one person and, on a separate sheet of paper, write a few sentences about his or her life.

Parent signature ______________________ (3)

Stuttering 26 Homework

Name ______________________ Date due ______________

With the help of a relative, search the Internet for famous people who stutter who do not appear on your *16 Famous People Who Stutter* brochure. Write down the names of three famous stutterers that you have not already read about.

1. ______________ 2. ______________ 3. ______________

Parent signature ______________________ (4)

27

The World Wide Web

Purpose

- To encourage children to research stuttering and to become active and responsible participants in their own therapy and growth

Materials

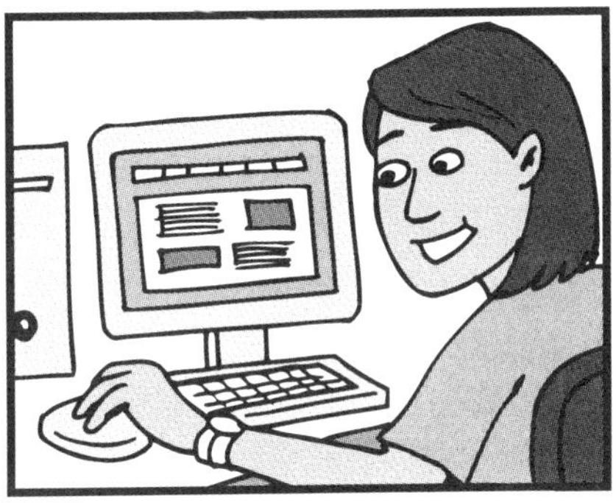

Internet-accessible computers
Stuttering Research: Stuttering Facts handout
Pencils

Directions

For some students it is important that they own their stuttering by being part of the fact-finding and discovery process. These students are curious about stuttering and want to be part of the process of exploring stuttering. Other students will become more involved in therapy by being encouraged to research stuttering.

Pass out copies of the Stuttering Research: Stuttering Facts handout. This will guide students in discovering more information about stuttering. Then explain the assignment:

> We are going to begin a fun project in which we use the Internet to learn about stuttering. There is a lot of information available about stuttering. Much of this information is very good and interesting, but some of it is misleading or inaccurate. We will find some opinions, facts, and stories about stuttering that we agree with, and we may find some that we disagree with. Let's see what we can find about stuttering! Write down five things that you learned on the Internet, and then write the Web addresses you used.

Explain that there are several Web sites that are dedicated to stuttering that offer a lot of information. An excellent example is www.stutteringhomepage.com, which offers pages specifically created for children and teens who stutter and has its own internal keyword search. You may also encourage students to search for information on the Internet by using a search engine and to search using several important keywords, such as "stuttering," "PWS," "stuttering information," or "stuttering facts."

Most popular search engines, such as www.Google.com, offer advanced search options. Under these advanced options you may search using exact phrases—which weeds out Web pages that may be unhelpful. When searching with an exact phrase, such as "facts about stuttering," all of the Web pages that come up in your search will include the exact phrase you entered. Some phrases to use are "information about stuttering," "stuttering facts," "facts about stuttering," "children who stutter," and "stuttering therapy." To search using exact phrases, go to www.Google.com and click on "Advanced Search," find the field (box) that indicates "exact phrase," and type your phrase in that field. Then click the "search" button. Google will then find all of the Web pages that include the exact phrase you entered.

Different students bring vastly different computer abilities to speech class. You may need to work closely with your students to help them conduct their Internet searches. As students find interesting Web pages and information, help them fill out the Stuttering Research: Stuttering Facts handout.

When the research is completed, sit down with the group and have each student share the information they found on the Internet. Discuss the topics. One fourth-grade student found a Web site that was written by a man who stutters and lives in Florida. This student was surprised to find out that people who stutter may live outside of New York City. It turns out that this student had been to Florida several times but had never met another person who stutters there. As a result of this discussion, I devoted some time in future speech classes to activities that explored stuttering throughout the world. We went back to the computer lab and learned about stuttering organizations in different states and countries.

If students find information that is inaccurate, discuss it with them. As an example, there are many Web sites that offer a cure for stuttering. When students find these sites, I bring up the concept of "snake oil." I explain:

> When America was first founded, some people tried to sell potions referred to as snake oil that promised to cure a range of problems. This happens even today. These potions are often expensive and make big promises, but they do not work.

More Ideas

Kuster (2004) recommends visiting many Web sites to learn about stuttering. See her article called "Internet Treasures for Kids and Teens Who Stutter" for a complete listing. Some of the sites offer free online books or coloring books written for children who stutter. Kuster suggests the following free books:

- *Sometimes I Just Stutter*
- *Jeremy and the Hippo*
- *Boo Goodnight to Halloween*
- *Angel Loves To Talk*

The easiest way to find these free books is to go to a search engine such as Google and type the title of the book within quotation marks (i.e., "Sometimes I

Just Stutter") and click on "search." By typing the title of the book within quotation marks, Google will complete an exact phrase search. After completing the search, click on a link that offers the book for free.

Homework

After students complete a Stuttering Research: Stuttering Facts handout in class and are comfortable with the Internet, assign this handout as homework under the supervision of an adult relative or caregiver.

Stuttering Research: Stuttering Facts

Name ______________________________ Date __________________

Directions: Go to www.stutteringhomepage.com and search it for stuttering facts. Or go to an Internet search engine, such as www.Google.com or www .Yahoo.com, and look for information about stuttering. Some helpful phrases to use for your searches are "facts stuttering," "stuttering information," or "stuttering questions answers." Write down five things you learned about stuttering and write down the Web address (URL) for each fact.

1. ____

____

Web address (URL): ____________________________

2. ____

____

Web address (URL): ____________________________

3. ____

____

Web address (URL): ____________________________

4. ____

____

Web address (URL): ____________________________

5. ____

____

Web address (URL): ____________________________

28
You Are the Expert

Purpose

- To offer students the opportunity to educate peers and teachers about stuttering
- To encourage students to talk openly about stuttering with peers and teachers

Materials

Silly Putty
The Best Stretching Award and various other stuttering awards (Appendix A)
Stuttering Challenge (copies for an entire classroom of students)
Pencils

Directions

Note: This activity will take a few sessions of student preparation and then about 45 minutes to present to a class.

In You Are the Expert, you and your students teach a class of children abou stuttering. The activity is intended for students who have already been provided ample opportunities to learn and talk about stuttering and to practice speech tools. Before proceeding with this activity, you need to engage students in many of the activities taken from the Learning the Facts section (i.e., Facts–Activity 24 and Famous Role Models–Activity 26), the Uncovering Feelings section (i.e., Stuttering Interviews–Activity 30, Questions and Answers–Activity 33, Dear Abby–Activity 34, and Do You Read Me?–Activity 35), and the Practicing Speech Tools section (i.e., Stretching–Activity 9, Bouncing–Activity 10, and Pausing–Activity 11).

Before discussing this project with students, talk to appropriate teachers and make a list of ones that you feel would be strong choices for hosting a presentation on stuttering. Ideally, students would present to their home classrooms, but you may find other teachers (i.e., a science teacher or art teacher) who might be enthusiastic and accommodating. Look for teachers who are eager to make this project a success. When you are ready to begin, announce:

> We are going to begin a project in which we go into a classroom and teach an entire class about stuttering. *We* are all experts on stuttering. What are some things you would like to share with your classmates and teachers about stuttering? We could talk to a class about stuttering facts; teach the class our speech tools using Silly Putty, bouncy balls, and our abacus; or challenge class members to compete for a stuttering award. What else can we do?

Students may respond to hearing about this project in different ways. Although some students may be excited, others could be hesitant to present in front of a class. Each student and group of students will need different levels of support and guidance. You may find your students taking the lead in this project, or you may find that you are taking the lead. Use your best judgment about how much to push students. Be sure to let them know that you will be with them during this presentation as a co-presenter.

Present a list of appropriate classrooms for this project and ask students to decide on one, or, if you believe that a certain class is the best choice, simply announce that you have chosen the first class to speak to about stuttering. What follows is just one of the many possible outlines you might use during a classroom presentation.

- Give a short introductory speech, explaining that the presentation is on stuttering.
- Teach one speech tool, such as stretching, to the class.
- Engage the class in competing for stuttering awards.
- Educate the class about stuttering by giving the class the Stuttering Challenge (quiz on stuttering).
- Discuss the results of the Stuttering Challenge.

Help your students prepare for the presentation. You may assign each student parts to present, or you may take the lead during the presentation while calling frequently on your students to share their "expertise." During speech class, review the Stuttering Challenge so students are fully prepared with the answers. They may need to review the Stuttering Facts handout (from Activity 24). See also the answer key at the end of the Directions section in this activity.

Using the outline above, the presentation may proceed as follows. Explain to the class:

> We are here today to teach you about stuttering. Who knows what stuttering is? (Call on students, discuss their comments, and then proceed.) Stuttering is when some people get stu-stu-stu-stuck like this on their wwwwwords. For some, stuttering feels like a traffic jam in their mouth. Even though they want their words to move, the words are stuck like cars in traffic.
>
> Many people throughout the world stutter. Boys stutter, girls stutter, men stutter, and women stutter. Besides the presenters, does anyone know a person who stutters? Does anyone have relatives or friends who stutter? (Call on students and discuss their comments and then proceed.)
>
> Sometimes stuttering is very hard for children in school because they feel very uncomfortable talking in class. How would you feel if your words got stuck when you tried to give an answer in class or when you tried to read in class? (Call on students and discuss their comments and then proceed).

> There are several tools or strategies that stutterers have to help them talk. Let's discuss tools for a moment. Who can think of some tools that a police officer uses? (Call on students.) Who can think of some tools that a doctor uses? (Call on students.) Who can think of some tools that stutterers can use? (Call on students).
>
> One of the tools we use to help us stutter more smoothly or more easily is called stretching. We will now show you how to stretch words using Silly Putty (take out the Silly Putty and show it to the class). Who can think of a good word for us to stretch on? (Call on students to provide the words—it will keep them engaged.)

At this point each student who stutters takes a turn demonstrating to the class how to stretch while using the Silly Putty. You or a student may wish to write down the words on a chalkboard or poster board and underline the first letter or initial blends. Ask a child who stutters to, "Please tell the class why you practice stretching only on the first sound of words." The student then replies, "Because we mostly stutter on the first sound of a word, not the second sound of a word."

Now ask, "Who would like to try stretching with the Silly Putty?" After a few students from the class try stretching, take out the Best Stretching Award (Appendix A) and ask, "Who thinks they can win the best stretching award?" Announce, "My students who stutter will closely listen to your stretches to make sure you do it right. At the end your teacher and I will decide who should win the best stretching award." If classroom students do not stretch correctly (i.e., stretching on the second sound of a word), ask speech students to show them how to do it. This shows the class that students in speech class really are experts on stuttering. Then consider using the Longest and Shortest Stuttering Awards (Appendix A) because these awards lend themselves to stretching. Sometimes it is helpful to offer small prizes for the winners of awards. (It is best to check with the classroom teacher to request permission to award prizes, especially food.) Work through as many awards as you feel is productive and fun.

If time permits give each student a copy of the Stuttering Challenge handout and explain:

> This challenge is very special and fun. If students "pass" the Stuttering Challenge, the class will be rewarded with a doughnut party. (Check ahead with teachers in case they prefer a different kind of reward.) Passing means that you tried; it is okay if you don't know the answers. In fact the Stuttering Challenge covers some information that you will not know. (Of course, you want all students to pass except in situations of poor behavior.). You will learn all the answers when we discuss the challenge. We need to follow the same rules for this challenge as we do when taking a test: Don't talk to other students during the test and turn your paper over when you are finished.

Hand out the Stuttering Challenge and ask students to complete it quietly. Then discuss the test by reading through the questions and asking students to provide their answers. For example, call on a student to read the first question: "If a boy named James plays with children who stutter, will James 'catch' their stuttering? Yes or No?" Call on other students to explain their answers and then provide them with the correct answer. A student might say, "I think you can catch stuttering because my friend started stuttering when he played with another boy." You could respond by saying, "If stuttering were truly 'catchable,' then everybody in here should now be stuttering because the student presenters all stutter." Most students will relate to this type of reasoning.

Use the discussion time to educate the class about stuttering. For example, Question 9 asks for the names of three famous people who stutter. This question allows the presenters to teach the class about famous people who stutter. When you get to Question 12, ask students to volunteer to read the short story they wrote about a personal teasing experience. Hearing students who do not stutter talk about being teased often helps students who stutter acknowledge and discuss their own teasing experiences.

When you are through discussing the Stuttering Challenges, collect them and explain that you and the classroom teacher will look at them and decide if the class has passed and earned a reward. At this point briefly confer with the classroom teacher before announcing, "Congratulations—everybody passed." Thank the class for their time and interest in stuttering.

Answer Key for the Stuttering Challenge

1. false 2. c 3. b 4. a 5. c 6. b 7. no 8. yes
9. See *16 Famous People Who Stutter* brochure 10. stretching (and stretch-outs), bouncing (and bounce-outs), voluntary stuttering, pausing

More Ideas

When working with an individual child who stutters, consider asking him to include a good friend in the presentation. This will require including the friend in some therapy sessions to help prepare.

You may use many other activities from this book during the classroom presentations. For example, use Stuttering Interviews–Activity 30 to encourage open discussion about stuttering. Students from the class take turns being interviewed by the presenters in front of the whole class. Presenters ask questions such as, "What do you think causes stuttering?" and "What would you do if your child stuttered?" You can also have classroom students prepare questions about stuttering to ask the presenters and then ask these questions while interviewing the presenters. You may refer to this activity as "Ask the Expert" or "Interview the Expert."

Stuttering Challenge

Name: ______________________________ Date ____________________

Circle the correct answers.

1. If a boy named James plays with children who stutter, will James "catch" their stuttering?

   Yes or No

2. What part of a word do you stretch on to smoothly start a word?

   a. The middle of a word

   b. The second letter

   c. The first sound

3. How many people stutter in the United States?

   a. 3

   b. 3 million

   c. 300

4. If there are 8 children who stutter in a school, on average, how many of the will be girls?

   a. 2

   b. 5

   c. 8

5. When a child who stutters speaks, she or he will

   a. stutter on every word.

   b. stutter once a year.

   c. stutter sometimes.

6. Most people begin stuttering

   a. the second they are born.

   b. between the ages of 2 and 8.

   c. after watching a scary movie.

7. Is there are cure for stuttering?

   Yes or No

8. Are people who stutter as smart as people who do not stutter?

   Yes or No

9. Write the names of three famous people who stutter (don't worry about spelling).

   1. ______________________________

   2. ______________________________

   3. ______________________________

10. Name two speech tools that a person who stutters can use to help himself or herself.

   1. ______________________ 2. ______________________

11. Read the following story:

You Can't Play
by Kevin

My name is Kevin and I stutter. I like playing kickball and basketball with the children on my street. One of the boys, Jeff, always makes fun of me because of the way that I talk. Jeff says things like, "Hhhhhhhear c-c-c-comes sssssssssstutter boy." Sometimes the other children tease me too, and sometimes my friends tell Jeff to be quiet. Once when I came out to play, Jeff said, "You can't play because you stutter." So I went home. I need some help. What should I do?

What should Kevin do? Write three things that Kevin could do to solve his problem.

   1. ______________________________

   2. ______________________________

   3. ______________________________

12. Have you ever been teased about something? Write a short story describing a time that you were teased.

____

____

____

____

____

____

____

____

____

13. Think of two reasons why we should *not* tease other people. Write them below.

   1. ______________________________

   2. ______________________________

Uncovering Feelings

Many children have developed fears, negative feelings, and negative atitudes toward their stuttering. Starkweather and Givens-Ackerman (1997) have pointed out that it is common for school-age children to believe that

1. dysfluent speech is the worst thing you can do;
2. people who are dysfluent aren't very smart/worthwhile/attractive;
3. stuttering is really a shameful thing to have; it means that you are bad in some way;
4. you should never mention stuttering to another person;
5. stuttering is mysterious and frightening; and
6. stuttering is a kind of personal weakness. (p. 112)

These negative self-perceptions are so debilitating that many speech–language pathologists believe that working on attitudes and feelings is the most important aspect of therapy for school-age children. Stuttering often becomes so negative and debilitating for children that their feelings surrounding the disorder become more of an impediment to social communication than do actual moments of stuttering.

In describing his own therapy approach during a discussion on the Stutt-L electronic mailing list, Starkweather (2003) wrote, "[I] spend a lot of time working on the emotional aspects of the disorder. That is what clears the deck for direct work on stuttering itself" (para. 4). One adult stutterer has written, "Changing your attitude on stuttering is more than half the battle" (Johnson, 2003, p. 6). Therapy approaches that do not guide children in identifying and discussing their feelings about stuttering are simply "inadequate" (Cooper, 1979, p. 85).

Few people attempt to openly discuss stuttering with children who stutter. As a consequence students are often reluctant to seek guidance or help when confronted with teasing or other stuttering-related difficulties. When you present opportunities for students to talk about stuttering, being a person who stutters becomes less shameful and less debilitating. Activities such as Stuttering Interviews–Activity 30 and Do You Read Me?–Activity 35 enable students to talk openly with their teachers, relatives, and peers about stuttering. This helps to demystify stuttering not only for the child but for others as well.

There are many emotions and feelings about stuttering that are common to most stutterers. However, bear in mind that each child will hold her own feelings and beliefs about stuttering, and these require individualized goals. There are students who will show significant emotional reactions toward their stuttering, students who will show little negative reaction, and many who are somewhere in between. The activities in this section will help students talk about stuttering, express how they feel, and react more positively to stuttering.

Note. Reproducible materials, such as homework and handouts, are located at the end of the description of how to facilitate an activity. Reproducible materials that are used in more than one activity are included in the appendixes.

29 Draw a Picture of How You Talk

Purpose

- To assess how students feel and think about their stuttering
- To help students express how they feel about their stuttering

Materials

Draw a Picture of How You Talk handout
Pencils (or pens, crayons, markers, or colored pencils)
Homework

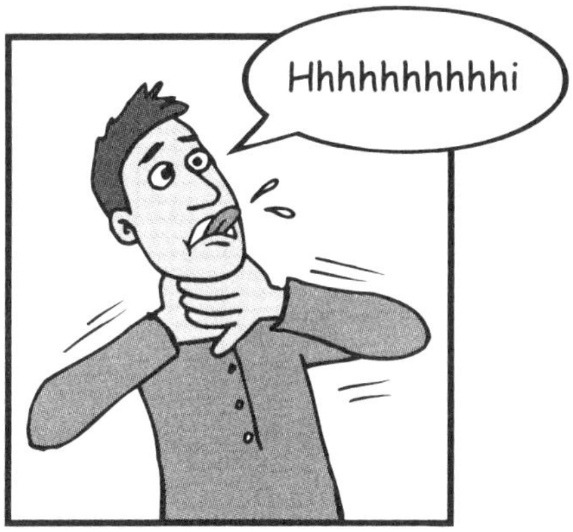

Directions

Many clinicians have encouraged children to draw pictures of how they talk to help them explore and express their feelings about stuttering (see Chmela & Reardon, 2001; Guitar & Reville, 2003; Murphy 2000, 2003; Reed, 1999; Walton & Wallace, 1998; Williams & Dugan, 2002). Drawings have also been used for assessment purposes (see Stewart, 1997; Wilson, 2004) and to treat adult clients.

Begin this activity by passing out the Draw a Picture of How You Talk handout. Provide students with appropriate drawing utensils. Do not go into a lengthy explanation of what you are expecting students to draw. Say, "I want you to draw a picture that shows your stuttering." Then turn away from the students and occupy yourself in your own work while students complete their drawings. If they ask, "What am I suppose to draw?" reply, "Draw a picture of your stuttering." If the student asks again, say, "Draw anything that shows us your stuttering." For students who do not understand the term stuttering yet, you may need to change the language you use. For example, say, "Draw a picture of your bumpy (or sticky) speech."

After students draw their pictures, engage them in a group discussion. Ask each person, "How does this picture relate to your stuttering?" One fifth-grade student drew a picture of himself eating an ice-cream cone. When asked to share what his picture had to do with stuttering, the student responded that every time he orders ice cream he is really scared to speak and often asks his older brother to order for him so that he does not stutter. One student drew a picture of himself playing in his backyard and explained that the children who live next door tease him about stuttering when adults are not around. Another student drew a picture of herself just standing. When asked how this picture related to stuttering, the child pointed to her throat in the picture and stated that when she stutterers, it feels like she is choking. One student drew a picture that demonstrated a positive attitude toward his stuttering. The picture consisted of himself rapping and saying, "Stuttering is c-c-c-cool."

This activity gives students the opportunity to express some aspect of their stuttering and also allows the clinician to better understand each student's particular stuttering problem. When students hang their completed drawings on the wall or take them home or back to their classrooms, they are given the opportunity to share stuttering with their peers, family, and teachers.

More Ideas

The Web site www.stutteringhomepage.com offers a "Pictures of Stuttering Gallery" that contains many pictures drawn by children who stutter. After completing the activity above, students may visit this picture gallery to look at the ways other children have drawn or depicted their stuttering. One quick way to find this gallery is to go to www.Google.com and search on "Pictures of Stuttering Gallery."

For students who may be reluctant to participate in this activity, consider adapting it. Try having students draw pictures of feelings. For example, instead of asking students to "draw a picture of stuttering," try having them draw a picture of anger, frustration, sadness, fear, happiness, or joy. For example, if students are assigned the task of drawing a picture that depicts frustration, engage them in a discussion about what causes them to feel frustrated. You may use these discussions about general feelings to lead into discussions about stuttering.

Homework

These homework assignments will be helpful in assessing how students view stuttering and how people in your students' lives respond to their stuttering. For example, one homework assignment asks children to draw a picture depicting what other people do when the child stutters. A student once responded by drawing a picture of himself hiding in his bedroom while his four sisters were standing at his door teasing him about stuttering. This alerted me to an unproductive situation at home. I was then able to meet with the student's parents and discuss the negative impact that teasing has on children who stutter. Keep in mind that many of the homework assignments in this book may also be used as additional speech class activities.

Draw a Picture of How You Talk

Name ______________________________ Date __________________

Stuttering (29) Homework

Name ______________________ Date due ______________

Take home your completed Draw a Picture of How You Talk handout and show it to your family. Explain to them how it relates to stuttering.

How did you feel showing your picture to your family? ______________________

____

____

____

____

____

Parent signature ______________________ (1)

Stuttering (29) Homework

Name ______________________ Date due ______________

What do other people do when you stutter? Use a separate piece of paper and draw a picture of one thing that people do when you stutter.

Parent signature ______________________ (2)

Stuttering (29) Homework

Name ______________________ Date due ______________

How would you like to change how you stutter? Use a separate piece of paper and draw a picture showing you with a different stutter.

Parent signature ______________________ (3)

Stuttering (29) Homework

Name ______________________ Date due ______________

Think of one thing about stuttering that you like. On a separate piece of paper, draw a picture of it.

Parent signature ______________________ (4)

Stuttering 29 Homework

Name ______________________ Date due ______________

Take home your completed Draw a Picture of How You Talk handout. Look at your picture. What is one thing you would change about this situation if you could? ____

____

____

____

____

____

Parent signature ______________________

(5)

Stuttering 29 Homework

Name ______________________ Date due ______________

Next time you are teased about stuttering, how would you like to respond? On a separate piece of paper, draw a picture of yourself responding to being teased.

Parent signature ______________________

(6)

30
Stuttering Interviews

Purpose

- To provide students with opportunities to calmly discuss their stuttering in open conversations
- To demonstrate to students that most people do not react negatively when talking about stuttering
- To demonstrate to both the interviewer and the person being interviewed that talking about stuttering is not only allowed but encouraged

Materials

Stuttering Interview 1
Stuttering Interview 2
Sample of Stuttering Interview 2
Pencils
Clipboards
Homework (including Stuttering Interview 3)

Directions

It is not uncommon for stutterers to have negative feelings about their stuttering and to project these feelings onto others (Guitar, 1998). An actor who stutters, Nicholas Brendon, who stars as Xander Harris on the television show *Buffy the Vampire Slayer,* has discussed this issue of projecting negative feelings. He said, "The truth is that people were generally nice to me, but that's not what I noticed. I couldn't help feeling people thought I was a moron, and my self-imposed insecurity constantly bedeviled me" (Moran & Shoop, 2001, para. 4). By talking to others about stuttering, children create relationships in which listeners will feel comfortable asking questions and stutterers will feel comfortable responding to stuttering inquiries.

Stuttering interviews may be assigned numerous times throughout the course of therapy to offer children opportunities to openly discuss their stuttering with others.[5] Encourage students to treat stuttering interviews as casual conversations. Many people being interviewed, such as teachers and relatives, want to react to stuttering in a sensitive and thoughtful manner, but often do not know how. This gives them the opportunity to ask how they should be responding to stuttering.

---

[5] The stuttering interviews in this activity have been adapted from *Successful Stuttering Management Program (SSMP) for Adolescent and Adult Stutterers, Second Edition,* by D. H. Breitenfelt and D. R. Lorenz, 2000, Cheney: Eastern Washington University. Copyright 2000 by D. H. Breitenfelt and D. R. Lorenz. Adapted with permission.

Stuttering Interview 1. Begin by handing each student a copy of the first interview form. Then explain:

> It is not easy talking to other people about stuttering. Today we are going to practice this. An interview is a good way for you let other people know that you stutter and that you are working on your speech. You are also showing people that it is okay to talk about stuttering. You will be helping to educate others about stuttering, and you will also learn what other people think about stuttering. And remember, *you* are the stuttering expert!

Give students the opportunity to role-play Stuttering Interview 1 before conducting actual interviews (see Sample of Stuttering Interview 2 for an example of a completed stuttering interview). Students may role-play with another student or with their clinician. While practicing interviews you will want to help students become comfortable and flexible with this assignment. For example, a student reads you the first question from Stuttering Interview 1: "What do you think causes stuttering?" You may respond, "I really do not know what causes stuttering; maybe you can tell me." This answer may confuse some students because they are not expecting their interviewee to ask something of them. But it is often the case that people being interviewed about stuttering *will* pose a question to the student because they are generally curious and interested. You need to encourage students to answer any questions asked of them and not feel the need to rush through the interview. Students may respond to this question in a number of ways. Those who are new in speech class may say, "I stutter because I tripped and banged my head when I was younger." Returning students may say, "No one really knows why people start stuttering." Many students are not accustomed to talking openly about stuttering and will need to be challenged a bit during role-playing situations to do so.

The introductory paragraph at the top of Stuttering Interview 1 and Stuttering Interview 2 is optional. Explain that students may choose to read the paragraph to the person they wish to interview, or they may simply explain the purpose of the interview in their own words. Also, explain to students that when conducting a second interview with someone (as many students wish to do), there is no reason to read the introductory paragraph again.

After students role-play Stuttering Interview 1, ask them who they would like to interview. Many students will choose their mother or another comfortable person to interview first and this may be assigned for homework. After students complete their first interview, ask them to choose a more challenging person to interview, such as a teacher, the principal, or a school staff member. Then arrange a time for the student to conduct the interview. I attend the first of these interviews (or first few interviews) to help students take their time and learn how to use the interview to trigger conversations about stuttering. For example, if a teacher mentions that she always wanted to know more about stuttering, I whisper to the student, "Ask your teacher why she finds stuttering so interesting." Students do not have to write down the answers to questions that come up during conversation, but are welcome to do so. After students become comfortable with conducting interviews, ask them to arrange their own interviews. Explain:

> Now that we have done an interview together, I want you to make a list of three other people you want to interview. They can be teachers, staff members, relatives, friends, or neighbors. After you make the list, it is your job to go up to the people you have chosen and ask them if you can set up a time to interview them about stuttering. For example, if you wish to interview your science teacher, let her know that you want to interview her about stuttering for a speech class assignment. If you have trouble setting up a time, ask me for help.

In the schools it is often possible to give students a hall pass and ask them to seek out their potential interviewees within the school. Students may either conduct interviews right then or schedule a time to return. In my school there are many staff members at any given time who are taking their preparatory periods and may be approached about interviews. If I know that all of the third-grade teachers are taking their "preps," then I will inform students that they may only approach third-grade teachers at this time. In this example, I will typically stand in the third-grade hallway to observe the students. I also make it clear that students should only approach teachers who are not working with children and who are not in meetings. I might ask, "What should you do if a teacher looks busy?" to which students reply "come back another time." I provide students with clipboards to write on during interviews that take place at school. This is practical but also lends the activity a level of formality and professionalism that many students find inspiring and comforting. Every school and site is different. Do your best to enable students to independently set up and conduct interviews.

After students complete their interviews, discuss them in speech class. Students are often surprised by the responses they receive. For example, one student was certain everyone he interviewed would attribute the cause of his stuttering to worrying. This student was amazed to discover that his teacher and principal did not consider him to a person who "worries too much." Other students have been pleasantly surprised when teachers tell them that they are both brave and strong for talking so openly about stuttering.

Some people being interviewed will not understand that the purpose of these interviews is for stutterers to talk about stuttering. On occasion an interviewee may ask the student if he can fill out the interview form and return it to the student. Explain to students that the point of the interview is to talk to other people openly about stuttering. You may tell students, "If you leave the interview form, then you will not be able to practice talking about stuttering with that person." Students should be instructed not to leave an interview with someone but to read all questions aloud to the person being interviewed. You may even role-play such scenarios so that students become accustomed to saying, "I can't leave this interview form with you. Can we schedule a time when I may ask you the questions?"

Stuttering Interview 2. Stuttering Interview 2 offers students a different set of questions to ask. This second interview also gives students the opportunity to discuss stuttering a second time with someone they have already interviewed if they have a desire to do so. Students should be given an opportunity to role-play Stuttering Interview 2 before it is assigned to use outside the therapy room.

More Ideas

Interviewer's Attitudes. After students complete an interview, ask them to turn over their interview forms and write a sentence or two on the back that describes the attitudes of the person they interviewed. You might say, "Turn over your interview form and write several sentences describing, in your own words, what Mr. Phillips feels about stuttering." This allows students to think about the discussions they have just had.

After an interview, one fourth-grade student turned over his paper and wrote the following: "Ms. McGuire said that stuttering isn't a bad thing in life, so you shouldn't have to worry about it. She said I could be a good speaker like Martin Luther King Jr."

Using Speech Tools. Another thing to consider is that interviewing others about stuttering may be highly stressful for some children and may precipitate increased moments of stuttering. Because of this, ask students on occasion to use speech tools during this activity. This way students may practice managing their speech during a practical situation. When students are asked to use speech tools, role-play the situation first in speech class. It is often the case that students are so concerned with the content of the interview that they forget to use the tool and need to be reminded. If you are with the child during the interview, you can remind him. Because the main purpose of stuttering interviews is to talk openly about stuttering, speech tools should be assigned on a limited basis. You might ask students to give their first two interviews without speech tools and then use speech tools during the next two interviews.

Homework

When asking students to complete stuttering interviews with family members or friends for homework, remind them that the purpose of the activity is to talk openly about stuttering. On occasion a student has returned to speech class with an interview that was completed in an adult's handwriting. Students need to write all answers themselves (unless they are delayed in writing and require an adult's assistance). For children who have delayed writing skills, contact the family and explain that although the family may help them write the answers, the child still needs to ask the questions. Let parents know that the purpose of this activity is to encourage open two-way discussions about stuttering.

Note. Two of the homework assignments require students to use Stuttering Interview 3. This form does not have preprinted questions on it, to allow the students to write in their own questions. Photocopy this interview form and send it home with Homework Assignments 5 and 6.

Stuttering Interview 1

Excuse me, my name is ______________________, and I am a stutterer working on my speech. I am also learning what other people think about stuttering. Would you mind if I took a few minutes of your time and asked you four questions about stuttering?

Name of person you interviewed: ______________________

1. What do you think causes stuttering? ______________________

____

____

____

____

2. What do you think a stutterer should do to manage his or her stuttering?

____

____

____

____

3. Do you know anyone else who stutters? What is their stuttering like?

____

____

____

____

4. Do you feel uncomfortable or embarrassed when you talk to a stutterer?

____

____

____

____

Thank you very much.

Stuttering Interview 2

Excuse me, my name is ______________________, and I am a stutterer working on my speech. I am also learning what other people think about stuttering. Would you mind if I took a few minutes of your time and asked you four questions about stuttering?

Name of person you interviewed: ______________________

1. What would you do if your child stuttered? ______________________

____

____

____

____

2. How do you think you would feel if you stuttered in front of a group of people or on the telephone?

____

____

____

____

3. Do you feel that stutterers can be classroom teachers? ______________________

____

____

____

____

4. What would you like to know about my stuttering? ______________________

____

____

____

____

Thank you very much.

Sample of Stuttering Interview 2

Excuse me, my name is Michael Carrol, and I am a stutterer working on my speech. I am also learning what other people think about stuttering. Would you mind if I took a few minutes of your time and asked you four questions about stuttering?

Name of person you interviewed: Miss Elizabeth Reynolds

1. What would you do if your child stuttered?
   She would take him to a speech teacher.

2. How do you think you would feel if you stuttered in front of a group of people or on the telephone?
   She wouldn't feel embarrassed. She said that people should judge you for what you say, not how you say it.

3. Do you feel that stutterers can be classroom teachers?
   Yes, because knowledge is in your head, not in your mouth.

4. What would you like to know about my stuttering?
   How do you handle it and how do you feel about yourself?

Thank you very much.

Stuttering Interview 3

Excuse me, my name is ______________________, and I am a stutterer working on my speech. I am also learning what other people think about stuttering. Would you mind if I took a few minutes of your time and asked you four questions about stuttering?

Name of person you interviewed: ______________________________

1. ______________________________

2. ______________________________

3. ______________________________

4. ______________________________

Thank you very much.

Stuttering 30 Homework

Name ______________________ Date due ______________

Your speech teacher will assign you Stuttering Interview 1 or 2 for homework. Use it to interview one person in your family. Write down the answers and bring the completed interview back to speech class.

Parent signature ______________________ (1)

Stuttering 30 Homework

Name ______________________ Date due ______________

Your speech teacher will assign you Stuttering Interview 1 or 2 for homework. Use it to interview a neighbor or friend of the family. Write down the answers and bring the completed interview back to speech class.

Parent signature ______________________ (2)

Stuttering 30 Homework

Name ______________________ Date due ______________

Take Stuttering Interview 1 or 2 and interview a teacher, principal, or school staff member. Write down the answers and bring the completed interview back to speech class.

Parent signature ______________________ (3)

Stuttering 30 Homework

Name ______________________ Date due ______________

How do you feel about doing stuttering interviews? ______________________

____

____

Is there anything you would want to change or add to the interview form?

____

____

Parent signature ______________________ (4)

Stuttering 30 Homework

Name ________________________ Date due ________________

Think of four things that you would like to ask others about stuttering. Write the four questions on Stuttering Interview 3.

Parent signature ________________________ (5)

Stuttering 30 Homework

Name ________________________ Date due ________________

Interview someone at school using the four questions you wrote on Stuttering Interview 3. Write this person's answers on the interview form.

Parent signature ________________________ (6)

Stuttering 30 Homework

Name ________________________ Date due ________________

Take a stuttering interview form and interview a friend. Write down the answers and bring the interview back to speech class.

How did it feel to interview your friend? ______________________________

____

____

____

____

____

Parent signature ________________________ (7)

31
You Feel That Way Too?

Purpose

- To give students an opportunity to express their own feelings and experiences with stuttering
- To provide students with opportunities to consider the experiences of other people who stutter

Materials

Stuttering story handouts
Stuttering poem handouts
Write Your Own Stuttering Story handout
Write Your Own Stuttering Poem handout
Pencils
Homework

Directions

Note: This activity is meant to take two sessions (one session for stories and one session for poems).

Many clinicians, especially those involved with the self-help movement, encourage children to read stories and poems about stuttering and then write about their own experiences.

Stuttering Stories. For students in elementary school, begin by choosing a story from the stuttering story handouts (beginning on page 217) for the group to read together, or, you may have students look through the stories and choose their own. Some of the stories are more appropriate for younger or less mature children, whereas some work better with older or mature children. For students in middle school or junior high school, there are additional stories and poems in Appendix C that are suitable for this age group. Use the stories you think will work best with your students.

You or a student reads aloud a chosen story and then the class discusses it. After reading "Oh Nuts" by Lucy Reed, you may wish to discuss how Lucy ended up telling her teacher something that was untrue to avoid stuttering. To make sure students understand what Lucy did, you may ask, "Why did Lucy lie to her teacher? What caused Lucy to change her words?" Then ask, "Have you ever told someone something that wasn't true because it was easier than stuttering?" or "Do you ever change your words like Lucy did?" For more discussion ideas, look through the homework assignments that follow this activity—they will help you consider ways to discuss the stories with your students.

Most of the stories and poems presented in this book will elicit an emotional reaction from students. For example, students may say, "I also don't like getting teased either" or "I am glad when I don't stutter." Students may also see the positive side of many of the readings and comment, "Stuttering is okay" or "When my mouth feels stuck I use my stretching."

Students will begin to share similar experiences after they have read stories about stuttering. Encourage them to do so. A student may return to therapy and say, "Remember that story we read last week about the boy getting teased? That happened to me today."

After reading and discussing a few stories, pass out the Write Your Own Stuttering Story handout and ask students to write their own stories about stuttering. For more mature students, you may offer them lined paper instead of the handout. Give students very few directions with this assignment so as not to influence them. You may simply say:

> Write a story that tells us something about your stuttering. You may write about being teased, about stuttering in class, about how your family treats your stuttering, about a funny stuttering story, or about any other part of your stuttering.

Then have students read their stories to the group. After each student reads his story, discuss it. After discussions, ask students if they would like to share their stories with others by hanging them up for display. Many students are eager to decorate their stories and display them in speech class or a classroom. Ask, "Is there anyone in particular you would like to share your story with?" Suggest making photocopies of the stories and giving them to teachers and family members. Revisit this activity as often as you feel is helpful and productive.

Stuttering Poems. Reading and writing stuttering poems offers students another avenue for expressing their feelings about stuttering and considering the experiences and feelings of others. Just as with stuttering stories, read through a few of the poems at the end of this activity (beginning on page 219) and engage students in discussing them. Then have students write their own poems on the Write Your Own Stuttering Poem handout and present them for discussion.

Typically I do not spend time defining and explaining the concept of poetry. Students usually come to speech class having already been exposed to poetry because it is part of their curriculum. Also, I find that students tend to learn easily by example.

You may learn a lot about your students by reading their poems. For example, one year I had two students who were in therapy together. Toward the end of the year, one child wrote a poem that read:

> Stuttering is fine.
> If people don't like my stuttering, then they are the ones with a problem.

The other student wrote a poem that read:

Stuttering is the worst.
Stuttering is really bad.
I wish someone would just take my stuttering away.
Some people won't even listen to me.
I want it to go away.

Other children who stutter saw these two poems hanging in the speech room and began a lively conversation comparing them. During the conversation, students expressed different opinions such as, "Stuttering *is* really bad," "It *is* okay to stutter," "People ignore me too when I stutter," "I wish I didn't stutter." One child even asked the author of the first poem, "Do you actually like your stuttering?"

During therapy sessions in which students are encouraged to bring a guest, many cannot wait to take their stories and poems off the wall or out of their folders to share with guests. Occasionally, students will ask if they can hang their stuttering stories and poems in their classrooms; this is a great way to open a dialogue on stuttering between students and teachers.

More Ideas

The popular Web site www.stutteringhomepage.com offers a kid's section that provides children the opportunity to read stories, poems, plays, and other writings by children who stutter. Click on "Just for Kids" and then help students explore the various links, such as "Good Stuff by and for Kids" and "Teasing." Choose stories, poems, and other materials to read and discuss.

After students read and discuss a few stories, you may assign speech tools to be used during readings and discussions. Keep in mind, the primary focus of this activity is discussing stuttering. If you find that practicing speech tools inhibits discussions, you may wish to practice them another time.

After students write their stories and poems, let them draw pictures to go along with their tales. Students may draw their pictures at the bottom of the page or on the back of their handouts.

Sisskin (2002) recommended using "wish lists" to determine what students would like to change about their stuttering. Ask students to write a story or poem in which they list several things that they wish were different about their stuttering. For example, students may wish that their parents did more to stop teasing or that other students did not complete their thoughts. Sisskin suggests using open-ended questions to elicit a child's wishes. For example, ask students, "What would you wish to change about your stuttering?" or "What would you like to change about the way other people treat your stuttering?"

Have students keep a journal to write down experiences about stuttering. You could ask students to write one journal entry a day about a stuttering experience.

Let students know that the journal is theirs, and they may share entries with their speech teacher and peers only if they wish to do so.

Homework

Each story and poem presented in this section has homework pertaining to it. As with all the homework assignments in this book, you may assign some as homework and use others for additional speech class activities. Cut lines separate stories and poems. Make photocopies of the pages you wish to use and cut out the chosen stories and poems.

Cerena

by Ryan Tatarniuk

My name is Ryan Tatarniuk, and sometimes I have trouble talking. Here is a little story about what happened to me in Grade One. In my class there was a girl named Cerena. One day when I was going home from school, Cerena heard me talking when I was having bumps and sticks. She started calling me names. She said, "Ryan doesn't know how to talk." I felt mad and sad because she was teasing me, so if it happens again, I will use a stretch in my speech to stop bumps and sticks. The End

Oh, Nuts

by Lucy Reed

One weekend I ate a lot of pistachio nuts—those little green nuts with the red shells. On Monday morning my fingertips were still colored red from the dye on the shells. My teacher asked me, "Why are your fingers red?" I knew I would get stuck if I tried to say "from eating nuts," so I said "paint." She said, "Paint? Are you sure it isn't from eating those red nuts?" I said, "No, it's paint." I felt silly for not telling her the truth because I knew that she knew I was making it up.

I Like Speech Class

by Jesse Dolce

I get to have a lot of fun in speech class. There is a tool kit we use with a lot of neat stuff in it like bouncy balls and Silly Putty. Sometimes kids tease me when I go to speech class, but they don't know that I get to play games. I like speech class the most when I get to bring my friend, Sarah, with me. She gets to play games with the group, and I teach her about my speech tools.

One time in my classroom, a kid was teasing me about my speech. He called me "Stutter Face." Sarah told the mean kid how much fun speech class was. Then the mean kid asked if he could come to speech class too. Maybe if he is nice and stops teasing me, I will take him to speech class.

Stuttering Is Like Walking

by Christos Pena

Stuttering is just like walking. Every day you walk and every day you stutter. Stuttering is no big deal. Just look at James Earl Jones, the actor who plays Darth Vader from *Star Wars.* He stuttered so much that he almost quit talking in high school. But James Earl Jones never stopped talking, and now he is a famous actor who stutters. My advice to you is simple: Don't give up!

Team Captain

by Izzy Zinman

Every day I play basketball in an after-school program. I love playing and am pretty good, but a couple of the kids tease me about my stuttering. When the mean kids tease, the nice kids sometimes join in. The gym teacher is always busy and does not stop the teasing unless it gets really bad. I never raise my hand to be team captain because that would mean I would have to talk. Then I would get teased even more. The gym teacher asked me once to be captain, but I said no. It would have be been fun to be captain, but getting teased is no fun at all.

I Still Stutter

by Leslie Furmansky

In third grade I thought to myself, "There is no way I will stutter in the fourth grade."

In sixth grade I thought to myself, "There is no way I am going to stutter when I begin junior high school." Junior high school came, and I was still stuttering. I thought to myself, "Okay, you have 3 years to stop stuttering. There is no way I am entering high school stuttering."

High school came and I was still stuttering. I thought to myself, "This is it. I'll make myself practice my speech all the time and I'll stop stuttering."

Trying not to stutter didn't work for me. I am in college now and I am still stuttering. My speech pathologist in college suggested that instead of trying not to stutter, I try stuttering in different ways. This is working better. Now I know that even when I stutter, I am still succeeding.

My Greatest Fear

by Leslie Furmansky

When I was in junior high school, I used to volunteer in a classroom with children with multiple handicaps. As a volunteer my job was to interact and become a friend to the students. I also assisted with activities and helped the teacher. Occasionally I would take walks with the students while the teacher stayed in the classroom. My biggest fear was that a child would have a medical emergency, and I would need to get someone's attention or if no one else was around, call 911 by myself. The problem was that I wasn't sure that if there were an emergency, I would be able to call for help. I imagined getting stuck in a big stuttering block. I could feel myself pushing and pushing, but the words wouldn't come out. That was my greatest fear—not being able to help the students in need.

My Mouth Got Stuck

by Eric DeLeon

One time when I was in school, I was sitting at my desk during quiet reading time. All the kids were reading and the teacher was working at her desk. I looked up from my book and saw a bird fly right into a classroom window. The bird must not have seen the window. I looked around the room, but no one else had seen it happen. I thought the bird might be hurt, so I raised my hand. The teacher asked, "What is it, Eric?" Just then my mouth got stuck. I wanted to say, "A bird just flew right into the window," but nothing came out. I didn't want to stutter, so I just said, "Never mind." After class I went up to the teacher's desk and told her what happened. The teacher was mad at me and asked, "Why didn't you tell me before?"

Stuttering Isn't So Bad

by Stephanie Saunders

Stuttering is good;
Stuttering is bad.
Stuttering makes me happy,
And it makes me sad.
I am happy when I don't get stuck.
But when my words won't come out,
I am sad and out of luck.

Stuttering is like . . .

by Tyler Morris

Stuttering is like . . .

A car stuck in the mud.
A rocket that won't take off.
A bird that wants to fly,
But never makes it to the sky.

Stuttering is like . . .

A car that can't go too fast.
A runner that cannot run.
A boat that will not sail.
My words get stuck in the word jail.

Stuttering Poem
by T. J. Polak

Stuttering is embarrassing.
Stuttering isn't fun.
Stuttering can get you in trouble
When you're on the run.
Stuttering isn't easy.
Stuttering can really stink.
Stuttering can make you queasy,
But it can also make your think!

My Dad
by Leslie Furmansky

I use to be scared of meeting a new teacher.
My dad would say, "You can do it!"

I use to be scared of reading in front of my class.
My dad would say, "You can do it!"

I use to be scared giving a class report.
My dad would say, "You can do it!"

I use to be scared of acting in the school play.
My dad would say, "You can do it!"

I use to be nervous when I had to speak.
My dad would say, "You can do it!"

I use to get nervous and ask my dad if I could back out of having to speak.
"No! You can do it!" he would say.

Now I know that I can do it (but I still like my dad telling me).

Stuttering
by Zhi Ying Liang

Stuttering is the worst.
Stuttering is really bad.
I wish someone would just take my stuttering away.
Some people won't even listen to me.
I want it to go away.

Stuttering
by Ahmed Rabbo

Stuttering is fine.
If people don't like my stuttering, then they are the ones with the problem.

Stuttering Well
by Matthew Law

Sometimes I stutter hard,
Sometimes I stutter soft.
Sometimes when I stutter a lot,
Kids say I stutter badly.
But my mom says I stutter well.

Stutter
by Michael Caggiano

I am my stutter;
My stutter is me.
I hate it, despise it.
Wish I could rectify it.

I used to wonder, why me?
Out of all the people
I had to be the one.
Do you know how it feels?

It's like a hand
Clamped over your mouth,
When you most want to speak;

When the air in your lungs
Just stops and won't even form words.

My stutter defines me.
It makes me, hurts me,
Confines and confronts me.
It is who I am.

What Letting Go Means To Me
by Shaina

Letting go means I like to talk now.
Letting go means telling friends that I stutter.
Letting go means that I just talk a little different.
Letting go means I raise my hand in class.
Letting go means telling jokes to my friends.
Letting go means laughing more.
Letting go means practicing my speech.
Letting go means I talk more now.
Letting go means I don't mind my stutter.
Letting go means I know I am like everyone else.
Letting go is fun.

Write Your Own Stuttering Story

Name ________________________ Date ____________________

Write Your Own Stuttering Poem

Name ______________________________ Date ____________________

Stuttering 31 Homework

Name ______________________________ Date due ____________________

Read "Cerena" by Ryan Tatarniuk. When Ryan gets teased he uses his speech tools to help him stop stuttering. What else could Ryan do when he gets teased?

1. ____

2. ____

3. ____

Parent signature ______________________________ (1)

Stuttering 31 Homework

Name ______________________________ Date due ____________________

Read "Oh Nuts" by Lucy Reed. Sometimes we say things that really aren't true because we are scared of stuttering. Think of a time that you have said something that wasn't true just so you would not have to stutter. Write about this below. ______________________________

____

____

____

____

____

Parent signature ______________________________ (2)

Stuttering 31 Homework

Name ______________________________ Date due ____________________

Read "I Like Speech Class" by Jesse Dolce. Jesse liked bringing a friend to speech class.

Who would you like to bring to speech class? ______________________________

What are two reasons you would like this person to come to speech class?

1. ____

2. ____

Parent signature ______________________________ (3)

Stuttering 31 Homework

Name ______________________ Date due ______________________

Read "Stuttering Is Just Like Walking" by Christos Pena. Christos wrote, "Stuttering is no big deal." What do you think this means and do you agree or disagree? Explain your answer. ______________________

____

____

____

Parent signature ______________________ (4)

Stuttering 31 Homework

Name ______________________ Date due ______________________

Read "Team Captain" by Izzy Zinman. Izzy's gym teacher did not stop the other children from teasing him. Who are three people Izzy could have told about this problem?

1. ____________ 2. ____________ 3. ____________

What could Izzy say to them about his problem? ______________________

____

____

(5)

Parent signature ______________________

Stuttering 31 Homework

Name ______________________ Date due ______________________

Read "I Still Stutter" by Leslie Furmansky. When will you stop stuttering?

____

Leslie wrote, "Trying not to stutter didn't work for me." How do you try not to stutter? Write three ways below.

1. ______________________
2. ______________________
3. ______________________

Parent signature ______________________ (6)

Stuttering 31 Homework

Name ______________________ Date due ______________

Read "My Greatest Fear" by Leslie Furmansky. Leslie's greatest fear was that she would not be able to call for help because of her stuttering. What is your greatest speaking fear? ______________________________

____

____

____

____

Parent signature ______________________ (7)

Stuttering 31 Homework

Name ______________________ Date due ______________

Read "My Mouth Got Stuck" by Eric DeLeon. Eric wanted to tell his teacher about the bird but decided not to because he might stutter. What are three things that Eric could have done when his mouth got stuck?

1. ______________________________
2. ______________________________
3. ______________________________

Parent signature ______________________ (8)

Stuttering 31 Homework

Name ______________________ Date due ______________

Read "Stuttering Isn't So Bad" by Stephanie Saunders. Write one good thing and one bad thing about stuttering.

1. ______________________________
2. ______________________________

Parent signature ______________________ (9)

Stuttering 31 Homework

Name ______________________ Date due ______________

Read "Stuttering is like . . ." by Tyler Morris. Tyler compares stuttering to a rocket that won't fly and a car stuck in the mud. What is your stuttering like? Complete the poem below.

Stuttering is like . . . ______________________

Stuttering is like . . . ______________________

Stuttering is like . . . ______________________

Parent signature ______________________ (10)

Stuttering 31 Homework

Name ______________________ Date due ______________

Read the poem by T. J. Polak. T. J. said, "Stuttering isn't fun" and "Stuttering stinks." Think of something good about stuttering and write it here.

____

____

____

____

Parent signature ______________________ (11)

Stuttering 31 Homework

Name ______________________ Date due ______________

Read "My Dad" by Leslie Furmansky. Leslie wrote that when she was having a hard time talking, her father would say, "You can do it." What do your parents or your relatives say to you about stuttering? ______________________

____

____

____

____

Parent signature ______________________ (12)

Stuttering (31) Homework

Name ______________________ Date due ______________

Read the poem "Stuttering" by Zhi Ying Liang. Zhi Ying wrote, "I wish someone would take my stuttering away." Can someone take Zhi Ying's stuttering away? Explain your answer. ______________________

____

____

____

Zhi Ying started his poem by saying, "Stuttering is the worst." Below is the beginning of a poem that starts with the line, "Stuttering isn't so bad." Complete the poem on a separate piece of paper.

Stuttering isn't so bad . . .

Parent signature ______________________ (13)

Stuttering (31) Homework

Name ______________________ Date due ______________

Read the poem "Stuttering" by Ahmed Rabbo. Ahmed said that even though he stutters, it wasn't a problem. Ahmed thinks that people who don't like stuttering have a problem. What do you think? ______________________

____

____

Parent signature ______________________ (14)

Stuttering (31) Homework

Name ______________________ Date due ______________

Read the poem "Stuttering Well" by Matthew Law. Mathew wrote that kids say he stutters badly, but his mother says he stutters well.

What does stuttering well mean? ______________________

____

List two words that you use to describe your stuttering.

1.______________________ 2. ______________________

Parent signature ______________________ (15)

Stuttering 31 Homework

Name ______________________ Date due ______________

Read "What Letting Go Means to Me" by Shaina. What do you think letting go means? ____

____

____

____

Complete the following poem.

Letting go means ____

Letting go means ____

Letting go means ____

Letting go means ____

Parent signature ______________________ (16)

- - - - - - - - - - - - - - - - - - -

Stuttering 31 Homework

Name ______________________ Date due ______________

Read the poem "Stutter" by Michael Caggiano. Michael wrote that stuttering feels "like a hand clamped over your mouth when you most want to speak."

How does stuttering feel to you? ____

____

____

____

____

What do you think of Michael's poem? ____

____

____

____

____

Parent signature ______________________ (17)

32
It's Showtime

Purpose

- To provide students, through role-playing, with ways to handle teasing situations and stressful speaking situations
- To provide students with the opportunity to express their feelings and attitudes about stuttering and bullying situations

Materials

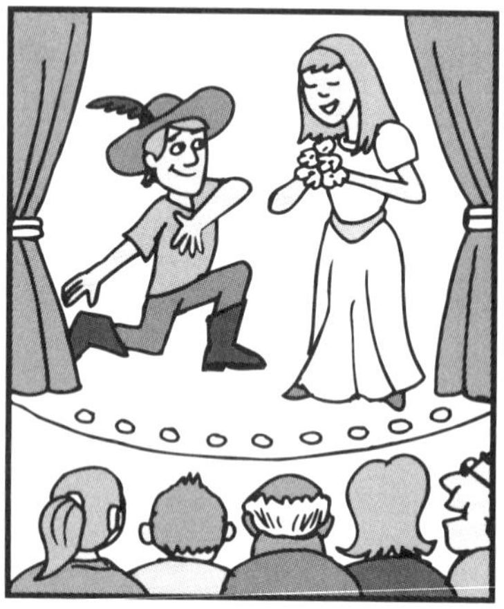

Stuttering Plays
Write Your Own Stuttering Play handouts
Prop-making materials for plays (i.e., paper, markers, and tape)
Homework

Directions

Many children who stutter report that being teased, mocked, or bullied is one of the worst parts about the disorder. Clinicians often use role-playing to help students face their fears and manage difficult situations.

Acting Out Plays. To begin this activity, explain:

> Today we are going to practice dealing with people who tease you and who are mean to you because you stutter. We will be acting out several plays about teasing. Let's see if we have any good actors among us!

Choose an appropriate play and hand out a copy to each student. Sometimes students do not understand that they should act the part of the character they are assigned, and they end up reading in a monotone. To prevent dull readings, assign yourself a role so that students observe you acting or even overacting instead of simply reading lines.

Students often enjoy arranging the therapy room in a special way for each play. For example, when practicing the Restaurant Play, students may wish to set the scene by using folders as menus, moving tables and chairs, and drawing a restaurant sign to hang on the wall. When acting out the plays, tell students performing in roles other than the "Stutterer," such as a "Cashier" or "Friend," it is okay if they happen to stutter.

You will notice that in Buying Ice Cream, the Stutterer and the Friend characters respond to a rude cashier by politely addressing his behavior three times. Whereas three polite reprimands may seem to be disproportionate to the act, children who stutter need opportunities to vent and voice their frustrations. This play provides students the opportunity to let their feelings and emotions out and to practice addressing other people's rude behavior through the dialogue. However, if you are working with a student with severe pragmatic or behavioral concerns, you may want to skip this particular play and focus on others.

After acting out the plays, engage students in discussing the many productive ways in which they may respond to inappropriate or uninformed comments about their stuttering. For example, when discussing the Classroom Teasing Play, students may disagree about whether or not they have the right to openly "stick-up" for themselves. They may need you to give guidance.

Students often want to act out plays several times, especially if each student is vying for the same part. Also, some students like to perform these plays with speech class guests as participants.

All of the plays except the last one (Advertising Play) have moments of stuttering written into the text. For example, in the Teasing At Lunch Play, the Stutterer character says, "Boy-boy-boy-boy, am I hungry." Moments of stuttering are written into most of the plays because some students will not stutter during role-playing situations, much the same way that actors who stutter, such as James Earl Jones, do not stutter when performing.

Using the previous example, as long as students stutter noticeably when reading aloud the word *boy,* you should not be overly concerned with how the student stutters. If the student stutters on boy by prolonging the first sound and saying "bbbbboy," you should not feel the need to correct him.

Writing Plays. After acting out several stuttering plays, encourage students to write their own, either individually or in small groups. Explain:

> Now that we have acted out several stuttering plays, I want us all to write a play together about stuttering. Let's think about these questions: When is speaking hard for you? When do you get teased about stuttering? What would you like to do differently when you are teased? What would you like to say to a teaser that you have never said before?

Call on students to answer these questions and to share their stuttering experiences. Review options students have when responding to teasing situations. Begin helping students write a play by steering the group toward one idea as the basis for the play. For example, one year students shared that they often got teased in the park when their parents were not within listening distance. The group then wrote a play about playing basketball in which a child who stutters was faced with a teasing situation. This play was a conglomeration of each child's experiences with stuttering and teasing.

When writing stuttering plays, some students have written parts for their nonstuttering friends so that these friends can help them deal with the teasing. In one of these plays, the friend's only line was, "Hey, leave him alone—it's okay to stutter."

For this writing assignment, use regular writing paper or pass out a version of the Write Your Own Stuttering Play handout. There are two versions of this handout: One is blank, and the other has two characters—a child and a teaser. This latter version is helpful for students who have difficulty organizing their writing into script form.

More Ideas

If you are a school clinician, you may take your students to the school auditorium or gym for these plays. Often I will bring several plays along with one or more additional activities and conduct the entire speech class in this location.

Homework

The homework assignments in this section ask students to write their own plays. For students who have difficulty working independently, help them begin their plays in speech class. It may also help if you attach a copy of a stuttering play to the homework so that parents and students have an example to use as a reference. For Homework Assignment 3, students may take home a copy of the Stuttering Facts handout (see Facts–Activity 24). This handout will help them include a few facts about stuttering in a play.

Stuttering Plays

Teasing At Lunch Play

STUTTERER: Boy-boy-boy-boy, am I hungry.

TEASER: Hey, stutter-face, you can't sit here.

STUTTERER: I can sit here.

TEASER: You can't sit here because you stutter.

STUTTERER: I *can* sit here because it's okay to stutter.

Playground Teasing Play

TEASER: Hey, everyone. Here comes stutter-face. Go-go-go-go play some where else, sssssstutter-face.

STUTTERER: Hey, it sounds like you stutter too.

TEASER: You sound stupid—you stutter.

STUTTERER: I stutter and I am also smart.

TEASER: Go play somewhere else stutter-head.

STUTTERER: I stutter and that's okay. I will play anywhere I want to play.

Buying Ice Cream Play

ICE-CREAM CASHIER: What can I get you both today?

FRIEND: Could I please have a waffle cone with chocolate ice cream, whipped cream, and sprinkles.

ICE-CREAM CASHIER (looking at stutterer): And what for you today?

STUTTERER: Ccccould I please hhhhave a wwwwwwwwww. . .

ICE-CREAM CASHIER (interrupts or cuts off the stutterer): You talk funny. What do you want?

STUTTERER: I-I-I-I-I don't talk funny. I ssstutter. Iiiit's okay to stutter.

FRIEND: We came here today to get ice cream, not to get hassled. It's not polite to make fun of people because they speak differently.

ICE-CREAM CASHIER: I'm sorry, I don't know many stutterers.

STUTTERER: When sssomeone is stuttering, iiiit is polite to gi-gi-gi-gi-give them the time they nnneed to talk.

ICE-CREAM CASHIER: Okay. What would you like today? Take your time.

STUTTERER: A wwwwaffle cone with vanilla ice cream, cho-cho-chocolate syrup, whipped cream, aaand a cherry, please.

Classroom Teasing Play

TEACHER (writing on the chalkboard with his back toward the class): Does anyone know what 5 times 5 is?

STUTTERER: I-I-I do.

TEACHER: Okay, what is the answer?

STUTTERER: Twu-twu-twu-twenty-five.

TEASER: Twu-twu-twu-twenty-five. You sound stupid.

STUTTERER: Teasing is not cool. You need to stop.

TEACHER (turning around and facing class): Who is talking?

STUTTERER: I wwwwas just telling Mike that teasing is not allowed.

TEASER: Hey, I wasn't teasing anyone.

STUTTERER: I have the right to speak in class without being teased. I stutter and that is okay.

TEACHER: Listen up, class. Teasing is not allowed.

TEASER (denying the charge): But it wasn't me.

TEACHER: **Nobody** is allowed to tease!

Coolest Stuttering Play

STUTTERER: Hhhhey, Dylan, llllet's go play some basketball.

DYLAN: Okay, there are some kids playing in the park. I think we can beat those guys.

STUTTERER (speaking to Teaser 1 and Teaser 2): Hey, you guys wanna play some ba-ba-ba-basketball against us?

TEASER 1: Check this out. Stu-stu-stu-stutter boy wants to play ba-ba-basketball with us.

TEASER 2: No, he doesn't want to play basketball; he wants to play stu-stu-stu-stutterball.

DYLAN: Yo, teasing is uncool—let's get out of here.

STUTTERER: No, Dylan. I want to stay and play bbbbbbasketball and teach these guys how to stutter.

TEASER 1 AND TEASER 2: You're gonna teach us how to stutter?

STUTTERER: Yeah—I 'm gonna teach you guys to stutter better. I (looking cool) ssstutter much cooler than you guys. Now lllet's play some bbbbbbasketball.

TEASER 1 AND TEASER 2: Well, okay, then. Let's play!

Restaurant Play

WAITER: Hello, I will be your waiter tonight. Are you ready to order?

BROTHER: Yes. I will have a cheeseburger, with french fries, and a large soft drink.

FATHER: I will have the same, and I also want a salad please.

STUTTERER: CCCCCCCCCould I . . .

WAITER: What do you want? Are you ready to order? I don't have all day.

FATHER: Please give my son the time he needs to order.

STUTTERER: I-I-I-I-I-I-I would like a lllllllarge soft drink and . . .

WAITER: Sir, what would your son like to eat? I can't understand him.

BROTHER: Of course, you can't understand him. You keep interrupting him.

STUTTERER: I-I-I stutter and I like to order for myself.

WAITER: Oh, you stutter. I don't know much about stuttering.

FATHER, BROTHER, AND STUTTERER (said jokingly): After we order we will tell you all about stuttering.

WAITER: Okay. What would you like?

STUTTERER: CCCCould I please have spaghetti and me-me-me-meatballs and a large soft drink.

WAITER: Right away!

FATHER, BROTHER, AND STUTTERER: Thank you!

Advertising Play

Stutterer: We have known each other a long time, and I wanted to talk with you about my stuttering.

Friend: Yeah, I know you stutter, but it's no big deal. I never wanted to bring it up because, well, it's just not an issue for me.

Stutterer: It's important to me that I tell you about my stuttering.

Friend: Okay, what do you want to say?

Stutterer: I have been stuttering since I was a little kid. When I stutter I know exactly what I want to say; it's just that sometimes I get stuck on saying the words.

Friend: Oh, I thought you weren't exactly sure what you wanted to say. Why do you get stuck like that?

Stutterer: I am not exactly sure why I get stuck on sounds and words. Different people will give you different reasons. I am working on my speech now, and there are also a few things that you can do to make speaking easier for me.

Friend: Like what?

Stutterer: It is best if you do not try to finish my words for me or guess what I want to say. By completing my words for me, you actually make speaking harder.

Friend: Oh, I thought I was helping you. Why does this make speaking harder for you?

Stutterer: When you complete my words for me, I feel rushed to speak. When stutterers feel pressure to speak, we tend to stutter a lot.

Friend: What else can you tell me about stuttering?

Stutterer (looks at watch): How much time do you have?

Write Your Own Stuttering Play

Name ______________________________ Date ____________________

Write Your Own Stuttering Play

Name ______________________ Date ______________

CHILD: ______________________

____

TEASER: ______________________

____

CHILD: ______________________

____

TEASER: ______________________

____

CHILD: ______________________

____

TEASER: ______________________

____

CHILD: ______________________

____

TEASER: ______________________

____

CHILD: ______________________

____

TEASER: ______________________

____

CHILD: ______________________

____

TEASER: ______________________

____

CHILD: ______________________

____

TEASER: ______________________

____

Stuttering (32) Homework

Name ______________________ Date due ______________

On a separate piece of paper, write your own play about stuttering. You may write about school, about a fun stuttering experience, about being teased, or anything else that relates to stuttering. Good luck!

Parent signature ______________________ (1)

Stuttering (32) Homework

Name ______________________ Date due ______________

Think about the last time someone teased you about stuttering. Write a play about this teasing experience. In the play you may respond to the teaser any way that you want.

Parent signature ______________________ (2)

Stuttering (32) Homework

Name ______________________ Date due ______________

What are some things that you would like to tell a teacher about your stuttering? Write a play in which you talk to your teacher about stuttering and about how you want him or her to respond to your stuttering. You may want to use the Stuttering Facts handout to help you remember some facts about stuttering.

Parent signature ______________________ (3)

33

Questions and Answers

Purpose

- To encourage students to discuss and reflect upon their stuttering
- To assess student progress and growth

Materials

Discussion Questions
Homework

Directions

Begin this activity by reading a discussion question aloud and encouraging students to talk about it. For example, ask, "What can you do if you feel you are about to stutter?" (This is Question 14 on the Discussion Questions page.) Students often respond with a range of different answers. Some students state that they would use their speech tools to help them work through the situation, whereas other students report that they choose not to speak when they anticipate stuttering. Encourage these conversations by asking students to consider each other's comments.

You may also use the questions as a way of assessing or measuring student growth and progress. For example, the first time students are asked, "Should teachers skip over you in class when you are stuttering?" some students will say "yes." Students frequently reconsider their answers later in therapy and may respond differently by saying, "No, they shouldn't do that" or "I would tell my parents or my speech teacher."

The first time students are asked, "Do you talk to your parents, friends, or teachers about stuttering?" some students have acted quite surprised and have responded with comments such as, "I would never talk to my friends about stuttering" or "I don't talk about stuttering." After participating in activities such as Stuttering Interviews and Do You Read Me? students may respond to this question by saying that speaking with others about stuttering is not such a big deal. This is a good time to remind students of how far they have come in therapy and how much their hard work is paying off. For example, say "Look at how much your hard work is helping you. You went from never talking about stuttering to making it look easy!"

The second question on the Discussion Questions page is, "If you could trade your stuttering for someone else's troubles, what would you consider to be fair trade?" This question was suggested by Rentschler (2004) as a good way to facilitate talking about stuttering.

More Ideas

Many of the questions easily lead into other activities. For example, when students consider Question 21, "Choose one thing to say about stuttering to someone in your family. What would it be?" the answer may easily turn into a letter-writing activity. When asked, "What are three things you can do when someone teases you?" student discussions have led to writing or acting out stuttering plays.

Consider having a "Question of the Day" in which speech class starts with discussing a question from the discussion questions.

Ask students to write and discuss their own discussion questions.

Homework

Some of the discussion questions are included as homework assignments. You may assign any discussion question for homework by writing the homework assignment yourself. You may also develop your own questions.

Discussion Questions

1. What would be different about you if you didn't stutter?
2. If you could trade your stuttering for someone else's troubles, what would you consider to be a fair trade?
3. Why do you stutter?
4. Would you take a pill to cure stuttering? Why or why not?
5. What are two jobs or professions that you *cannot* do if you stutter?
6. What would you do if a teacher lowered your grade because you stuttered during a presentation?
7. Should teachers skip over you in class when you are stuttering?
8. If you could say one thing to your stutter, what would it be?
9. What can you do when someone tries to finish your sentences?
10. Tell about a time when you were teased about stuttering.
11. What is the best (or worst) thing about stuttering?
12. What are three things you can do when someone teases you?
13. When do you avoid talking?
14. What can you do if you feel you are about to stutter?
15. What are three good and three bad things about stuttering?
16. What do you like or dislike about speech therapy?
17. What speech tools do you find useful or difficult?
18. Do you talk to your parents, friends, or teachers about stuttering?
19. What would you like your parents to know about stuttering?
20. What would you like your best friend to know about stuttering?
21. Choose one thing to say about stuttering to someone in your family. What would it be?

Stuttering 33 Homework

Name ______________________ Date due ______________

What are some questions about stuttering that you want to talk about? Think of three questions and write them below.

1. ____

____

2. ____

____

3. ____

____

Parent signature ______________________ (1)

Stuttering 33 Homework

Name ______________________ Date due ______________

When do you avoid talking?

1. ____

2. ____

3. ____

Parent signature ______________________ (2)

Stuttering 33 Homework

Name ______________________ Date due ______________

What would you like your parents to know about stuttering?

1. ____

2. ____

3. ____

Parent signature ______________________ (3)

Stuttering 33 Homework

Name ______________________ Date due ______________

What would be different about you if you didn't stutter? ______________

Parent signature ______________________

(4)

Stuttering 33 Homework

Name ______________________ Date due ______________

What can you do when someone tries to finish your sentences? ______________

Parent signature ______________________

(5)

Stuttering 33 Homework

Name ______________________ Date due ______________

Should teachers skip over you in class when you are stuttering? Explain your answer. ______________

Parent signature ______________________

(6)

34
Dear Abby

Purpose

- To enable students to consider how they have handled difficult situations in the past and how they could handle such situations in the future
- To assess how students manage difficult speaking situations

Materials

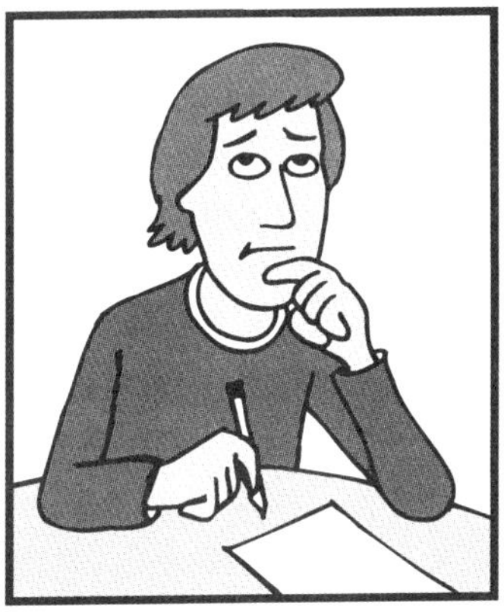

Dear Abby letters
Write Your Own Dear Abby Letter handout
Pencils
Homework

Directions

People who stutter are experts on stuttering (Murphy, 2000; Quesal, 1999; Reitzes, 2002; St. Louis, 2001) because they cope with their stuttering every day. Even when students have difficulty talking about their own stuttering, many will enjoy giving advice and discussing other people's stuttering problems. Begin this activity by reminding students that they are stuttering experts. Explain:

> Many people who stutter have a lot of questions about and problems with their stuttering. Some stutterers like to ask for help. We are going to read a few letters today written by children who stutter and who are asking for advice. Because you live with stuttering every day and are stuttering experts, let's see what kind of advice you can give them.

Reading and Discussing Dear Abby Letters

Assign one of the Dear Abby letters to read in class. Then engage students in a discussion about the letter. As a guide, you may look at the discussion of the letters that follows. You may assign speech tools after discussing a few letters.

Dear Abby Letters allow you to assess students by considering the advice they give each other. For example, if a student responds to a Dear Abby letter by stating that the best way to handle being teased is to stay home and pretend to be sick on certain days, then you know it is time to specifically target ways to react to teasing. Following is a discussion of each Dear Abby Letter:

My Name Is Christian and I Wish It Wasn't. "My Name Is Christian and I Wish It

Wasn't" often elicits strong emotional responses from students. Student responses have included, "Christian should not change his name and should use a speech tool such as stretching to help him," "Christian should break his name in half and say Chris-tian," "Christian should look in a mirror to see how he is stuttering," "Christian should not shorten his name because it is the same thing as changing his name," and "Christian should just shorten his name to Chris." After reading this letter one student explained that he was having great difficulty saying his full name, Michael, so now he just asks to be called Mike. Discussing this letter allowed this student to speak openly about the fear he had saying his own name. I was then able to provide more productive strategies to help him say his name.

When My Teacher Is Sick, I Get Teased. This is a story that often elicits strong feelings from children who stutter. Most often, classroom teachers try to create safe, tolerant classroom environments that respect children's differences. But when these teachers are absent or out of their classrooms, students who stutter may get teased and harassed by other students. I have worked with parents who chose to keep their child home from school on days when they knew a substitute teacher would be teaching the class. After reading "When My Teacher Is Sick, I Get Teased," students have felt a strong bond for Michael (the boy writing the story) and want to discuss their own teasing experiences and ways to help Michael and themselves.

My Science Teacher Skips Over Me. After reading this story students will respond in many different ways. Some of the typical responses are, "That happens to me too," "Sometimes the teacher cuts me off when I am stuttering," "I get stuck in the throat too," and "I don't like talking in class." Other students will get angry about this story and make comments such as, "You are allowed to stutter in class" and "I hate it when teachers don't let me talk." And, of course, many students have understanding and patient teachers and will say, "My teacher always lets me talk" and "I don't have this problem."

The Problem with Pepperoni Pizza. Children who stutter learn many ways to avoid moments of stuttering by changing words or avoiding talking. This is a story about avoidance behavior, and most children who stutter will be able to relate to it.

Talking on the Phone. This letter addresses a host of speaking-on-the-telephone challenges facing children who stutter, such as time pressure, talking to relatives, receiving unrequested and unhelpful speaking advice, and experiencing the embarrassment of stuttering.

The Big Brother. Children know that teasing hurts, and they know that they want the teasing to stop, but they do not always know their options. When reading "The Big Brother," students have made comments such as, "My friend's brother (or sister) teases me too" or "I get mad when I can't play." Students may disagree about how to handle the situation. For example, some want to "tell on" the teasers, whereas others worry about being a "snitch." Some students want to talk back to the teaser, and others feel unable to do so. This letter allows you to help students productively address teasing.

I Want To Be Normal. A major focus of the activities in this book are to help children view stuttering and the way that they talk as being acceptable and normal even if it is also frustrating and painful. In this letter Betty expresses frustration at feeling different from everyone else. Her story stimulates students to discuss the frustrations involved in stuttering and the feeling of being different from other children.

Speech Class. On occasion students will openly come to you with the question, "Sometimes my speech tools don't work—what should I do?" Because students want to please their clinician, they might be reluctant to ask such a question. The Speech Class letter engages children in this difficult discussion.

The Kids on the Block. Students need to know that they have many options for handling teasing situations. Many stutterers do not know that they are allowed to stand up for themselves when teased because that would mean they would need to acknowledge that they stutter. This letter allows students to explore the options available for dealing with bullies and teasers.

Write Your Own Dear Abby Letter

After reading and discussing several Dear Abby letters, pass out the Write Your Own Dear Abby Letter handout and ask students to write their own letters. Explain:

> At some point or another all of us need to ask for help or advice. Think about what causes you trouble with your stuttering. Write a letter describing a difficult stuttering situation. In the letter, ask for help with this situation.

Then ask students to read their letters to the group so that they may offer each other advice and talk about the difficulties they face. If you are working in a one-on-one situation with a student, write your own letter asking for the student's help solving a general problem you are having while the student writes his letter. For example, you might write a letter explaining that you lent your bicycle to a friend who returned it with a broken wheel. In the letter ask your student to help you figure out the best way to respond to this problem. Be sure that your letter reflects a problem that the student can relate to.

More Ideas

Ask students to read a Dear Abby letter and then ask them to write a response to the letter before discussing it. The reason for this is that some students have an easier time being open about stuttering when writing rather than speaking.

Homework

The homework assignments ask students to read stories and discuss them (in writing). Be sure to pass out photocopies of the stories when you are assigning the homework.

My Name Is Christian and I Wish It Wasn't

Dear Abby,

My name is Christian, and I have been stuttering since I was 4 years old. I think what has made me stutter even more is the fact that I can't say my name because the "chr" is difficult for me to say. This made me less willing to talk to people because if I introduce myself I will stutter.

This has led me to fear introducing myself. I am 16 now and I still find it difficult. Some said it was going to go away but it hasn't; it just keeps getting worse.

My question is, Do you think I should change my first name to something I can say or just keep trying until I can say it? Please help me with an answer.

When My Teacher Is Sick, I Get Teased

Dear Abby,

My name is Michael. I am 10 years old, and I am having trouble in school. My teacher doesn't let anyone tease during class. At the beginning of the year, she told the class that teasing is not allowed and that we are all different in some ways. But when my teacher is sick and we have a substitute teacher, there are two boys who sit close to me who tease me about stuttering. They copy the way I talk. They say, "C-c-c-c-can I go-go-go-go-go to sssspeech class too?" When they tease me everyone laughs and our substitute doesn't seem to hear them tease me. What should I do?

My Science Teacher Skips Over Me

Dear Abby,

I am in the sixth grade, my name is Nancy, and I am 13 years old. My science teacher, Ms. Gonzalez, calls on a lot of students to answer questions during class. I always know the answer, and she used to call on me a lot. A few weeks ago Ms. Gonzalez called on me and I stuttered very hard. I tried to say *electricity*, but nothing came out. It sounded like I was choking, and I could feel my throat getting tighter and tighter.

Ms. Gonzalez then called on Rachel and didn't let me answer the question. Now when I raise my hand in science class, Ms. Gonzalez acts like she doesn't see me and calls on other students. I really want Ms. Gonzalez to call on me again. I don't know what to do. Please give me some advice to help with my problem.

The Problem with Pepperoni Pizza

Dear Abby,

My name is Kenny. I am 12 years old, and my favorite food is pepperoni pizza. Only, every time I say *pepperoni,* it comes out "pe-pe-pe-pe-pepperoni." When I go out for pizza after school, I have many different plans and ways to get pepperoni pizza without having to say it. Sometimes I just point to a slice of pepperoni pizza when the guy asks me what I want. Sometimes I tell my mother to order for me while I use the bathroom—Mom knows what I want. And sometimes, when I have to talk, I just order plain pizza rather than risk stuttering on the word *pepperoni.* I like plain pizza—it is good—but I would much rather eat pepperoni pizza. What should I do?

Talking on the Phone

Dear Abby,

My grandparents live far away, and I don't get to see them much. We call them several times a year on all of the big holidays. My mom always passes around the phone and says, "Now don't talk long—this is costing us a lot of money." By the time it is my turn to talk, I feel like I can barely say a word. One time I could barely say "hello." I got stuck on the "h" sound and just kept trying to push it out.

My grandparents are happy to talk with me and love me very much, but I can never get a word in. They keep saying things like "Talk faster," "Slow down," "Take a big breath," "Try and relax," and "Don't be upset." Every time I stutter with them on the phone, they just start talking over me. Or even worse, just when I get going, my mom comes and says, "Your turn is over—say good-bye." Sometimes I don't even want to have a turn talking to my grandparents because it always makes me feel bad. I could sure use some help. Do you have any suggestions for me?

The Big Brother

Dear Abby,

My name is Josh. I like to go over to my friend Brian's house after school to do my homework and to play video games. Brian knows that I stutter, and he never teases me. Sometimes Brian even sticks up for me when other kids tease me.

Brian has an older brother named Andy who teases me when their mother isn't home or in the room. When we play video games, Andy won't give me a turn and says things like, "Stu-stu-stutter boy can't play because he ssssstutters."

I don't like being teased by Andy, but I like being friends with Brian. What should I do?

I Want To Be Normal

Dear Abby,

Why did it have to be me? My name is Betty and I have stuttered since I was 5 years old. I don't want to stutter. I want to be like everyone else. I want my words to glide like the ice skaters on TV. I want my lips to move like a skier swooshing down a mountain. I don't want to be scared of talking. I don't want to look at my feet when the teacher calls on students to read in class. But instead, my words get stuck, and I end up just wanting to run away from talking. I want to know what it is like to be normal. And I want everyone else to spend a day stuttering so that they know how it feels. Can anyone help me?

Speech Class

Dear Abby,

My name is Jorge. I am 13, and my speech teacher teaches me "tools," such as stretching and pausing, to help me with my stuttering problem. Sometimes for speech homework my speech teacher asks me to go home and teach my mom and dad how to use speech tools.

My parents want me to use my speech tools all the time. My speech tools help me, but sometimes I don't like using them. Pausing helps me to stutter a lot less, but pausing can be hard to practice, and sometimes I would just rather stutter. I am not sure what to do about this. I like that my speech tools help me, but I also like just talking without having to think about speech tools. Please help me figure this out.

The Kids on the Block

Dear Abby,

My name is Brandon and I have a teasing problem. There are a bunch of kids on my block who tease me about stuttering. They even call me bad words (curse words) that I don't want to repeat. My mother watches me play from the window at home, but she doesn't hear the names that other kids call me. There is this one girl, Amy, who teases me the most. She gets everyone else to call me names and be mean to me. Once when I was stuttering a lot, she got a few kids to sing a song about me—they called it "Stutter Stupid Face." Amy's class is across from mine in school. Amy doesn't tease me much in school because she will get in trouble. What should I do?

Write Your Own Dear Abby Letter

Name: ______________________ Date: ______________

____
____
____
____
____
____
____
____
____
____
____
____

Write Your Own Dear Abby Letter

Name: ______________________ Date: ______________

____
____
____
____
____
____
____
____
____
____
____
____

Stuttering 34 Homework

Name ______________________ Date due ______________

Read "My Name Is Christian and I Wish It Wasn't." What do you think? Should Christian change his name? Write at least three sentences about this below. ____________________

____

____

____

Parent signature ______________________ (1)

Stuttering 34 Homework

Name ______________________ Date due ______________

Read "When My Teacher Is Sick, I Get Teased." What should Michael do? Write at least three sentences about this below. ____________________

____

____

____

Parent signature ______________________ (2)

Stuttering 34 Homework

Name ______________________ Date due ______________

Read "My Science Teacher Skips Over Me." Write two things that Nancy could do to help solve her problem.

1. ____________________

2. ____________________

Parent signature ______________________ (3)

Stuttering 34 Homework

Name ______________________ Date due ______________

Read "The Problem with Pepperoni Pizza." Kenny needs some help deciding how to order food. What should he do?

____

____

____

____

Parent signature ______________________

(4)

Stuttering 34 Homework

Name ______________________ Date due ______________

Read "Talking on the Phone." Sometimes it is hard for people who stutter to talk on the phone. What are two things you can do to make talking on the phone easier?

1. ____

2. ____

Parent signature ______________________

(5)

Stuttering 34 Homework

Name ______________________ Date due ______________

Read "The Big Brother." What should Josh do so that he can continue going over to Brian's house to play? ______________________

____

____

____

____

Parent signature ______________________

(6)

Stuttering 34 Homework

Name ______________________ Date due ______________

Read "I Want To Be Normal." Betty sounds like she is in a lot of pain because of stuttering. What are two things that Betty can do to help herself?

1. ______________________________

2. ______________________________

Parent signature ______________________ (7)

Stuttering 34 Homework

Name ______________________ Date due ______________

Read "Speech Class." Jorge is confused about his speech tools. Should Jorge always have to use them? What should he do? ______________________________

____

____

Parent signature ______________________ (8)

Stuttering 34 Homework

Name ______________________ Date due ______________

Read "The Kids on the Block." Brandon is getting teased a lot and needs some help. What are three things that Brandon can do?

1. ______________________________

2. ______________________________

3. ______________________________

Parent signature ______________________ (9)

Stuttering 34 Homework

Name ______________________ Date due ______________

On a separate piece of paper, write your own Dear Abby letter and show it to your parents. We will discuss your letter in class.

Parent signature ______________________ (10)

35

Do You Read Me?

Purpose

- To encourage students to take responsibility for their stuttering by providing them with the opportunity to discuss stuttering with others
- To educate teachers about stuttering

Materials

About My Stuttering: Sample Letter handout
About My Stuttering blank handout
The Child Who Stutters: Notes to the Teacher handout (Appendix B)
Pencils
Homework

Directions

Adults who stutter commonly attribute part of the unhappiness they felt in school to the fact that teachers did not understand their speech problem. It is vitally important to educate teachers about stuttering and the impact that it may have on a student's school experience. Begin by explaining:

> Today you are going to write a letter to a teacher to tell him or her about stuttering. Not everybody understands what stuttering is and why you talk the way that you do. Your teachers want to help you, but they often do not know the best way. Let's write a letter that tells a teacher about your stuttering and how he or she can help you and respond to your stuttering.

You may pass out the About My Stuttering: Sample Letter if you feel this would be helpful. This sample letter is included to provide students with an idea of what a letter about stuttering might look like. If desired, students may use the Letter About My Stuttering blank handout to write their stuttering letters. This form simply lends the letter a touch of formality, which students often appreciate.

Students are then asked to think of a few aspects of their stuttering that they want to share with their teachers. Some students will easily engage in the activity, whereas other students will express shock, fear, and even anger at such an assignment. Discuss the topic by saying, "Let's think of three things we can tell our teachers about stuttering." If students easily list three ideas, then you may suggest, "Wow, that was easy for you, let's think of two more." If students are significantly fearful of this activity, explain that they do not have to send the letters, only write them.

Within their letters some students have written statements such as, "Please give me the time I need to speak," "I wanted to tell you that I am a stutterer," and "My speech teacher and I are working on my speech." As a result of this activity, you are often able to identify and target difficulties that individual students face. One student wrote that he wanted his teacher to skip over him when he stuttered in class. During a discussion about this letter, the student explained that sometimes other children laugh at him when he speaks and that his teacher usually attempts to finish his sentences. The student expressed a reluctance to speak in class. This issue was then addressed in therapy. Some students have written comments that reflect strong and appreciative relationships with their teacher. These comments have included, "Thank you for being so nice when I talk" and "I like being in your class."

After writing a letter, students may then attach a copy of the handout adapted from a Stuttering Foundation of America brochure titled *The Child Who Stutters: Notes to the Teacher* (Scott & Williams, 2005) located in Appendix B. It is a rich source of information for teachers on stuttering in general, speech therapy, and how best to handle working with children who stutter in a classroom situation.

Then ask the students to deliver the letters to their teachers. Once I know a letter has been delivered, I will seek out the teacher and let her know that it is helpful for her to acknowledge the letter by speaking to the student (privately) about stuttering. You might suggest the teacher say, "Thanks for telling me about your stuttering" or "Is there anything I can do to help you with stuttering in class?" Explain to teachers that even if they are uncomfortable bringing up stuttering with the child, it is important that they appear comfortable, so they send the message to the student that talking about stuttering with their teacher is safe and acceptable.

More Ideas

After writing letters to teachers, students may then write to other people in their lives, such as relatives, friends, neighbors, and coaches.

Encourage students to attach copies of any of their speech class work to their letters, such as Dear Abby letters, pictures they have drawn about stuttering, or completed stuttering interviews. You may then guide students in discussing this work with their teacher.

Homework

Homework Assignments 1 and 2 ask students to write letters to family members about their stuttering. After you discuss first drafts of these letters with students, ask them to write a final copy of the letters. Then students deliver them or mail them to the appropriate relatives. Homework Assignment 3 is best assigned to students after teachers have had time to read the letter they have received. Hopefully, the teachers have attempted to discuss the letters in a meaningful way with their students. In this way students will be able to report comments or questions made by their teachers.

About My Stuttering: Sample Letter

Dear Mrs. Jacobs

I am writing you today to let you know that sometimes when I speak I stutter. There are several things that I want you to know about my stuttering.

- Please call on me in class as much as any other student. I like to speak in class.
- Please do not try to finish my words or sentences when I am stuttering. This often makes me stutter more.
- Please give me the time I need to talk.
- Please do not give me speaking advice. My speech teacher and I are working on my stuttering.

If you have any questions to ask me about stuttering, please do so. It is good to talk about stuttering. You may also ask my speech teacher, Ms. Lingren, about stuttering.

Sincerely,

David Barry

About My Stuttering

Dear ________________________________

Stuttering 35 Homework

Name ______________________ Date due ______________

On a separate piece of paper, write a letter to your grandparents or another relative telling them at least three things about your stuttering. Although your relatives probably know that you stutter, they may not know how you feel about stuttering. In your letter you may want to tell them how it feels to stutter, what you are working on in speech class, and how they can best respond to your stuttering.

Parent signature ______________________

(1)

Stuttering 35 Homework

Name ______________________ Date due ______________

Choose a friend to write to about stuttering. On a separate piece of paper, write the friend a letter that includes at least one paragraph about your stuttering.

Parent signature ______________________

(2)

Stuttering 35 Homework

Name ______________________ Date due ______________

How did you feel after giving your teacher the letter about stuttering? Do you think it helped? Explain. ______________________

____

____

____

____

____

____

____

Parent signature ______________________

(3)

36
Big News

Purpose

- To provide students with a way to advertise (let people know about) their stuttering
- To enable students to educate others about stuttering

Materials

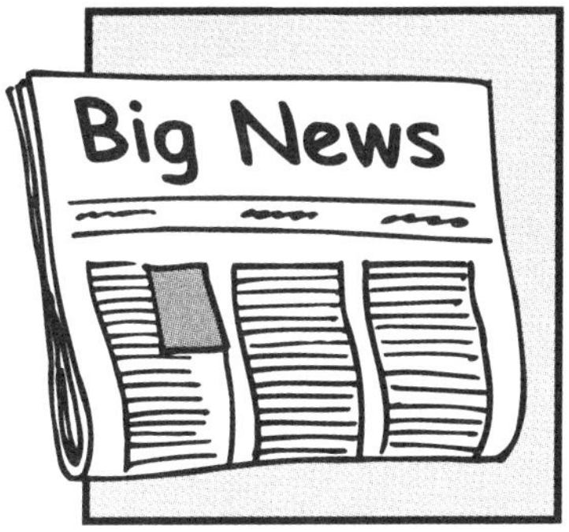

Sample stuttering newsletter (2 pages)
Materials for making a newsletter (pencils and paper or computer and printer)

Directions

Note: Planning and completing a newsletter will take several sessions. It is helpful if students can refer to their folders of completed speech class work to use in their newsletters.

By being open about stuttering, children learn ways to reduce their shame and feel comfortable with the way they speak. Begin this activity by explaining the concept of a newsletter:

> Newsletters help groups such as soccer teams, student councils, and chess clubs inform their members and their fans about upcoming events and how the club is doing. What kinds of things do you think a basketball team's newsletter might discuss?

Students typically begin listing ideas for sports newsletters, such as reports on recent games, dates of upcoming games, player biographies, and health and fitness articles. If your students are interested in music or dance, ask them what type of newsletter a music club or dance troupe might produce.

After students have a good idea what the purpose of a newsletter is, pass out copies of the sample stuttering newsletter and discuss it with your students. In this example three students decided that their first newsletter should include 10 pieces of advice for speaking with a stutterer, an educational stuttering quiz, some stories written in speech class, and 2 short articles that describe stuttering and speech class. Other newsletters have been much simpler and have contained one or two items. One group of students created a 6-page newsletter that included stories and poems about stuttering, facts about stuttering, Dear Abby Letters, student drawings depicting their stuttering, stuttering interviews with teachers, a few short articles defining stuttering and describing the purpose of speech class, and a question and answer section about stuttering.

Encourage and guide your students while working through topics and articles. You may inquire:

> Now that we have seen a newsletter about stuttering, what would you like to have in your stuttering newsletter? Is there a teacher or a principal you would like to interview about stuttering? I bet many students would like to read such an interview. What have you done in speech class that we could use in our newsletter? What are your ideas?

This activity may be as simple or as involved as you make it. I usually proceed by having students write their newsletter articles by hand and then typing and formatting the newsletter myself on a computer, using a program such as Microsoft Publisher. Teaching students how to format a newsletter could require several sessions and take too much time. You and your students *can* produce the newsletter by hand. When doing so, remind your students to write neatly and to "press hard when writing" so that their pencil or pen marks are clearly recognizable by a photocopy machine. After creating a newsletter, have students pass out copies to classmates, friends, and teachers. They may also be posted on bulletin boards in the school.

Homework

You will want to assign homework that leads to completing a stuttering newsletter. For example, if students decide that the newsletter will contain drawings of their stuttering, assign homework from Draw a Picture of How You Talk–Activity 29. If students want to include facts about stuttering in their newsletter, you may wish to write your own homework assignment, such as, "Review the facts about stuttering from your Stuttering Facts handout (see Activity 24) and choose three to include in the newsletter." Provide students with copies of the Stuttering Facts handout if they do not already have it.

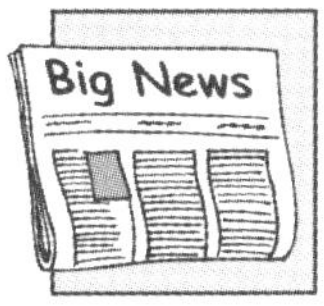

The PS 222 Stuttering Newsletter

A Speech Class Publication

Volume 1, Issue 1

Our First Stuttering Newsletter Is Here!

How To Speak with Children Who Stutter

10 Pieces of Advice

BY JAMIE GARDENER, STEVEN GARCIA, AND MICHELLE HUI

1. Please don't finish our sentences for us.

2. Please listen to what we are saying not how we are saying it.

3. Please don't give us advice like, "Just take your time" and "Try to relax." That is why we have a speech teacher!

4. Please be patient when speaking with us. Stuttering means that we need extra time to talk.

5. Please don't look away from us when we stutter. Try to make eye contact.

6. It is okay to ask questions about stuttering. We will do our best to answer them.

7. Teachers: Please don't let children tease us about stuttering.

8. Teachers: Please call on me at anytime to speak in class (Michelle and Steven).

9. Teachers: Please call on me only when my hand is raised (Jamie).

10. Teachers and students: Thanks for listening!

In this issue

Newsletter Staff

Jamie Gardener: Grade 5
Steven Garcia: Grade 3
Michelle Hui: Grade 4
Mr. Peter Reitzes: Speech Teacher

What Is Stuttering?

There are some children and adults who get "stuck" when they talk. This is called stuttering. Some children call it "bumpy" or "sticky" speech because their words do not come out smoothly. One child refers to stuttering as "mouth traffic" because sometimes she feels like her mouth is stuck in traffic.

Why Do Children Go to Speech Class?

1. To learn how to talk smoothly. (Michelle)

2. To talk about stuttering. (Jamie)

3. To have fun! (Steven)

PS 222
5555 10th Avenue
Brooklyn, NY 11330
(718) 555-8888
Fax: (718) 555-7777

Principal:
Debbie Murphy

Assistant Principal:
Mark Retzinger

Assistant Principal:
Wanda Heller

Take the Stuttering Quiz

BY JAMIE GARDENER

1. How many people stutter in the United States?
   a) 300
   b) 1,000
   c) 3 million

2. For every 4 boys who stutter, there is/are
   a) 1 girl who stutters.
   b) 4 girls who stutter.
   c) 10 girls who stutter.

3. Which two famous people listed below stutter?
   a) James Earl Jones (actor who played Darth Vader)
   b) Michael Jordan (basketball player)
   c) Marilyn Monroe (actress)

4. There are people who stutter in every country in the world.
   TRUE or FALSE

5. People who stutter are as smart as anyone else.
   TRUE or FALSE

6. You can "catch" stuttering like you catch a cold.
   TRUE or FALSE

7. Most people begin stuttering between the ages of
   a) 6 months and 1 year.
   b) 2 years and 8 years.
   c) 8 years and 12 years.

The Grocery Store

BY MICHELLE HUI

I am almost 10 years old. When I was younger, I always hated going to the grocery store because my father always wanted me to help him find things. He would say things to me like, "Michelle, I can't find the potato chips that are on sale; please go ask the manager where the potato chips are." I would rather walk around the store than ask someone a question. It seemed that whatever word I had to say, I would stutter on it. If my father asked me to go find the cereal, I knew I would stutter when saying the word "cereal."

I told my speech teacher about my fear of asking questions at the grocery store. So Mr. Reitzes took me, Steven, and Jamie to the grocery store, and we practiced asking questions. Mr. Reitzes asked first and when he said "potato chips," he stuttered so hard that it came out "pppppp-potato chips." Mr. Reitzes showed me that it is okay to stutter and ask questions. Now when I go to the grocery store, I ask questions when I need to find something.

Teasing Needs To Go!

BY STEVEN GARCIA

There are some children who tease me at school. They say things that are mean. They say, "You ta-ta-ta-ta-talk li-li-like a du-du-du-dummy." In speech class we talk about teasing a lot. My speech teacher wanted to invite one of the teasers to speech class to show him that stuttering is cool. I was scared of this but said okay. We invited a boy from my class who was teasing me. We taught him a lot about stuttering and taught him a few "speech tools" that we use to talk more easily. The boy thought speech class was really fun and he wants to come back. Mr. Reitzes said that if he stopped teasing me for one week he could visit speech again!

Answers to Quiz

1. c; 2. a; 3. a and c; 4. TRUE;
5. TRUE; 6. FALSE; 7. b

Stuttering 36 Homework

Name ______________________ Date due ____________

An adult woman who stutters, Lucy Reed, wrote a one-sentence story about stuttering. She wrote: "If I could think of *one* thing I wish someone had told me when I was in school, it would be, 'It's okay to stutter.' "

In our stuttering newsletter, it would be cool to have several very short stories by children who stutter. We could title this section "One Thing I Want To Tell You About Stuttering." Think of one thing that is very important to you that you want other people to know about stuttering. Write it below.

____

____

____

Why is this important to you? ______________________

____

____

____

Parent signature ______________________ (1)

Stuttering 36 Homework

Name ______________________ Date due ____________

Think of three things that we could put in the stuttering newsletter. Write them below.

1. ____

____

2. ____

____

3. ____

____

Parent signature ______________________ (2)

37
Post It

Purpose

- To enable students to advertise their stuttering
- To educate teachers, school staff, and peers about stuttering

Materials

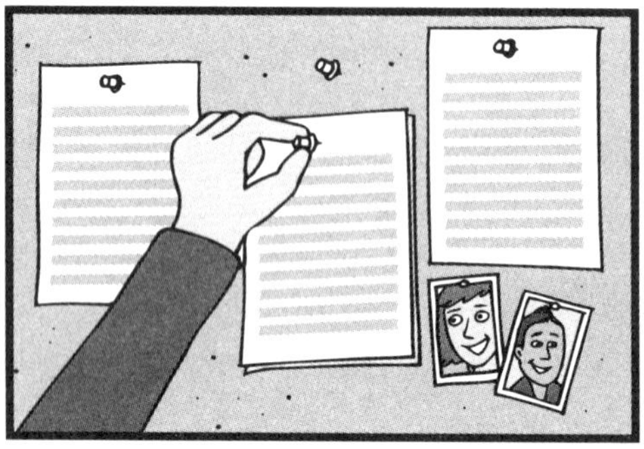

Copies of previously completed handouts (i.e., Stuttering Stories and Poems [in You Feel That Way Too–Activity 31], Stuttering Interviews, and Dear Abby letters)

Directions

Making a stuttering bulletin board offers children a way to reduce their shame and normalize who they are and how they speak. Teachers and students learn that stuttering is a topic that is open for discussion. This is an activity best undertaken after students have completed several of the other lessons in the Uncovering Feelings section.

Begin this activity by securing a bulletin board or wall space in your school. If you are a clinician in private practice, contact your student's school and explain that you and your client will be working on several projects about stuttering, such as a newsletter and stories about stuttering, to be posted for display. Schools take pride in their bulletin boards and should be open to your interest in helping your student "advertise" her stuttering. You may offer to come to the school and inaugurate the bulletin board by discussing stuttering with your client's class or with a group of teachers for staff development.

Explain to the students:

> We are going to make a stuttering bulletin board to help other students and teachers better understand stuttering. This will also help you show others that stuttering is interesting and nothing to be ashamed of. What would you like to share about stuttering? What have we done in speech class that we can post on our bulletin board?

Some students may initially be embarrassed or fearful of making a bulletin board that highlights their stuttering. Most students will begin sharing your enthusiasm if this activity is presented as an honor and not as a duty.

One year students wanted to include Stutter Punch on their bulletin board (Stutter Punch is used to practice stretch-outs and bounce-outs. See Stretching–Activity 9). We decided to play Stutter Punch while having a teacher photograph the group. Students posted the photographs on their bulletin board and wrote captions describing what they are doing in the picture. One caption read, "In this picture I am practicing holding a stutter with my stutter punch before I stretch out of it."

After collecting the material to be displayed on the bulletin board, you will want to include students in constructing the bulletin board. This provides them with an opportunity to take ownership and pride in their work. Students often cannot wait to show their friends the completed bulletin board. I often ask students if they would like to invite a friend to help construct the bulletin board—this adds another layer of acceptance and fun to the project. When guests attend speech class, take the group on a "field trip" to show them the bulletin board. I try to have the bulletin board ready for parent–teacher conference night so that parents can see first hand that being open about stuttering is a fundamental aspect of stuttering management.

More Ideas

Suggest that students conduct several stuttering interviews and have them explain to the teachers, students, and staff members involved that these "special" interviews will be published on the school bulletin board.

A Collection of Successes. Typically, bulletin boards are periodically changed. When students take down the stuttering bulletin board, use the materials to start a stuttering scrapbook. A scrapbook is different from a student's folder because it will include highlights from each child within a group, rather than just one child's work. As therapy continues add completed projects to the scrapbook.

Homework

Just as with the Big News activity, you will want to assign homework that leads to completing this activity. The two homework assignments that follow ask students to read stories about stuttering and then write their own stories for inclusion on the bulletin board. You may also revisit homework assignments from previously covered activities. For example, assign homework that asks students to draw pictures of stuttering (see Draw a Picture of How You Talk–Activity 29), respond to discussion questions about stuttering (see Questions and Answers–Activity 33), and write responses to Dear Abby letters (see Dear Abby–Activity 34). Display completed homework on the bulletin board.

Stuttering 37 Homework

Name ______________________ Date due ______________

Directions: Read the following story. On the stuttering bulletin board, we will have an area titled "Feeling Better." In this area we will put stories about things that have happened to us that made us feel better about stuttering. On a separate piece of paper, write your story.

Feeling Better

by Lucy Reed

The worst thing I remember about school is having to read aloud. It was something I dreaded every day. My words would get so stuck that I would hold my breath and feel like I was going to faint. I always felt like the whole class was looking at me. One day the teacher asked me to read the word *work.* I still remember the word. I just knew that I was going to get stuck on it if I tried to say it, so I said I didn't know the word. The teacher knew I really knew the word, and I felt bad for telling her I didn't know it when I really did. That day on the way to lunch she stopped me and kindly asked me if I really didn't know the word or if I said I didn't know it because I couldn't say it. I told her I knew it, but I couldn't say it. I felt a lot better after that.

Parent signature ______________________ (1)

Stuttering 37 Homework

Name ______________________ Date due ______________

Directions: Read the following story. Then for the stuttering bulletin board, write a story titled "What I Want To Tell Other Children Who Stutter." Use a separate piece of paper to write this story.

Nobody Told Me

by Lucy Reed

When I was in school, a lot of the other girls wanted to be friends with me. I thought it was weird that anybody would want to be friends with me because I stuttered. I thought that I didn't deserve to have friends because I stuttered. Now that I am grown up, I realize that friends like you because of the kind of person you are, not because of how you talk. I wish someone had told me that when I was in school.

Parent signature ______________________ (2)

38

Talking About Feelings and Emotions

Purpose

- To help students express how they feel about stuttering
- To provide students with vocabulary to describe their feelings

Materials

Game (i.e., Candyland, checkers, Uno)
Feelings Word List handout
Homework

Directions

The Feelings Word List contains vocabulary words that will help students discuss and express how they feel about stuttering. One way to facilitate this activity is to use a board game such as Candyland or Chutes and Ladders (for younger students) or checkers or Uno (for older students). Explain (example below uses Uno):

> Before you take a turn with Uno, you will be given a vocabulary word. You need to use the word in a complete sentence. After using the word in a sentence, you then get to take your Uno turn. The first word I will choose is *angry.* I get angry when I am late for a movie. Now you will each get a turn to use the word angry in a sentence.

As shown above, give an example of the first vocabulary word in a complete sentence before students take their turns. Each child uses the assigned word before you introduce the next word. Notice how I did not mention stuttering in the sentence using angry. If you relate every word to stuttering, students will often find the game stale. During this activity it is best to let students be the ones to bring stuttering into the discussion. After students understand the activity, you may wish to give sentence examples only for particularly challenging vocabulary.

You may want to gently influence this activity by giving examples of sentences such as, "I am *scared* to speak in front of large crowds," "I want to be *fearless* in facing my problems," or "It *hurts* when people tease me."

For some students this is an ideal time to invite speech class guests or friends. While working with a student named James who showed almost no awareness of his stuttering, I always included a friend or classmate in the session. During one session James and his guest used their vocabulary words to discuss feelings such as being angry with a sibling or being tired of doing homework. When given the word *crazy,* James' guest said in a serious manner, "James' bu-bu-bu-bu-bu is a crazy way to talk." James' classmate did not say this in a mean or teasing manner but in a calm and factual way. James pointed to his throat and said, "It's not crazy—it's painful in my throat when I talk like that." On his next turn James was given the vocabulary word *annoying* and used it to say that he found his "bu-bu-bu" to be annoying. This was the first time during therapy that James was able to discuss his stuttering in an open and reflective way. Bringing a guest to speech class helped James to talk openly about his stuttering.

The Feelings Word List is only a suggestion of words you may use to encourage students to discuss how they feel. You may always choose your own words or change the suffixes of the words on the provided list (i.e., changing *annoyed* to *annoying*).

Do not be alarmed if students do not mention their stuttering during this activity. You are providing them the opportunity to talk openly about feelings with you. This impresses upon them that they are allowed to trust you with their problems. You are also providing students with valuable vocabulary that they may use later in therapy to describe their stuttering. Even if students do not talk directly about stuttering, you are providing them with a foundation for success.

More Ideas

For older students you may pass out the word list and have students choose their own words. You may or may not need to provide sample sentences.

Make up a "word wall" (a popular vocabulary-building instrument in many schools) in which words are written on large note cards and displayed for reference on classroom or office walls. When using a word wall for the activity above, students are encouraged to go to the wall before each turn to choose a vocabulary word. If the word wall uses Velcro or pockets to hold the words, the student may return with the word card itself. If the word cards are not removable, the student announces the word he would like to use.

Homework

Homework Assignments 1 through 4 contain short stories. These stories feature a few of the vocabulary words included in this activity and will show students how these words may be used to describe stuttering.

You may wish to create your own homework assignments that focus on vocabulary words that you feel would benefit your students. Also, if students never bring up the topic of speaking or stuttering during a therapy session, I might assign homework from this activity and say, "I'd like at least two of the sentences you write tonight to be about stuttering (or speaking)."

Feelings Word List

- Ache
- Admire
- Afraid
- Angry
- Annoyed
- Anxious
- Ashamed
- Attentive
- Awkward
- Bad mood
- Believe
- Bold
- Bored
- Brave
- Calm
- Carefree
- Caring
- Cautious
- Cheerful
- Clever
- Comfortable
- Concerned
- Confident
- Confused
- Cooperative
- Cranky
- Crazy
- Cry
- Daring
- Decided
- Delighted
- Desire
- Despise
- Determined
- Discouraged
- Disgusted
- Dissatisfied
- Doubtful
- Dream
- Eager
- Embarrassed
- Excited
- Explosive
- Exposed
- Fear
- Fearless
- Fed up
- Frustrated
- Furious
- Graceful
- Grouchy
- Guarded
- Guilty
- Happy
- Hate
- Hesitant
- Hope
- Hopeless
- Horrible
- Hurt
- Impatient
- Important
- Insecure
- Inspired
- Jealous
- Kind
- Know
- Laugh
- Love
- Mad
- Make a mistake
- Mean
- Misery
- Moody
- Motivated
- Mysterious
- Nervous
- Offended
- Outgoing
- Panicky
- Patient
- Peaceful
- Please
- Prefer
- Proud
- Relaxed
- Remember
- Resourceful
- Sad
- Safe
- Scared
- Shocked
- Shy
- Sick
- Skilled
- Smart
- Smile
- Spectacular
- Strong
- Supportive
- Surprised
- Sympathetic
- Tense
- Terrified
- Thankful
- Thoughtful
- Tired
- Trapped
- Ugly
- Understand
- Unkind
- Unpredictable
- Wish
- Worried

Stuttering 38 Homework

Name ______________________ Date due ______________

Directions: Read the following story. In Evan's story, the word *embarrassed* is in bold. Think about a time that you have been embarrassed. On a separate sheet of paper, write a story about it.

My Vacation in Florida

by Evan Posada

I went to Florida when I was 5 years old for vacation. We were in a park, and my mother was very thirsty. I saw a man selling drinks and ice cream in a cart. I kept trying to tell my mom that I saw someone selling water, but I was stuttering and couldn't get the words out. I was so **embarrassed** because a few people overheard me stuttering.

Parent signature ______________________ (1)

Stuttering 38 Homework

Name ______________________ Date due ______________

Directions: Read the following story. In Hali's story the word *knew* is in bold. Think of a time that you just knew you were going to stutter. On a separate sheet of paper, write a story about it.

New Year's Eve

by Hali Lapinski

On New Year's Eve I was at a party at my cousin's house. We were allowed to stay up late to watch TV and see the celebration going on in New York City. Everyone was eating food, and we were all playing games in the kitchen. I walked into the TV room, and I saw on the screen that it was almost the new year. Only 10 seconds to go! So I ran into the kitchen to tell everyone. But I just **knew** I wasn't going to be able to say it. And then it happened. As I opened my mouth to speak, nothing came out. Later that night my mom said, "How could we have all missed the countdown to New Year's?" I felt bad because I had not forgotten, but just couldn't say it.

Parent signature ______________________ (2)

Stuttering 38 Homework

Name ______________________ Date due ______________

Directions: Read the following story. a. Brett's story describes Quincy as being *brave* and *free.* Think about a time that you felt brave. Using a separate sheet of paper, write a story about it. b. Think about a time that you felt free. Using a separate sheet of paper, write a story about it.

The Boy Who Was Free

by Brett Greene

When I was in the third grade, there was a blond boy in my class named Quincy. He always raised his hand in class and repeated sounds loudly and rapidly. His hand would shoot up, and he would say, "I-I-I-I-I know the answer." I remember thinking quietly to myself: "He's like me." I had never heard anyone else stutter. I remember thinking how **brave** he was because I would never raise my hand. I would never let my classmates hear me stutter. I remember thinking, "He is **free** and I am not." Even in the third grade, I knew in my heart that it was better to just stutter, but I was too scared to show it.

Parent signature ______________________ (3)

Stuttering 38 Homework

Name ______________________ Date due ______________

Directions: Read the following story. In her story Brett is *afraid* to go to class because she might stutter while reading. Think about a time you have been afraid to go somewhere or do something because you might stutter. On a separate sheet of paper, write a story about it.

Snickers in the Background

by Brett Greene

When I was in the sixth grade, my class received a subscription to the daily newspaper. My teacher made us go around the room and read aloud every day. Every morning I felt sick and scared to read. I didn't want to be **afraid** to go to class, but I was. I couldn't hide. I *had* to read. I was a popular girl in class, and I desperately wanted to hide my stuttering, but it was impossible. I was trapped. I remember blocking as I read, afraid to lift my head as I heard snickers in the background. No one ever teased me to my face, but I remember people snickering and laughing as I struggled through my readings.

Parent signature ______________________ (4)

Stuttering (38) Homework

Name ______________________ Date due ____________

Write complete sentences using the following words.

Example: thankful—I am thankful that so many people love me for who I am.

1. worry ____

2. excited ____

3. terrified ____

4. wish ____

5. comfortable ____

Parent signature ______________________

(5)

Stuttering (38) Homework

Name ______________________ Date due ____________

Write complete sentences using the following words.

Example: shy—I am shy when it is my turn to talk.

1. hope ____

2. frustrated ____

3. ashamed ____

4. safe ____

5. admire ____

Parent signature ______________________

(6)

Stuttering 38 Homework

Name ______________________ Date due ____________

Write complete sentences using the following words.
Example: safe—I feel safe when I am with my parents.

1. shy ______________________

2. confident ______________________

3. nervous ______________________

4. horrible ______________________

5. calm ______________________

Parent signature ______________________ (7)

Stuttering 38 Homework

Name ______________________ Date due ____________

Take home the Feelings Word List and look over the vocabulary words. Choose five words that you want to use to describe your stuttering. Write five sentences below using those words.

1. ______________________

2. ______________________

3. ______________________

4. ______________________

5. ______________________

Parent signature ______________________ (8)

39
Below the Surface

Purpose

- To identify and express covert and overt aspects of stuttering
- To assess student growth and progress

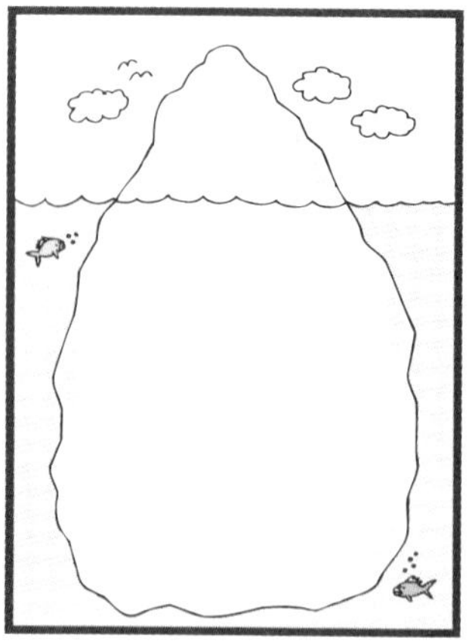

Materials

Stuttering Iceberg handout
Sample Stuttering Iceberg handout
Pencils (or pens or markers)
Homework

Directions

Stuttering has often been compared to an iceberg in which the most dangerous part of the problem lies below the waterline where it cannot be seen. It is commonly noted that although audible (and visible) stuttering behaviors found above the surface are certainly an important aspect of the disorder, often the most debilitating parts of stuttering are the feelings, emotions, and unproductive behaviors found and hidden below the surface. Lying below the surface are feelings of fear; shame; guilt; and avoidance behaviors, such as using word substitutions and avoiding speaking opportunities. Russ Hicks, a veteran of the stuttering self-help movement, has written about the therapeutic ramifications of the stuttering iceberg analogy. He wrote:

> What you are doing is teaching people to work *below* that waterline far beyond where the old fluency-shaping therapies go. It's not hard to produce fluent speech under controlled conditions, but the hard part is working on those emotions that form the bulk of the stuttering iceberg far beneath the waterline. . . . Yes, that's where the real progress will surely be made. (2002, para. 3)

Sheehan (1970) suggested that stutterers draw their own iceberg picture or diagram. This is done to detail a student's overt (audible) and covert (inaudible) stuttering behaviors. Begin the activity by passing out the Stuttering Iceberg handout. Explain:

> Stuttering is a lot like an iceberg. An iceberg is big enough to sink a great ship like the Titanic, but most of the iceberg is kept hidden away under water where people can't see it—that is the dangerous part. A ship might pass an iceberg and see only a little piece of ice and snow sticking out of the water, but the ship should be careful because of what is below the surface where you can't see it. Today you are going to draw a picture of your stuttering iceberg. Use words, short sentences, and even drawings to show your stuttering. Re-

member, above the waterline are the things people can see and hear; below the waterline are the things they can't hear or see.

Go over the Sample Stuttering Iceberg handout with students so they can visualize what is expected of them. You may need to help some get students started. If so, direct them to the area above the waterline and suggest that each student write a generic phrase such as, "Sometimes my words get stuck" or "I repeat words." Then direct students to the area below the waterline and ask, "How do you hide your stuttering from others? Who can suggest something to write that shows how you hide stuttering?" Typically students may make comments such as, "I don't talk in class" or "I start my sentences over again."

Encourage students to work independently by turning away and becoming involved in some task such as paperwork or reading. Students may be embarrassed or feel that they are completing the assignment the wrong way if you watch closely.

After completing their drawings, discuss the completed Stuttering Iceberg assignments. Talk about the covert feelings and beliefs as well as the overt behaviors. An example of what one student wrote below the waterline is, "My mother took me out of after school [activities] because other children were teasing me. She wouldn't let me stay."

When the student read the previous sentence aloud, she expressed shame with her stuttering, her inability to manage the teasing, and with being taken out of an activity that she enjoyed. After discussing the situation, the student came up with a way the situation might have been handled differently. She gave permission for me to contact her mother and discuss other ways she might help manage the after-school teasing. I arranged to meet with the student's mother, who reported that she did not want to talk to the school about her daughter's teasing because she did not believe the school would respond favorably. I let the mother know that it is the school's responsibility to provide a productive learning environment for all children. And to do so we often need input from parents. I also discussed the importance of teaching our children that teasing and bullying behaviors are not acceptable.

As with many activities in this book, you may use the Below the Surface activity as ongoing assessment. At an appropriate time in therapy, ask students to complete a second Stuttering Iceberg handout that will help you determine student progress. In this type of ongoing assessment, see if students have become more adept at describing their stuttering and whether they are beginning to change how they feel about stuttering.

Homework

The first homework assignment is most suitable for mature students.

Stuttering Iceberg

Name ______________________________ Date ____________________

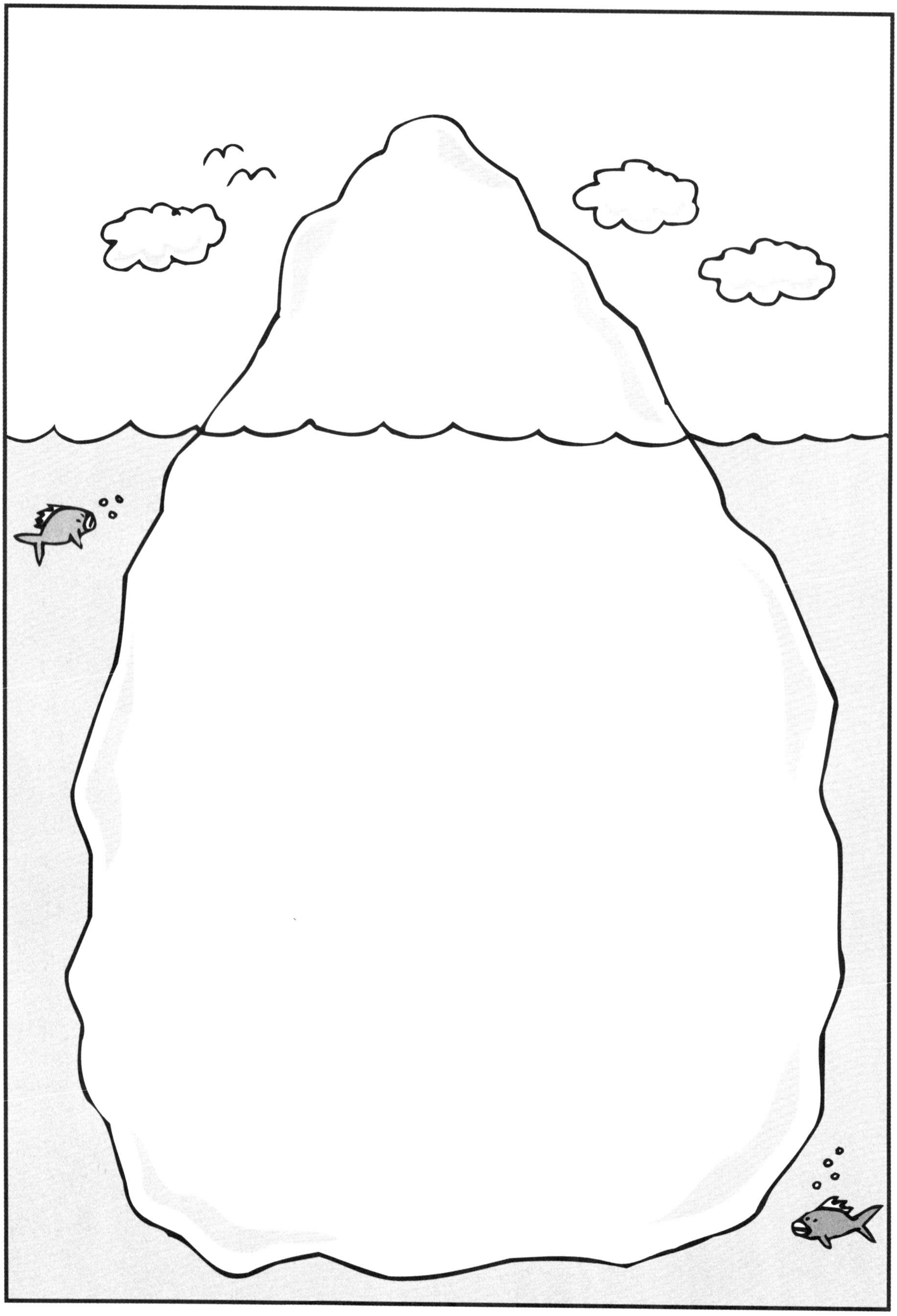

Sample Stuttering Iceberg

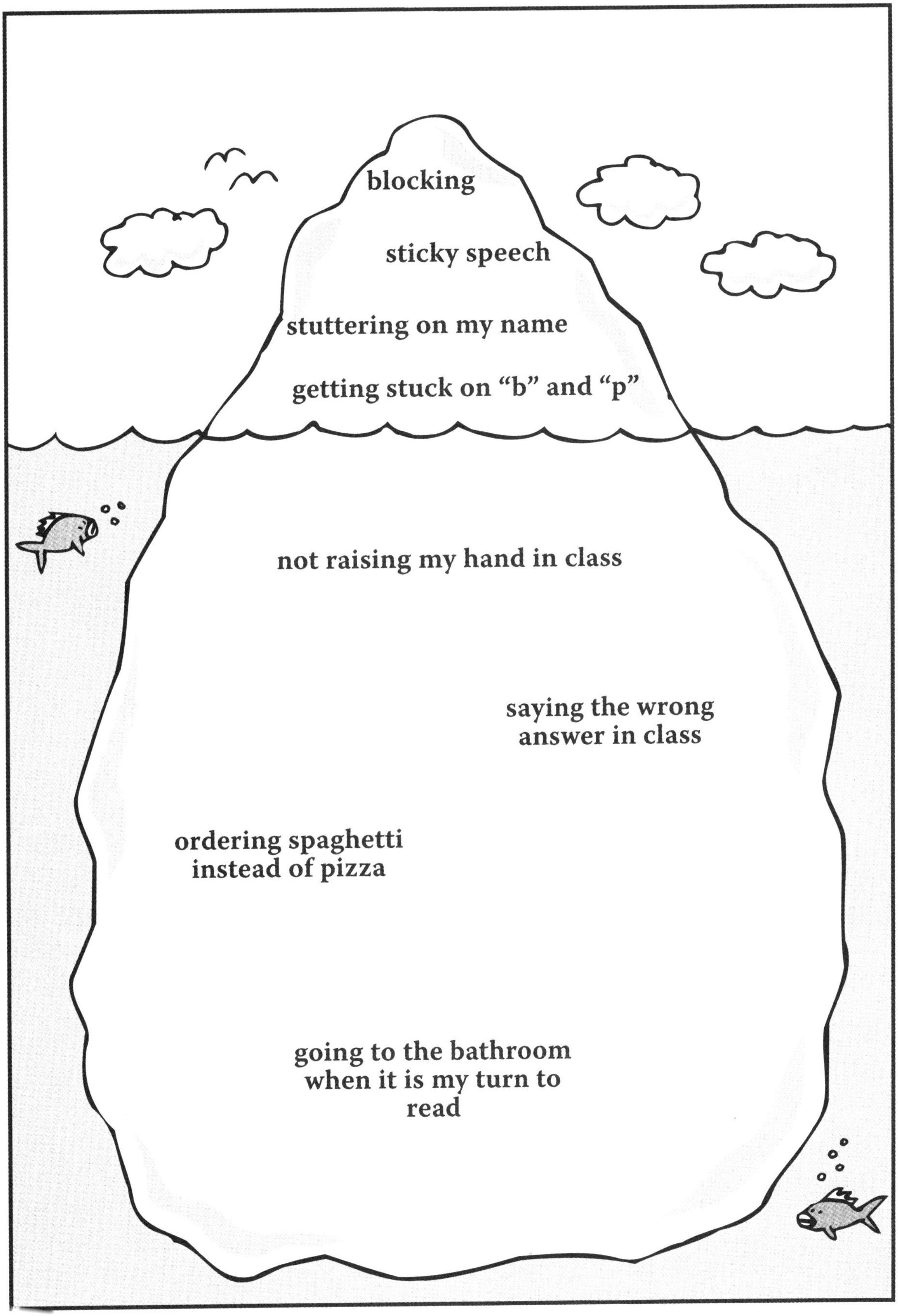

Stuttering (39) Homework

Name ______________________ Date due ______________

Take home your completed Stuttering Iceberg and show it to your parents or other adult relatives. Explain to them that stuttering is like an iceberg: Some stuttering can be seen and heard, and other stuttering is below the water and is hidden.

Think of one thing on the bottom part of your iceberg (below the water) that you wish was not there. When you find it, circle it and write a few sentences explaining why you don't like it there. ______________________

Parent signature ______________________ (1)

Stuttering (39) Homework

Name ______________________ Date due ______________

Take home your completed Stuttering Iceberg and review it. Which part of stuttering is harder for you to deal with—the part above the waterline or the part below the waterline? Explain your answer. ______________________

Parent signature ______________________ (2)

Targeting Language and Stuttering Goals

Although it is ideal for children who stutter to work together in a group, this is not always possible. Many clinicians work with few stutterers, are saddled with high caseloads, and must contend with the scheduling concerns of teachers. It is common practice for school clinicians to provide therapy to stutterers within groups that contain children with other speech and language difficulties (Manning, 2000; Williams & Dugan, 2002; Yaruss, 2002).

The activities in this section were included to enable clinicians to concurrently meet the needs of children who stutter and children with language difficulties. Many children who stutter also face co-existing speech and language difficulties. For these children, the activities in this section can target both stuttering goals and language goals.

Some of the language goals in this section include understanding and expressing figurative language, following and expressing directions, building vocabulary within categories, speaking with appropriate vocal inflection, speaking in complete sentences, turn-taking, initiating and maintaining eye contact, speaking with appropriate vocal intensity, and expanding vocabulary and categorization skills. The language goals listed within specific activities should not be considered an exhaustive list but are merely suggestions to help you consider ways to meet language needs. At the end of the activities, homework is included for children who stutter. Create your own homework assignments to specifically target the language needs of students.

As mentioned earlier in this book, it is important to recognize that the propensity for stuttering increases as the length and linguistic complexity of utterances increase. Zackheim and Conture (2003) found that when a child speaks above her mean length of utterance, the child is more likely to stutter. As you increase the expressive language demands placed upon students, you are creating the potential for increased stuttering. For example, if students are working on expressing two-level verbal directions, this can trigger more stuttering than expressing one-level directions.

At times you will want to challenge students who stutter by increasing the language demands placed upon them. This is wise when done appropriately and in ways that do not overly stress students. Students need to learn how to use their speech tools and control their stuttering in difficult and stressful situations. By carefully and thoughtfully increasing the linguistic difficulties of tasks, you are offering students a challenging, yet controlled, situation to practice their tools.

At other times you may wish to reduce the language demands placed upon students to reduce the potential for stuttering and to encourage easier use of speech tools. Students facing language formulation difficulties may be unable to focus on using speech tools. Although you want to challenge students in therapy, you also want to offer them frequent opportunities for success.

Conduct therapy that includes a combined group of students in a casual and open way. For example, explain to the group:

> Some of the students here are working on their speech because they stutter. Stuttering means they get stuck on their words when they talk. For example, children who stutter may say "ba-ba-ba-ball" or "sssssssports." Other students are here because they need help with things like following directions, using new words, asking questions, speaking with louder voices, or speaking in complete sentences. We will be working together on fun lessons to help us all meet our goals.

At any time during the sessions, you or students who stutter may explain speech tools and other aspects of stuttering therapy to the group. For those students who stutter and may be embarrassed in a combined group, the therapy room offers a safe environment to practice being open about stuttering. And all children, not just children who stutter, will occasionally come to speech class upset about something that happened at home or in school. When appropriate, discuss these situations with the entire group. For example, if a student is upset because someone was teasing her on the playground, ask her to share what happened. Students who stutter and those who do not may both have stories to tell about being teased or bullied. Engage students in problem solving these situations. Show students, through example, that stuttering will be discussed calmly and respectfully.

The activities in this section are beneficial for students who stutter who also need to work on concomitant language goals. Keep in mind that at times you will need to focus primarily on a child's stuttering. For example, when a student comes to speech class and is having a difficult day managing his stuttering, it is not the time to focus on increasing his language skills. This would be the time to reduce the language demands placed upon the child and to focus on stuttering-related goals.

After completing an activity in this section, you may wish to assign homework from other sections of the book to focus on areas and goals that may need review. For example, if a student demonstrates little difficulty talking about stuttering but needs more speech tool practice, assign homework from the activities that focus on speech tools.

Note: Reproducible materials, such as homework and handouts, are located at the end of the description of how to facilitate an activity. However, reproducible materials that are used in more than one activity are included in the appendixes.

40
20 Questions

Purpose for Children Who Stutter

- To practice speech tools
- To practice being open about stuttering with others

Purpose for Language Students

- To practice asking questions using complete sentences
- To practice expressing descriptors, such as colors, shapes, and sizes
- To practice turn-taking
- To practice categorization skills

Materials

Questions handout
Using Speech Tools with 20 Questions handout
Large tote bag or shoebox
Items to hide (office supplies; food items; clothing items; and other objects, such as coins, books, a deck of cards, sunglasses, and deodorant)

Directions

Twenty Questions may be played for an entire session or for several minutes at the beginning or end of a session. Gather a box or a bag to conceal objects and place several of the objects in it. Then introduce the activity by saying:

> Today we are going to play a game that will help us ask and answer questions. Before we begin I want each of you to think of three times that you ask questions. For example, I ask questions when I go to a store and want to know the price of something. I may ask a store employee, "How much are your double A batteries?" When do you ask questions?

Have each student name three occasions when he asks questions. This helps the students understand the usefulness of this activity. Then begin the actual game by announcing:

> I have many things hidden in this box (bag), but I have chosen one thing for you to guess. Each student can ask one question about what is in the box. I will call on you when it is your turn. Sometimes I will help you by providing different questions to ask. For example, I may say to you, "Ask me, 'Do you eat it?' or ask me, 'What do you use it for'?" After you ask a question, I will answer it. Then you will get one guess at what is in the box. We will keep taking turns until someone correctly guesses the item.

Many students will be able to think of their own questions, but for those who cannot, you may pass out copies of the Questions handout, which provides students with some sample questions.

As the game continues, give each student an opportunity to play the role of the teacher. Often I will take an object out of the box and put it into a smaller box. Then I will hand this smaller box to the student playing the teacher. This is done so that the student playing the teacher does not see all of the hidden objects; he just sees the one object he needs for his turn.

Once students who stutter are comfortable with this activity, ask them to continue the game while using speech tools. (You will need to explain the reasons and purposes for using speech tools to children who do not stutter.) You may pass out copies of the Using Speech Tools with 20 Questions handout that shows students exactly when to use a speech tool. Instead of using the handout, you can assign pausing and model a question while using pausing, such as "What, do you use, the item, in the box, for?" You may also suggest that students bounce-out (or stretch-out) of the first word of each sentence or any words that they stutter on.

Although this activity is an excellent way to make working on speech tools enjoyable, it also may be used to target a wide range of language goals. For example, you may target categorization and vocabulary goals by hiding different objects within categories in a box. After guessing all of the items in the box, ask students, "How do these go together?" or "How are they the same?" During the next session you may choose to use different items to continue targeting categorization and vocabulary goals.

Many students demonstrate difficulty asking and answering questions, and this activity provides them with the opportunity to practice this skill. You may ask students to formulate their own questions or to use questions that you provide and model.

More Ideas

Try using noun picture cards instead of objects.

Play Headbanz, a commercially available game that is similar to 20 Questions and may be purchased for approximately $20.00 in many toy stores, educational stores, and catalogs. When playing Headbanz, each student is given a headband (like a visor) that has a place to hold a picture card. A student takes a card and puts it on the headband so that he cannot see it (the card is above his head). The student then has to ask questions to guess what is on the card.

In 20 Questions it is helpful for students who stutter and for students with language difficulties to be asked to repeat all of the "hints" or clues before guessing the item. If the object in the box is a pencil, the student may end up repeating the following:

"It is yellow. It is long and thin. And you write with it." This allows students to consider all hints before guessing.

Twenty Questions can also offer students an opportunity to practice taking notes. As clues or hints are given, each student is assigned the task of writing down the clues. Using the previous example, a student would write, "It is yellow. It is long and thin. You write with it." It is important that students write each hint after it is given. If a student asks, "What color is it?" and they are told "purple and green," all students should immediately write down this clue.

Questions

1. Where do you find it?
2. What do you use it for?
3. How big is it?
4. Is it alive?
5. What color is it?
6. Can you eat it?
7. What shape is it?
8. What is it made of?
9. What letter does it start with?
10. What does it rhyme with?

Using Speech Tools with 20 Questions

Questions Using Pausing

1. Where, do you, find it?
2. What, do you, use it for?
3. How, big, is it?
4. Is, it, alive?
5. What, color, is it?
6. Can, you, eat it?
7. What, shape, is it?
8. What, is it, made of?
9. What, letter, does it, start with?
10. What, does it, rhyme with?

Questions Using Stretching, Bouncing, or Voluntary Stuttering

1. Where do you find it?
2. What do you use it for?
3. How big is it?
4. Is it alive?
5. What color is it?
6. Can you eat it?
7. What shape is it?
8. What is it made of?
9. What letter does it start with?
10. What does it rhyme with?

41
Barrier Games

Purpose for Children Who Stutter

- To practice using speech tools in a challenging speaking situation
- To practice being open about stuttering with others

Purpose for Language Students

- To practice following directions
- To practice speaking in complete sentences
- To practice using appropriate vocal intensity
- To practice turn-taking

Materials

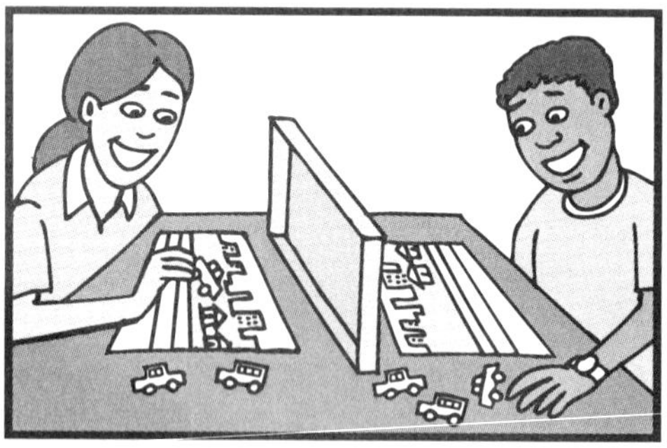

Barriers (such as cardboard dividers or the boxes for board games that can stand on edge)

Duplicate sets of magnetic games with common scenes and magnetic pieces

Directions

Choose magnetic board games with common themes, such as a neighborhood, a school classroom, a grocery store, a house, or an airport. Each game comes with many relevant magnetic pieces. An airport scene might come with different colored planes, helicopters, and mechanics.

Two students or teams sit across from one another at a table. Give each opponent an identical magnetic board with identical pieces. (A student seen individually for therapy will enjoy playing this game against you.) Place a barrier, such as a board game box, between the players so that they cannot see each other's boards. You may also use a barrier that is higher, such as a small chalkboard, so students cannot see each other's faces. Tall barriers emphasize the importance of using verbal, not visual, language. They are also challenging for those who stutter and for students with language difficulties because they require them to verbalize instructions without being able to use body language, such as pointing. Explain:

> I am going to give you some directions to follow. Each person has to follow the directions and put their pieces in the right places. The goal of this game is for each team to end with boards that look exactly the same. At the end of the game, we will remove the barrier and compare the two boards. If you follow the directions correctly, then each board will look the same.

Give students a direction to follow. For example, if using an airport game, you may say, "Put the red airplane to the left of the blue airplane." Some students require one-level directions, whereas other students may be able to follow two- and three-level directions with several modifiers. After students become accustomed to following your directions, explain:

> Each student will now have a turn to give directions to the group. It is very important that you give specific and exact directions. If you say, "Put the blue plane here," the other team won't know where to put the plane because they can't see your board, and they won't know what you mean. It is important that the person giving the directions also follow them so that the boards look the same at the end. Students take turns giving each other directions.

After playing one barrier game without using speech tools, play a second game asking students who stutter to use an assigned speech tool. You or your students may explain speech tools to students who do not stutter. Begin by giving directions while modeling the assigned speech tool. For example, if you have assigned pausing, you may say, "Put, the blue, car, on the, red bridge, next to, the red car."

Then give a few more examples using the chosen speech tool before allowing students to take turns giving each other directions. If students forget to use the speech tool, or use it in an incorrect manner, stop and review it.

More Ideas

Draw My Picture. This type of barrier game requires students to describe and draw simple pictures, such as a smiley face, a house, or a design such as a rectangle with a circle in the middle of it. Prepare these basic drawings ahead of time. Students will then take turns describing the picture to the other players, and those players have to draw the picture. The major difference in this barrier game is that the student giving the directions will not be drawing the picture he describes (because the picture has already been given to him). Provide one student with a basic drawing as described and provide the other students with paper and pencils. Set up the barriers. Begin with very simple drawings before moving on to more challenging drawings. Incorporate speech tools into this game when you feel students understand how to play. If you would like to have colorful drawings for this activity, give students crayons, markers, or colored pencils. Students are then required to give directions using color modifiers (i.e., "Draw a purple circle inside the red square").

42
Let's Talk

Purpose for Children Who Stutter

- To practice pausing
- To practice being open about stuttering with others

Purpose for Language Students

- To practice conversational turn-taking skills
- To practice maintaining and expanding topics of conversation
- To practice asking and answering questions

Materials

Index cards
Pencils
Homework

Directions

In this activity students who stutter will practice pausing. It is best for these students to have had plenty of practice with pausing—the activity is not meant for students who are just learning pausing. You will need to briefly explain pausing to the entire group. For example, say (while using pausing): "Some of the students in speech class today stutter, and they will be working on speaking a little slower then usual. We call this pausing. I am using pausing right now." Then explain to students who stutter (while still using pausing):

> Today, we are going, to be having, conversations, in speech class. Let's, use our pausing, while we talk. Listen, closely, to my speech. I, will be using, pausing, after the first word, in every sentence, and then at least, one, or more times, in the sentence. If, I speak, and forget, to use pausing, give me, the thumbs up sign, to let me know, that I need to remember, to use pausing. If, I hear you, forgetting to use pausing, I will, give you, the thumbs up sign, to remind you, to use pausing.

I prefer using thumbs up rather than thumbs down because thumbs up is a positive signal and will appear as a simple reminder and not as punishment. Remember, you need to use pausing the entire time that your students are expected to do so (except when you want them to catch you forgetting to use the tool). Give your students a natural-sounding model in which you pause for a fraction of a second after the first word of each sentence and then after every two, three, four, or five words.

Continue the activity with the group by announcing:

> There are many things that we can talk about in speech class. We can talk about baseball, animals, our last vacation, or anything else that we are interested in. I am going to give each student five note cards. On each note card you are to write one topic that you would like us all to talk about. For example, one of my note cards will say "pets" on it because I love talking about dogs, cats, and other pets. My second note card will say "favorite places to eat" because I really like going out to eat for dinner." Think of five things that you would like to talk about. Make sure that all of the things you write down are topics the entire class could talk about. For example, don't write "My Uncle George" because nobody here is going to know your uncle. I will collect your cards and mix them up. Then we will pick one off the top of the deck to talk about.

Pass out index cards and pencils to each student. When students have completed their cards, check topics to make sure they are appropriate. Then shuffle the cards into a pile. You or a student chooses the first topic off the deck and reads the card. Ask, "Who wrote this card?" Then instruct the student who wrote the card to begin by talking about the topic. If the card picked says "video games," then say, "Susan, you wrote this card—what would you like to tell us about video games?" Then engage students in a conversation on this topic.

You will need to remind students who stutter to use their pausing. You may attempt to do so by simply making eye contact with them and saying, "Remember to pause" or "Remember the thumbs up."

When you take a turn during the class conversation, continue to use pausing. Then begin to speak much faster, in an exaggerated way, so that students can catch you forgetting to pause. This will help your students remember to use their pausing, and it is fun and motivating to give students the chance to catch you. If students recognize that you are speaking quickly on purpose, this is fine. A student may say, "You are trying to talk too fast." You may simply say, "Yes, I am; it is my job to help you pay attention to how I talk and to how you talk—good listening!" If students who do not stutter want to catch you forgetting to pause, that is fine, but I typically do not allow students who do not stutter to catch students who do stutter. If this occurs, you may say, "You may catch me but not other students."

Once you and your students have completed the note cards for this game, save them and use them during future speech classes. I like to begin each speech class with a short conversation. Take out the note cards and work through one or more topics before moving on to another activity.

More Ideas

Category Topics. When the class is preparing the note cards, try limiting the possible topics of conversation. As an example, explain to students:

> Every student here goes to gym class. Think of all the fun things you have done in gym class. I will give each student three note cards. Write down the three things you have enjoyed doing most in gym class. Then we will mix them up and choose one to discuss.

The King of Pausing–Revisited. Instead of having a group discussion, ask each student to choose a topic card to present to the class. It is important that students choose a topic that they are able to discuss at length. It is also helpful if students are excited about this topic. This will challenge them when using pausing. Students who stutter will then compete to see who is able to use pausing for the longest amount of time without having to be cued or reminded. Time each student. Using a stopwatch will add to the excitement of this contest. You could even suggest goals for the group by saying, "Let's see who can get into the 2-minute pausing club today. That means that you were able to pause during 2 whole minutes without being reminded." As the game continues increase the amount of time students are challenged to use pausing. Make sure you start with a time goal that students can reach. If using pausing without cues for 2 minutes is too difficult for a student, start with a 1-minute challenge.

You may easily include children who do not stutter in this game. Explain to the group:

> Even if you do not stutter, it is good practice to work on slowing your speech the same way that many good speakers do. For example, sportscasters often speak with frequent pauses so that they are clearly understood. Try to use pausing when talking about your topic. If you have any trouble, there are pausing experts here who can help you.

If students who do not stutter have difficulty using pausing, give them a few extra opportunities during this assignment, especially if it is their first time. If children who stutter think this unfair, you may remind them that they have had a lot more practice using pausing. This also gives students who stutter the chance to teach pausing to the other students.

Homework

When assigning the first homework assignment, mention to students that they should not list conversational topics that have been discussed in speech class. Homework Assignment 2 is meant to challenge students to think about stuttering. Sometimes students return to speech class with questions that have already been covered. Other times students will come back with very creative questions, such as, "Why do some children have relatives who stutter and some children don't?" To encourage creative questions, offer students a reward for the most creative stuttering topic.

Stuttering 42 Homework

Name ______________________ Date due ______________

Think of three things that you would like to talk about in speech class. Remember, you need to choose topics that other students will also be able to talk about.

1. ______________________________

2. ______________________________

3. ______________________________

Parent signature ______________________ (1)

Stuttering 42 Homework

Name ______________________ Date due ______________

In speech class we talk a lot about stuttering. Is there something about stuttering that you have thought about that we have never talked about in speech class? Think of a good stuttering topic to talk about during our next speech class and write it here. ______________________________

____

____

____

Parent signature ______________________ (2)

43
Joke Telling

Purpose for Children Who Stutter

- To practice speech tools
- To practice appropriate eye contact

Purpose for Language Students

- To understand and express figurative language
- To practice using appropriate prosody
- To practice speaking in complete sentences
- To practice appropriate eye contact
- To increase auditory memory abilities

Materials

Jokes
Index cards
Pencils
Homework

Directions

Joke Telling is an excellent opportunity to work with a combined group of students. Some students who stutter feel that they cannot be funny if they stutter. Students working on language skills will benefit from many aspects of telling jokes, including understanding and expressing figurative language, speaking with appropriate vocal inflection, and using appropriate eye contact.

Begin by telling students a few jokes (see Jokes page). I typically overemphasize the prosodic shifts and the body gestures inherent in telling jokes. Many students need this form of overacting to understand that telling jokes is about much more than simply reading lines. After you tell a few jokes, students may want to share their own jokes. Take the time to appreciate any jokes they may know. Then explain to students that they will each get a chance to tell a joke to the group.

When it is a student's turn, take her outside the therapy room to tell her the joke you have chosen from the jokes handout. (This prevents other students from hearing the joke.) Many students, especially those with pragmatic language difficulties, will benefit from hearing the clinician's model of the appropriate vocal inflection necessary for good joke telling. When outside the therapy room, the student should practice telling her assigned joke to you before returning to tell it to the group. Help the student stress appropriate prosodic features and body gestures that go along with the joke.

Using Stretching, Bouncing, Voluntary Stuttering, and Pausing. Students who stutter can now move on to using speech tools while telling jokes. It is common for students to report difficulty because of time pressures inherent in joke telling. Saying punch lines seems to be particularly difficult for some. Suggest that it is often helpful to have a goal or game plan that helps students focus on something specific. The following are possibilities:

- Stretch or bounce to smoothly initiate the joke and the punch line.
- Voluntarily stutter on the punch line to reduce the fear of saying it.
- Pause between words to reduce the frequency of stuttering.
- Initiate eye contact on the punch line while using a stretch or a bounce.
- Voluntarily stutter on assigned words to reduce the fear of talking.

You may practice a joke with a student by saying, "I want you to stretch on the first word in the joke. Here is how I do it: 'Wwwhat do you call a boomerang that doesn't work?' Now you stretch the first word of the answer."

The student says, "Yyyou call it a stick."

Give students choices and options during therapy. For example, ask students who stutter what speech tools they would like to use. Depending on the student and her ability to use speech tools, you may choose to write out the jokes on index cards and use commas to signify pausing and underlines to signify stretching, bouncing, or voluntary stuttering.

Incorporating Eye Contact. After practicing a few jokes using speech tools, begin to emphasize the importance of all students using appropriate eye contact during joke telling. This is an excellent time to take out the toy glasses from the Stuttering Kits. Many students will tell jokes without establishing any eye contact or only minimal eye contact. By wearing or holding the toy glasses, students who stutter have a fun reminder to use eye contact during moments of stuttering, and students with pragmatic language difficulties have a reminder that using eye contact is important during joke telling.

More Ideas

Help students search the Internet for more children's jokes. For example, go to a search engine such as Google.com or Yahoo.com and search using words such as "children" and "jokes." Advanced searches are helpful (see The World Wide Web–Activity 27 for assistance conducting advanced searches). Good phrases to use for advanced searches include "jokes for children" and "children's jokes." Also, popular children's Web sites such as www.Scholastic.com have joke pages.

Homework

Several of the following homework assignments ask students to tell jokes while using speech tools. At times, when you are not present to give a model, students will use the speech tool in a robotic or unnatural-sounding way. You may want to role-play these homework assignments to prevent this from occurring. It is suggested that, at first, students play the role of the family member listening to the joke, and you play the role of a student telling the joke. This way you model how to use speech tools in a natural-sounding way during joke telling. Then switch roles so that the student practices telling you the jokes while using speech tools.

JOKES

Why was the broom late?
It overswept!

How do you catch a monkey?
Act like a banana.

What do you get when a cow is in an earthquake?
A milk shake!

What do you call a dog at the beach?
A hot dog.

What do you call a deer with no eyes?
I have no ideer.

What kind of dance does a tissue do?
A boogy.

Why did the cookie visit the doctor?
It felt crummy.

Why do cows wear bells?
Because their horns don't work.

Why do hummingbirds hum?
Because they can't remember the words.

Why do birds fly south for the winter?
Because it's too far to walk.

What do you call a boomerang that doesn't work?
A stick.

Where do you find a turtle with no legs?
Right where you left it.

What did the teddy bear say when he was offered dessert?
"No thanks, I'm stuffed!"

What did the Pacific Ocean say to the Atlantic Ocean?
Nothing. It just waved.

Why do gorillas have big fingers?
Because they have large nostrils.

Why is 6 scared of 7?
Because 7-8-9!

What did the alien say to the garden?
"Take me to your weeder."

What do you say when you meet a two-headed monster?
"Hello, hello!"

What looks like half a cat?
The other half!

How do cats eat spaghetti?
The same as everybody else—they put it in their mouths!

What do you get if you cross a cat with a canary?
Shredded tweet!

Why did the golfer wear two pairs of pants?
In case he made a hole in one.

What is a ghost's favorite dessert?
Booberry pie.

What has milk and a horn?
A milk truck.

What animal can jump higher than a house?
Any animal—a house can't jump!

How do you catch a squirrel?
You go up in a tree and act like a nut.

When do you know that an elephant is under your bed?
When your face is against the ceiling.

What happens when a frog's car breaks down?
He gets toad away.

What's big and red and eats rocks?
A big, red rock eater.

What do you call a gorilla with bananas in his ears?
You can call him anything because he can't hear you!

Why was the skeleton afraid to cross the road?
He had no guts!

There are three kinds of people in the world.
Those who can count and those who can't.

What vegetable do you get when an elephant walks through your garden?
Squash!

What kind of hair does an ocean have?
Wavy hair.

What happens when you tell a duck a joke?
It quacks up.

What time is it when an elephant sits on your bed?
Time to get a new bed.

How do you stop an elephant from charging?
Take away its credit cards!

What do you give a sick lemon?
Lemon–Aid.

Why did the boy throw the clock out the window?
He wanted to see time fly.

Why are graveyards loud and noisy?
Because of all the coffin!

What do you call Dracula's dog?
A blood hound!

Why are basketball players never asked to dinner?
Because they're always dribbling!

What kind of car does Mickey Mouse's wife drive?
A Minnie van.

What did the parents say to their son who wanted to play the drums?
"Beat it."

What did the tie say to the hat?
"You go on a head and I'll hang around."

What do you call an ant in outer space?
An astro–ant.

How do you start a teddy bear race?
You say, "Ready, teddy, go."

What is a chicken's worst day?
Fry–day.

Why do bees buzz?
Because they never learned how to whistle.

What are the smartest kinds of bees?
Spelling bees.

How does a lion say hello to other animals?
"Pleased to eat you."

What do you call an elephant at the North Pole?
Lost.

What do you call a box full of ducks?
A box of quackers!

Why did the whale cross the road?
To get to the other tide.

What kind of bee is hard to understand?
A mumble bee!

Why do you have to oil a mouse?
Because it squeaks!

Why did the chicken want to join a rock 'n' roll band?
Because it had its own drumsticks.

What did the cake say to the ice cream?
"You're cool!"

Where do cows live?
In Moo York City.

What do you say to a cow that is in your way?
"Mooooooooove over!"

What kind of nails do carpenters hate to hammer?
Their fingernails.

Why don't bats live alone?
Because they like to hang around with their friends.

How does a pig go to the hospital?
In a hambulance.

Where does a frog go to get glasses?
A hoptomotrist.

Stuttering 43 Homework

Name ______________________ Date due ______________

Tell your parents the following jokes while stretching on the first sounds of all underlined words.

1. <u>What</u> looks like <u>half</u> a cat?
   <u>The</u> other half.
2. <u>How</u> do you catch a <u>monkey</u>?
   <u>Act</u> like a banana.
3. <u>Where</u> do you find a <u>turtle</u> with no legs?
   <u>Wherever</u> you left it.

Parent signature ______________________ (1)

Stuttering 43 Homework

Name ______________________ Date due ______________

Tell your parents the following jokes while bouncing on the first sounds of all underlined words.

1. <u>Why</u> did the cookie <u>visit</u> the doctor?
   <u>It</u> felt crummy.
2. <u>What</u> do you give a <u>sick</u> lemon?
   <u>Lemon</u>—Aid.
3. <u>What</u> time is it when an <u>elephant</u> sits on your bed?
   <u>Time</u> to get a <u>new</u> bed.

Parent signature ______________________ (2)

Stuttering 43 Homework

Name ______________________ Date due ______________

Tell a relative or friend the following jokes while pausing at all the commas.

1. What, happens, when you tell, a duck a joke?
   It, quacks up.
2. There, are, three kinds, of people, in the world.
   Those, who can count, and those, who can't.
3. Why, is, 6, scared of, 7?
   Because, 7, 8, 9.

Parent signature ______________________ (3)

Stuttering 43 Homework

Name ______________________ Date due ______________

Tell a friend the following jokes while stuttering on purpose on the first word of each punch line.

1. What do you call Dracula's dog?
   A blood hound!
2. Why are basketball players never asked to dinner?
   Because they're always dribbling!
3. What is a chicken's worst day?
   Fry–day.

Parent signature ______________________ (4)

Stuttering 43 Homework

Name ______________________ Date due ______________

Tell a relative the following jokes while stuttering on purpose on the first word of each question.

1. Why was the skeleton afraid to cross the road?
   He had no guts!
2. Where does a frog go to get glasses?
   A hoptomotrist.
3. What vegetable do you get when an elephant walks through your garden?
   Squash!

Parent signature ______________________ (5)

Stuttering 43 Homework

Name ______________________ Date due ______________

Think of any jokes you know. Write them below. You may ask a friend or relative for help if you do not know any jokes. You will share them with the group during our next class.

1. ____

____

2. ____

____

Parent signature ______________________ (6)

44
Pleased To Meet You

Purpose for Children Who Stutter

- To practice using pausing
- To practice using appropriate eye contact

Purpose for Language Students

- To practice following directions
- To practice speaking in complete sentences
- To increase pragmatic language skills, including appropriate eye contact and turn-taking

Materials

8 ½" x 11" paper
Pencils

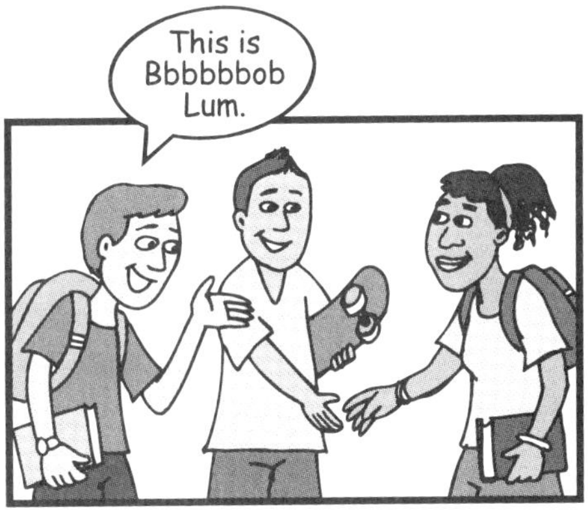

Directions

People who stutter often report that introducing friends and acquaintances to others is often stressful, and introductions are particularly challenging speaking situations. Using pausing can help students who stutter have some control in these difficult situations.

Begin by handing each student a piece of paper and a pencil. As you instruct students, follow all of the directions yourself so that you are participating fully in the activity. Explain (while using pausing):

> Today we will be learning about each other. Each student will have the chance to introduce another person to the class. During our introductions students who stutter will practice a speech tool that we call pausing. I am using pausing right now. As you can see, I am briefly pausing between some words in each sentence that I say. We use pausing to help us stutter less often.

Now that you have explained the speech tool aspect of this assignment, announce:

> Before we introduce one another, we need to write down a few things about ourselves. Listen closely so you can follow these directions. In the middle of your paper, draw a large square that takes up most of the paper.

The directions that follow often become confusing for students with language disorders. You may consider first reviewing relevant vocabulary, including *left, right, top, bottom* and *middle.* Then explain:

Put your pencil point on the top border of the square. The word *border* is used to describe the different lines that make up a square (it helps if you point to the borders). Now that your pencil point is on the top border, move it to the very middle of that top border. Draw a line straight down until your line touches the bottom border of the square. Now put your pencil point on the left border of the square in the very middle of that border. Then draw a line across the square until your pencil reaches the right border (see Figure 44.1)

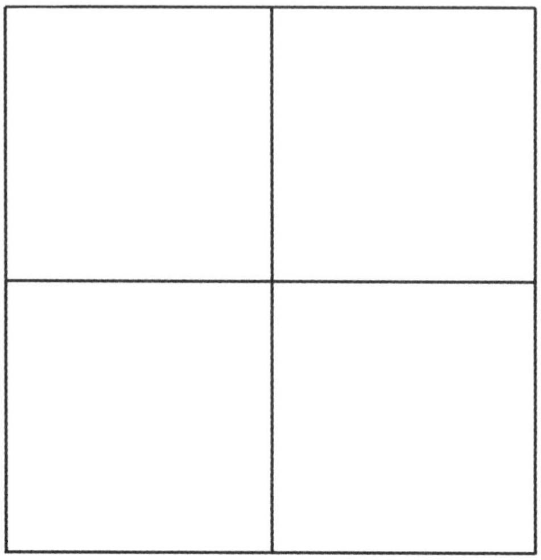

Figure 44.1 A blank game board

Now we are ready to start writing down information about ourselves. Don't tell or show anyone what you are writing; keep your boards to yourselves. Here is your first direction: In the top left square, write the names and ages of all your brothers and sisters (if a student does not have a sibling, instruct her to write the names and ages of other young relatives or of friends). In the bottom right square, write the names of your favorite toys and games. In the top right square, write two things that you are very good at doing. For example, I am very good at playing chess and swimming, so I will write that. In the bottom left square, write down something that you wish you could do better. Now for the last thing: At the very top of your page, above the board you have just completed, write your name. Now that you are finished, pass your board to the person on your left-hand side. (See Figure 44.2 for an example of a completed board.)

Jose

Eric–10 Rosa–4	Playing kickball Playing video games—good at baseball and wrestling video games
Playing soccer and running faster	Checkers Uno Stratego

Figure 44.2 A completed game board

Once every student has passed his completed board to the person on his left and has received another person's board, it is time to begin the introductions. Be sure to demonstrate strong models of pausing and eye contact. Announce that you will be the first one to introduce a student to the group. While you are introducing a student, it is best to have students turn over their papers so that they are attending to the class and not preparing their introductions. As an example, using the completed board from Figure 44.2, you would explain (while using pausing):

> I now have Jose's board. I will introduce Jose to the class. Notice that while I am introducing Jose, I will be making eye contact with everyone in the room. Watch how my eyes move from person to person to show that I am speaking to everyone. I will begin now. Jose has two siblings—a brother, Eric, who is 10, and a sister Rosa, who is 4. Jose likes to play checkers, Uno, and Stratego. He is very good at playing kickball and playing video games, especially video baseball and video wrestling. Jose wants to be better at playing soccer, and he also wants to be able to run faster.

Now give each student a turn to present his introduction. Explain, "Remember, students who stutter will be using pausing during these introductions. And let's be sure that we all make good eye contact with everyone in the group just as I did."

If a student does not attempt to make eye contact while speaking, stop his introduction in a friendly way and say something such as, "There are five people in this room, and you are talking to the table. Please speak to the class." If this is said in a lighthearted way, students will find it amusing and not punishing. It also helps to show students ways to organize the information they have. For example, you may say, "Introduce your person one square at a time. First look to see the names and ages of your person's brothers and sisters. Then look up, make eye contact with someone, and tell us." After a student does so, say, "Now look down at the board and see what your person is good at doing. Then look up and make eye contact with someone else and tell us."

Some students who stutter will have great shame surrounding their speech and will be upset at the prospect of making eye contact. Start them off slowly by asking them to try making eye contact only one or two times during the activity. For students who are particularly fearful of making eye contact, ask them to simply use pausing and attempt eye contact another day.

More Ideas

You may wish to simplify the board-making directions. Instead of having students draw a board, instruct them to fold their paper in half twice so that when they open the paper, there are four squares of equal size.

Repeat the activity but change the requests for information. For example, give the following directions and have students introduce each other again:

1. In the top right corner, write the names of your two favorite movies.
2. In the bottom right corner, write the name of the job you want to have when you grow up.
3. In the top left corner, write the name of one special place that you go with your family.
4. In the bottom left corner, write the names of your three favorite foods.

Play *Guess Who I Am.* This is a fun activity to play with a group of students, and it fosters a friendly and open speech class environment. Ask students *not* to put their names on the top of the boards. Then collect the completed boards. Choose a board and introduce the person as "the mystery person." Students have to guess who is being introduced. The more students in speech class, the more fun this game is. This activity is a fun way to introduce guests or new students to the group.

45
Listen Up

Purpose for Children Who Stutter

- To practice speech tools
- To practice being open about stuttering

Purpose for Language Students

- To practice speaking in complete sentences
- To practice expressing plurals and tenses correctly
- To practice appropriate vocal inflection

Materials

Checkerboard and checkers
Game-playing pieces, such as the car and thimble from Monopoly
Sample Sentences page

Directions

Begin by putting the checkerboard on the table and giving each student a game-playing piece (token). Instruct students to put their tokens on any square in the first row. Then explain:

> The object of this game is to move your game piece one space at a time from one side of the checkerboard to the other. You may move forward, backward, and sideways, and your game piece may share a square with another player. The first person to reach the other side and return is the winner. Each red and black checker piece will represent a land mine or obstacle.

To shorten the game, you may say, "The first person to reach the other side is the winner."

> We will now place the checkers on different squares on the checkerboard. You will need to move your game piece around these obstacles to get to the other side. When you are moving, if your hand or game piece touches a checker, you lose that turn.

Start putting the red and black checkers on different squares and encourage students to help you. Most checker games have 12 red and 12 black checkers. You may use all 24 checkers or fewer. Sometimes as students are putting the checkers on the board, they will attempt to trap a game-playing piece so it cannot move by completely surrounding it with red and black checkers. If this occurs, simply tell students that it is against the rules of the game to completely trap a player's game piece. Now continue to explain directions:

> Before you get a turn to move, you will have to repeat a sentence. Children who stutter will repeat the sentence while using a speech tool (you may wish to explain to children who do not stutter what speech tools are). For example, I may ask you to stretch the first word of the following sentence, "After speech class I go to gym." Or I may say, "Pause after every several words in this sentence, 'My, favorite sports, are, baseball, football, and soccer.' " If you remember to use the speech tool when repeating the sentence, you get to move one space.

Repeating sentences is helpful for students with language difficulties because it provides them with strong clinician models that target any number of specific language needs. For example, students who have difficulty expressing irregular plurals often have difficulty repeating irregular plurals. A student who says "childs" instead of "children" may hear the sentence, "The children are playing" and continue to repeat it incorrectly by saying, "The *childs* are playing." Listen Up helps students learn correct language usage by repeating appropriate models. In the previous example, when a student hears the word children and repeats it as childs, he will quickly learn to adjust when he realizes that advancing in the game requires an exact repetition of the sentence. It helps to remind students to, "Say exactly what I say without changing anything."

Students with difficulty using appropriate prosody will benefit from being asked to repeat statements or questions while modeling your vocal inflection. For example, you may say:

> I am going to ask a question, and I want you to pay very close attention to how I make my voice go higher at the end of the question. I want you to repeat both the words in the sentence and how I say the sentence. Try repeating this question with the same voice that I use: "Do you know where Burger King is?" (Model an exaggerated vocal inflection here to signify that a question is being asked.)

See the Sample Sentences page for a few ideas of sentences to use during this activity. This page is for you to read from, not to hand out to students. You may wish to break sentences in two if they are too long for a particular group. Instead of asking students to repeat, "I have one chipped tooth, but the rest of my teeth are fine," say, "Repeat these two sentences, 'I have one chipped tooth' (student repeats) 'but the rest of my teeth are fine' (student repeats)." Most of the sentences can be broken up this way. Remember to assign Speech Tools for those who stutter.

More Ideas

Use other games such as Candyland or Stratego. Play these games using their regular rules, but before students take a turn, they are asked to repeat a sentence in the manner that you request.

Sample Sentences

Verb Tense

Yesterday I walked home, and today I will walk home.

Yesterday I played outside, and today I will play inside.

Last week I ate pizza, and today I will eat candy.

Last week I ran home, and today I will run home.

This morning I caught the ball, and now I will catch the ball.

This morning I washed my face, and now I will wash my face.

For lunch I drank milk, and now I will drink water.

During math I wrote a lot, and now I will write some more.

Yesterday I swam, and today I will swim.

Yesterday I jumped a lot, and today I plan on jumping.

This morning I threw the ball, and this afternoon I will practice throwing.

Irregular Plurals

There is a mouse in my house and many mice in my backyard.

One child is very slow, but the rest of the children are fast.

This woman likes red clothes, but those women like blue clothes.

I have one chipped tooth, but the rest of my teeth are fine.

I have one red fish and three blue fish.

I brought one leaf to school, but I have many leaves at home.

One person is not enough to play, but four people should work.

My teacher is a man, and my baseball coaches are men.

One foot is cold, and both feet are wet.

My mother needed a loaf of bread, and my aunt gave her two loaves.

Three thieves broke into the bank, but only one thief was caught.

My room has two broken shelves and one good shelf.

I played the happy elf in the play, and my friends played the mean elves.

A fireman came to my school, and then three more firemen came.

One knife is dull, but three knives are sharp.

46
Verbal Sequencing Activities

Purpose for Children Who Stutter

- To practice using speech tools in challenging speaking situations
- To practice being open with others about stuttering

Purpose for Language Students

- To practice following directions
- To learn new words within categories
- To practice sequencing and ordering information

Materials

Making Ice Cream handout (includes list of materials needed)
Making a Pie Pan Aquarium handout (includes list of materials needed)
Homework

Directions

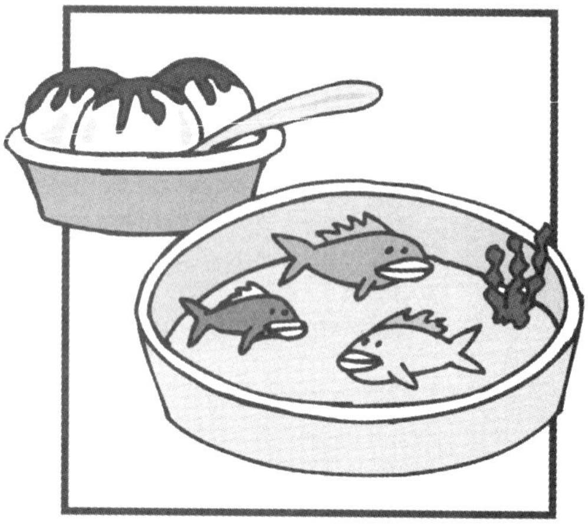

There are many verbal sequencing activities, such as preparing food, doing arts and crafts, and explaining sports and games that will motivate students to talk. Students become excited during the following activities and will often interrupt one another and attempt to speak at the same time. Students who stutter will benefit from using their speech tools under these conditions. Children with language impairments will benefit from the opportunities they receive to take turns speaking, sequence and organize language, use new vocabulary, and learn words within categories. Below is a description of three activities that offer challenging, fun opportunities for children who stutter and children with language difficulties.

Making Ice Cream. Making ice cream during speech class is just one of the many fun food preparation activities you may use to engage students. This activity is an ideal time to invite guests to therapy. Rare is the child who would turn down the opportunity to make (and eat) ice cream. It is best to check with parents and teachers before beginning the activity to make sure that students do not have food allergies that may be of concern.

Prepare by setting out the necessary materials listed on the Making Ice Cream handout. Pass out copies of the handout. Help students make the ice cream as directed. As you are making the ice cream, you and your students can take turns reading the directions aloud. At this point, do not assign speech tools. If you follow the directions, this recipe will work and the ice cream will get cold enough to freeze. After eating the ice cream and cleaning up, have students verbally explain or retell the steps of the activity. Students who stutter are asked to do so while using a speech tool. For example, if the assigned speech tool is pausing, explain: "Now, that we, have made, ice cream, please, tell us, all of, the ingredients, using, pausing." After a student has done this, ask a different student to, "Tell me, everything we needed, to do, to make, ice cream, while using, your pausing. It, is important, to go, step, by step, and include, all of the, important information."

Students with language disorders will benefit from retelling and sequencing the events in this activity while also recalling the relevant vocabulary. You may also challenge students to express the directions in different tenses. For example, you might say, "Explain how we could make ice cream again next week." Then help the student get started by saying: "To make ice cream next week, we will need to have all the ingredients and materials ready. First thing we will do is put the rock salt and the ice in a Ziploc bag. Then we will mix them together. Now you tell me the rest." During subsequent therapy sessions, you can have students teach the lesson to another group.

Pie Pan Aquarium. Making pie pan aquariums is a fun arts and crafts activity that is used to engage students in practicing their speech tools while also meeting language goals.

Again, have all materials set out and ready to use (see Making a Pie Pan Aquarium handout). Pass out copies of the handout. Begin making the aquarium as directed while taking turns reading the directions. At the end of the session, challenge students to list the materials or explain the directions as they did when making ice cream. Students who stutter are asked to use an assigned speech tool.

Sports and Games. There are many ways to encourage students to talk about their favorite sports or games while using speech tools. Pick a sport or game for discussion that students enjoy. One year a group of students often played handball together before school. These students became very excited when asked to describe the rules of handball. As students took turns and explained the rules, some began stuttering quite a lot with much struggle and little control. These students were then asked to retell the rules of handball while using pausing. The use of pausing dramatically decreased the frequency of stuttering and increased the students' communicative abilities by helping them take control of their speaking situation.

Explaining and organizing the rules of sports and games can meet many goals of students with language difficulties. These students will have the opportunity to work on language skills, such as speaking in complete sentences, using different tenses, and increasing word-finding skills.

In the community in which I work, many students grow up playing soccer and basketball and know very little about baseball and kickball. I like teaching kickball to students by taking them outside to the schoolyard as a special treat. We learn the rules and may invite friends to impress upon them how "cool" speech class is. Then, when we return to class, students are asked to explain the rules of kickball.

Homework

The first homework assignment in this activity calls for the student to bring in a favorite game to be played in speech class. The student is expected to explain the directions before playing while using a speech tool. Speech tools may also be assigned when playing the game. If a student brings in a deck of cards and teaches the class how to play Go Fish, you may ask students to practice stretching or bouncing on a word before taking a turn.

Making Ice Cream

Ingredients for Ice Cream

5–6 teaspoons sugar
1 cup Half-and-Half or milk
1/2 teaspoon vanilla extract or flavoring
Any extra ingredients, such as candy, fruit, or nuts (to taste)

Supplies

1/4 cup rock salt
1 large bag of ice
1 pint-size Ziploc bag
1 gallon-size Ziploc bag
Several plastic grocery store bags
Bowls or paper cups
Spoons
Measuring cup
Measuring spoons

Directions

1. Put the ice and the rock salt in the gallon-size Ziploc bag. Seal the bag tightly.
2. In the pint-size Ziploc bag, add the milk or Half-and-Half, the sugar, the vanilla, and any extra ingredients, such as candy or fruit. Tightly seal the bag.
3. Put the bag with the ice-cream ingredients into the larger bag that has the rock salt and ice in it.
4. Put the gallon-size bag into a couple of grocery store bags (to prevent leaking and to prevent hands from getting too cold).
5. Shake for approximately 8 to 12 minutes.
6. Open up the ice-cream bag, scoop into bowls or cups, and eat!

Fun Tip: Shaking the ice cream makes your fingers very cold. Bring in an old baseball mitt or a pair of gloves to wear while shaking the ice cream. Students share the mitt or gloves as they take turns shaking.

Making a Pie Pan Aquarium

Things You Need

1 aluminum pie pan per student
1 piece of blue construction paper per student
Fake grass (i.e., the kind found in Easter baskets)
2–3 fish pictures for each student (see Fish Pictures handout)
Plastic wrap—a piece for each student several inches larger than the pie pan
1 rubber band per student (large enough to stretch around the outside of the pie pan) or tape
Pencils and crayons
Scissors
Glue

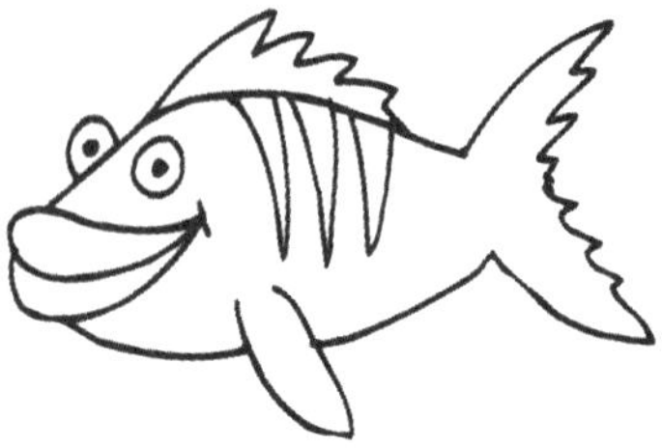

Directions

1. Give each student a pie pan and explain that it will be the fish tank for the aquarium.
2. Give each student a piece of blue construction paper. Put the pie pan on top of the blue paper (so that the bottom of the pan is touching the paper) and trace around it using a pencil so that you have a circle the same size as the inside of the pie pan.
3. Cut out the circle and throw away the scraps.
4. Glue the circle to the inside of the pie pan to represent water.
5. Glue a little grass onto the blue paper to represent seaweed on the floor of the ocean.
6. Color and cut out fish pictures (approximately 2–3 per student).
7. Glue each fish to the blue paper.
8. Cover each pan with a piece of plastic wrap so that there is a 1" to 2" overlap around the pie pan.
9. Pull the plastic wrap tightly over the pie pan and stretch a rubber band (or attach tape) around the pan so that it goes over the excess plastic wrap and holds it to the pan.

Fish Pictures

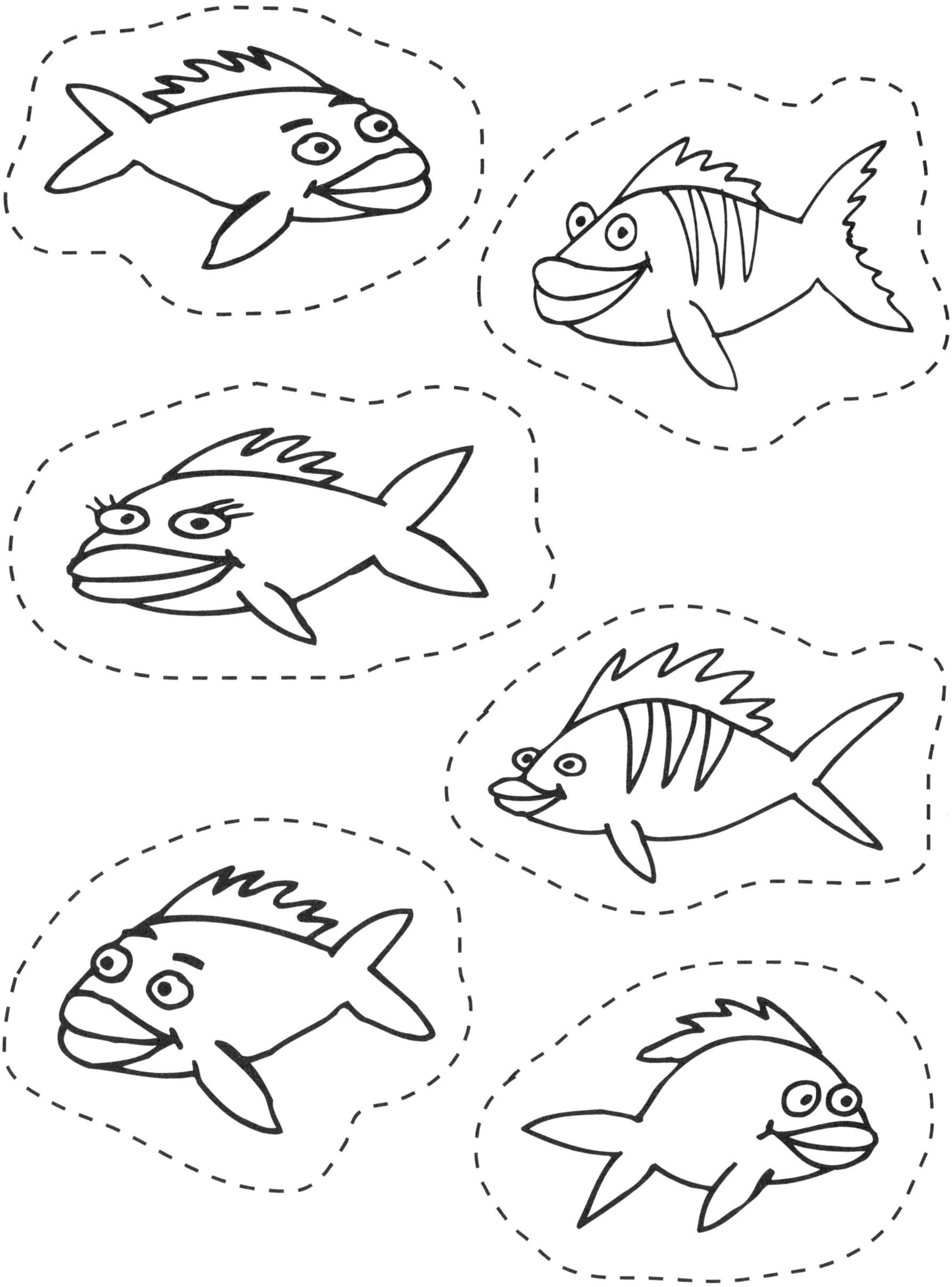

Stuttering 46 Homework

Name ______________________ Date due ______________

Choose a card game or a board game that you play at home and can bring to school. Write the directions (how to play) below. Use a separate sheet of paper if necessary.

In speech class you will tell the directions to the class, using the speech tool of your choice. Then we will play the game.

Parent signature ______________________

(1)

Stuttering 46 Homework

Name ______________________ Date due ______________

Think of something you make to eat at home. Write the directions (recipe) below. Use a separate sheet of paper if necessary.

In speech class you will read the directions to the class, using the speech tool of your choice.

Parent signature ______________________

(2)

47
Having Fun with Errands

Purpose for Children Who Stutter

- To practice using speech tools with teachers and school staff members
- To practice being open about stuttering with others

Purpose for Language Students

- To practice following directions and recalling information
- To practice speaking and asking questions in complete sentences
- To practice using appropriate eye contact

Materials

None

Directions

Speech–language pathologists in schools often have errands that need to be carried out during the day, such as returning books to teachers or picking up materials from various offices or classes in the school. Save many of your errands for students to give them the opportunity to practice using speech tools while speaking to teachers, principals, and staff members.

Completing errands is an excellent opportunity for stutterers to work on their speech under situations that are more challenging than in the therapy room. Students with language difficulties will benefit from completing errands, such as having to follow directions in a real-life situation rather than during a game. Students enjoy the freedom and responsibility of helping their speech teacher by running errands.

First, students role-play errands before completing them. When assigning speech tools to children who stutter, model the speech tool during the directions. For example, when assigning pausing, you may say, "Go, to room, 110, and give, Ms. Benito, this book, for me. Using, your pausing, say, 'Mr. Reitzes, says, thank you, for letting him, borrow the book.' "

Role-play this situation by having the student briefly leave the room and then come back in and talk to you as if you are the other teacher. Repeat role-playing situations until students understand the directions. If students who stutter remember what to say but forget to use the assigned speech tool, exclaim, "That was great, but you forgot to use your tools! Try it again." You may wish to role-play the part of the student to demonstrate a strong model of the tool.

When assigning voluntary stuttering, you might say:

> I-I-I-I wwwant you to go to the office and pick up mmy mail. Please ask the secretary for my mmmmmail whi-whi-while voluntarily stuttering on the fffffirst word that you say. You could say, "Eeeexcuse me, could I please have Mr. Reitzes' mail?" I-I-I am asking you to stutter on purpose so that you may practice getting your stuttering out in the open right away.

You may assign students to work individually during errands, but it is often helpful for two students who stutter to work together—one is the speaker and the other is the observer. It is also helpful to provide a mentor to a new student by pairing him with a veteran student. Assign a pair of students two errands. The mentor would complete the first errand to model the request and the assigned speech tool. This allows students who stutter to support one another, to feel safe, and to remind each other what the assignment is. The new student would then complete the second errand while being observed and supported by the veteran student.

One year a student thought that the voluntary stuttering assignments during errands were too hard and unfair. We made a quick deal that changed the student's attitudes toward these assignments. The student agreed to stutter on purpose during errands if I agreed to pick her up for speech class while voluntarily stuttering on her name. Thereafter, every time I picked this student up for speech class, she greeted me with a smile and waited for me to stutter on her name.

Completing errands is a good way to meet the needs of students with language difficulties. For example, for students who have difficulty following directions you may say, "Please deliver these report cards to room 209 and then come back to speech class."

If the student is able to follow this direction, increase the difficulty level for the next assignment by turning the task into a two-level direction, such as: "Please deliver these speech class report cards to room 300. Then ask the art teacher if you may borrow a roll of tape for speech class."

To challenge a student who has difficulty asking questions, you might say,

> Go to the science room and ask Ms. Lorenz if your speech class can borrow a few books. Ask if she has books on African animals and tropical fish. You may say, "Excuse me, Ms. Lorenz, my speech teacher would like to borrow a few books. Do you have any books on African animals and tropical fish?"

If a student is unable to remember the assignment and formulate the questions in the therapy room during role-play, then she will be unable to do so on her own. The student will need to either practice the assignment some more or you will need to simplify it.

I make sure to send students on errands to teachers and staff members who are particularly helpful and sensitive to children with special needs. Make sure that when you assign errands they are at appropriate times for the teachers involved.

More Ideas

Consider scheduling students who stutter for therapy at times that enable them to pick up your next group of students. This way your students who stutter are able to practice their speech tools and strategies while speaking with teachers.

48
Idioms

Purpose for Children Who Stutter

- To practice using speech tools
- To practice being open about stuttering with others

Purpose for Language Students

- To understand and express figurative language
- To practice pragmatic language skills including turn-taking and eye contact
- To practice using appropriate prosody and vocal inflection
- To practice speaking in complete sentences

Materials

Idiom Plays handout
Pencils

Directions

Begin this activity by using a few idioms in conversation. You may say, "I skipped breakfast this morning and am as hungry as horse" or "I wanted to go on the roller coaster this weekend but I didn't—my brother said I was a scaredy-cat." A few students will understand these idioms. They may even say, "Those are expressions" or "That is figurative language. We work on that in class." Explain the idioms you just used. You may say, "When I say that I am hungry as a horse, that is an expression that means I am *really* hungry" and, "When my brother says that I am a scaredy-cat, he means that I am scared to do something. Have you ever seen cats get scared? The hair rises high on their backs, they bunch up and raise their backs up high, and they often jump backward." Then ask students if they know of any idioms.

After discussing a few idioms, give each student a copy of the Idiom Plays handout. Assign roles to students. The plays each have two characters, so if you have more than two students in the session, they will need to take turns reading. Make this activity light and humorous by helping students exaggerate and "act out" idioms when reading the plays. Just as during Joke Telling–Activity 44, overact or exaggerate the vocal inflection and body gestures that accompany specific idioms. After reading a play, ask students to tell you what the idiom really means. If students are not sure, give them another example using the same idiom or simply tell them what the idiom means.

After reading a few idiom plays, begin incorporating speech tools into this activity by asking students who stutter to choose a speech tool to practice. If the chosen speech tool is stretching, students who stutter are instructed to underline the first word in every sentence of the chosen idiom plays. These words will be stretched. Keep in mind, once students become comfortable using speech tools, they may not need to use commas and underlines to remind them to use their tools. This will help them use their speech tools more independently.

Students who do not stutter are instructed to simply read the plays in a normal manner. On occasion, students who do not stutter will be intrigued by the speech tools and will want to learn them. If this occurs, you or your students who stutter may teach the speech tools to the other students.

Idiom Play 1

STUDENT 1: Wow! Look outside. The rain is really coming down hard.

STUDENT 2: Yeah, it is really **raining cats and dogs.**

Idiom Play 2

STUDENT 1: When we go on our school trip tomorrow, let's go on all of the roller coasters and the fastest rides.

STUDENT 2: I don't want to go on the roller coasters or the fast rides. Let's go on the merry-go-round.

STUDENT 1: What's wrong? Are you a **scaredy-cat?**

Idiom Play 3

STUDENT 1: Hi. I usually don't go around giving things away, but I like your face. If you give me $10, then tomorrow I will come back and give you a $300 gold watch.

STUDENT 2: How do I know that you will come back with the watch?

STUDENT 1: Well, because I promise to come back.

STUDENT 2: No, I won't give you ten dollars because this **seems a little fishy** to me.

Idiom Play 4

STUDENT 1: Thanks for lending me your video game last week.

STUDENT 2: You are welcome, but I would like it back now.

STUDENT 1: Well, there is a problem. I accidentally lost the video game.

STUDENT 2: Oh, I am so mad at you that **I could spit fire.**

Idiom Play 5

STUDENT 1: I can't believe that we missed our bus home today.

STUDENT 2: The worst part was that we were so late getting to the restaurant that we missed eating dinner.

STUDENT 1: Yeah. **I am so hungry that I could eat a horse.**

Idiom Play 6

STUDENT 1: I hope our teacher doesn't find out about the party we are planning for her.

STUDENT 2: How could our teacher find out about the party? Nobody is going to tell.

STUDENT 1: I hope everybody keeps quiet. I don't want anyone to **spill the beans.**

Idiom Play 7

STUDENT 1: When I came home from the hospital after breaking my foot, everybody was trying to help me.

STUDENT 2: How did they help you?

STUDENT 1: My mother brought me my meals in bed and my brother and sister sat with me and played games.

STUDENT 2: It sounds like everybody was **bending over backward** to help you.

Idiom Play 8

STUDENT 1: Hey buddy, I need the $10 back that I lent you last week.

STUDENT 2: I'm sorry, but I don't have your money yet. I will get it soon.

STUDENT 1: Of course you have my money, I just saw your mother give you $20. Now **cough it up.**

Idiom Play 9

STUDENT 1: I forgot to bring a drink to school today.

STUDENT 2: I brought a drink but forgot my sandwich.

STUDENT 1: Maybe we should share?

STUDENT 2: Sure, **I'll scratch your back if you scratch mine.**

Idiom Play 10

STUDENT 1: I am so mad at William for tripping me during lunch today. But just wait—I've got something planned for him.

STUDENT 2: What do you have **hidden up your sleeve?**

STUDENT 1: Well, tomorrow at lunch I'm going to sneak up behind him and scare him.

Idiom Play 11

STUDENT 1: My parents just bought a new computer.

STUDENT 2: Is it cool? What does it come with?

STUDENT 1: It is really fast, comes with many video games, and looks cool. Just wait until you see it. It will **knock your socks off.**

Idiom Play 12

STUDENT 1: My parents just bought a new car, but they are having a lot of problems with it.

STUDENT 2: What's wrong with the car?

STUDENT 1: The stereo is broken, the brakes need to be replaced, the motor is bad, and even the horn doesn't work.

STUDENT 2: It sounds like your parents really got stuck with a **lemon.**

Idiom Play 13

STUDENT 1: How is your knee doing after you slipped and fell on it last week?

STUDENT 2: After taking my medicine and putting ice on it, my knee **feels like a million dollars.**

Idiom Play 14

STUDENT 1: I would really like be the first person to wish our teacher a happy birthday.

STUDENT 2: You should get to school early so you are the first student that she sees. You know what they say: **The early bird catches the worm.**

Idiom Play 15

STUDENT 1: That new student in Mr. Brown's class looks really mean.

STUDENT 2: The new kid might look mean but maybe he's really nice. **Don't judge a book by its cover.**

Idiom Play 16

STUDENT 1: I was playing with my dog when I was supposed to be reading, and we knocked over a lamp and broke it.

STUDENT 2: I always tell you, don't **horse around.** Now you are in trouble.

Idiom Play 17

STUDENT 1: I can't believe you borrowed your brother's brand new camera without telling him.

STUDENT 2: He will only find out that I borrowed the camera if you **rat on me.**

Idiom Play 18

STUDENT 1: I thought you put all your toys away before we went to the park.

STUDENT 2: I did put all of my toys away before we left, but now they are all over the floor.

STUDENT 1: Somebody has been playing with your toys. I think I **smell a rat.**

Idiom Play 19

STUDENT 1: Have you been to the corner deli recently?

STUDENT 2: Yeah, I was there last night. The shelves are almost empty, the floors are dirty, and it smells bad.

STUDENT 1: The deli has **really gone to the dogs.**

Idiom Play 20

STUDENT 1: We are planning a surprise party for my uncle. It is his birthday soon.

STUDENT 2: Don't tell him! The party is a surprise. **Don't let the cat out of the bag.**

49
Trust Building: The Blindfolded Walk

Purpose for Children Who Stutter

- To foster trusting and cooperative relationships among students
- To demonstrate to students that stutterers may be leaders and speak with powerful voices (Yeoman, 2003)
- To practice being open about stuttering with others

Purpose for Language Students

- To practice following directions
- To practice verbally giving directions
- To practice expressing spatial and directional vocabulary
- To practice speaking with an appropriate vocal intensity

Materials

Blindfolds (you may use strips of old sheets or scarves)
Sidewalk chalk

Directions

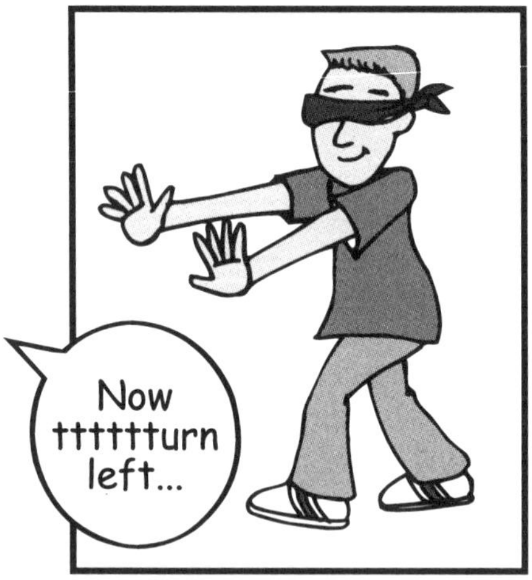

Trust-building activities are frequently used in the stuttering community at various support group workshops and in group therapy programs, such as the Successful Stuttering Management Program (SSMP). One of the most popular trust-building activities is the blindfolded walk. In this activity a student is blindfolded and verbally guided through an obstacle course or natural environment by one or more students who are not blindfolded. The blindfolded student is encouraged to walk slowly and to listen carefully to the directions of the guides. Guides may touch the student only to offer them balance or for other safety reasons.

The blindfolded walk is an excellent activity for stutterers because success is determined by the ability of students to give accurate directions. These activities stress the importance of what students say, not how they say it. Students who stutter will be particularly challenged as guides because they will not be able to compensate for stuttering through body gestures. Guides who stutter will also be unable to avoid specific words or use word substitutions because doing so may lead the blindfolded student into an object or in the wrong direction.

This activity is also very good practice for language students. Students who demonstrate difficulty expressing and sequencing directions will benefit from experiencing how important it is to give specific, clear directions. Students learn a lot when they realize that a simple mistake, such as directing a blindfolded partner to turn left instead of right, will mean the difference between succeeding and not succeeding.

It is important that you take strong safety measures, such as walking very closely alongside students to offer support if needed. You may also obtain the help of other adults to add an extra measure of safety. Be sure to teach the appropriate vocabulary words to students before attempting this activity. You cannot expect students to use vocabulary such as *left, right, forward* and *backward* outside the therapy room if they cannot use these words inside the therapy room. During the sessions leading up to this activity, I often engage students in activities such as Barrier Games–Activity 41 so they practice using the appropriate directional vocabulary.

Begin by choosing a safe environment, such as a your school's blacktop area or lawn. With your students, construct a very simple maze. If using a blacktop area, you can draw a maze with sidewalk chalk that contains only three or four turns. If on a lawn or field, use cones or other markers to construct a path. Explain:

> Today we are going to practice some of the direction words we have been using in the speech room. First, we will draw a maze together using sidewalk chalk. Then we will blindfold one student; each student will get a chance to be blindfolded. The blindfolded student will then be guided through the maze by his partners—we will call them *guides.* The guides may only touch the blindfolded student if it looks like he is losing his balance; we don't want anyone to fall. The guides will give directions to guide the blindfolded student through the maze. For safety reasons it is important that the blindfolded student walk very slowly.

Be the first guide so that you may demonstrate to students what is expected of them. Carefully tie a blindfold around the first student's head to cover her eyes. Use simple directions such as, "Make a right turn and walk forward until I say 'stop.' " If the maze has diagonal turns, give directions such as, "You are about to turn left—imagine that there is a clock in front of you—turn toward 10 o'clock." Walk closely beside your students to offer assistance or to help the guides formulate directions. If guides are having difficulty formulating directions, instruct the blindfolded student to stop and wait until the guide is ready. This can be fun if you exclaim, "Halt" as if you are in the army.

At first play this game without having students who stutter use speech tools. They will usually realize that even though they are stuttering, they are able to successfully and safely guide students through the course. Begin assigning various speech tools once students become comfortable with the activity.

Students with language difficulties often need assistance in giving directions. It is common for these students to confuse basic direction words, such as left and right, during this game.

More Ideas

After students demonstrate that they are able to complete simple mazes, increase the difficulty of the maze by introducing obstacles to be avoided, such as cones in a gym. As you increase the difficulty of this activity, you need to be even more careful to ensure the safety of your students.

This is an excellent opportunity to create a word wall or vocabulary list of important spatial and directional words. You may ask students to review these words at the beginning of the session before going out for a blindfolded walk.

50

Scavenger Hunt

Purpose for Children Who Stutter

- To practice using speech tools in a challenging speaking situation
- To practice being open about stuttering with others

Purpose for Language Students

- To practice following directions
- To practice writing directions
- To practice using spatial and directional terms
- To practice turn-taking

Materials

Clinician created scavenger hunts
Scavenger Hunt example
Write Your Own Scavenger Hunt handout
Pencils

Directions

Scavenger hunts are ideal activities for speech–language pathologists working in the schools. While students who stutter are working on using speech tools, students with language impairments can work on following directions, learning and using spatial and directional terms (i.e., *left, right, after, before, between, through, on, next to,* and *closest*), and speaking and writing in complete sentences. Those who speak with low vocal intensity will need to speak loud enough to be heard in a hallway or building. Students enjoy this activity so much that their friends have often stopped by the speech office and asked to be included in the "detective game."

Scavenger hunts involve written directions that students need to follow to get them from a starting point to an ending point. A common scavenger hunt might ask students to follow written directions to get from the speech room to the gym (see Scavenger Hunt example). The scavenger hunt may start by saying, "Begin at the bottom of Stairway A. Walk up Stairway A until you reach the third floor. Then turn left and walk until you reach the second water fountain." The fun part is that students do not know their final destination until they get there. At the bottom of the scavenger hunt, students write down their final destination once they arrive there and return to speech class to see if they were correct.

You will need to create several scavenger hunts that are specific to your setting. Begin by giving each student a scavenger hunt. Review hallway rules, such as "no running" and "no yelling," and explain to students that they are to stay within the building at all times. Also tell students that they are not to ask for help or accept help or enter into classrooms during this activity. Students complete their scavenger hunts individually or in small groups and then return to class.

After completing a few scavenger hunts, students are asked to write their own scavenger hunts. Give each student a Write Your Own Scavenger Hunt handout and explain:

> Now you are going to write your own scavenger hunts. Be very specific in your writing. Include as many steps as you need to get from your starting point to your ending point. When you are finished, I will follow your directions *exactly* as you read them to me. Let's see if you can get me from your starting point to your ending point.

Allow each student a turn to read his directions to you as you follow the commands. During the reading of their directions, students who stutter are assigned a speech tool. All students come along for "testing" the scavenger hunt, but only the assigned student may speak.

Follow the directions exactly as they are read. If the student accidentally instructs you to walk the wrong way, do so. Students find it amusing when you follow the directions by pretending to walk into walls or by walking right past the scavenger hunt destination. This lets students know that their directions need to be specific.

More Ideas

For students who stutter who are ready for a more challenging assignment, ask them to use two speech tools during a single reading of directions. For example, you may ask a student to, "Use your pausing and if you stutter, use a bounce-out to move through the stutter."

Students often earn free time or "choice time" in their classrooms. Talk to classroom teachers and ask them if during choice time students may work on writing scavenger hunts for speech class.

Scavenger Hunt Example

Name ______________________________

1. Start at room 310 (the speech room).
2. Make a right and go down the stairs until you get to the second floor.
3. Make a right turn and walk straight through the doors that say Exit 7.
4. Walk slowly down the hallway.
5. Make a left after you pass the girls' restroom and walk through the large yellow doors.
6. Walk slowly down the hallway and stop at the fire extinguisher.
7. What classroom do you see between the fire extinguisher and the boys' restroom?

What classroom have you found? ____________________

Write Your Own Scavenger Hunt

Name ______________________ Date ______________

1. Start at room ______________________

End at ______________________

Part 3

Appendixes

A
Reproducible Forms

Stuttering Homework

Name ______________________ Date due ______________

Parent signature ______________________

Stuttering Homework

Name ______________________ Date due ______________

Parent signature ______________________

Speech Class Guest Pass

You have been invited by ______________________________ to attend

speech class as a special guest on ________________ at ________________

in room ________________.

– – – – – – – – – – – – – – – – – – –

Speech Class Guest Pass

You have been invited by ______________________________ to attend

speech class as a special guest on ________________ at ________________

in room ________________.

Please bring three questions to speech class to ask about stuttering.
Write them below.

1. ____

____

2. ____

____

3. ____

____

Scorecard

Name: ________	Name: ________	Name: ________	Name: ________	Name: ________

Scorecard

Name: ________	Name: ________	Name: ________	Name: ________	Name: ________

Scorecard

Name: ________	Name: ________	Name: ________	Name: ________	Name: ________

The

LOOOOOOOOOOONGEST

Stuttering Award

Presented to:

____

by

____

The SHORTEST Stuttering Award

Presented to:

____

by

____

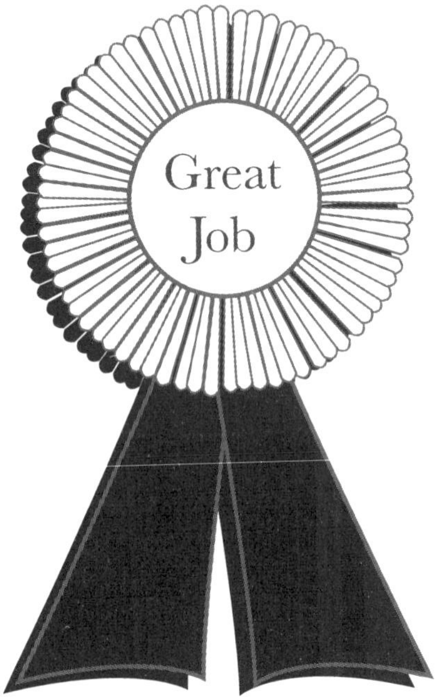

THE COOLEST STUTTERING AWARD

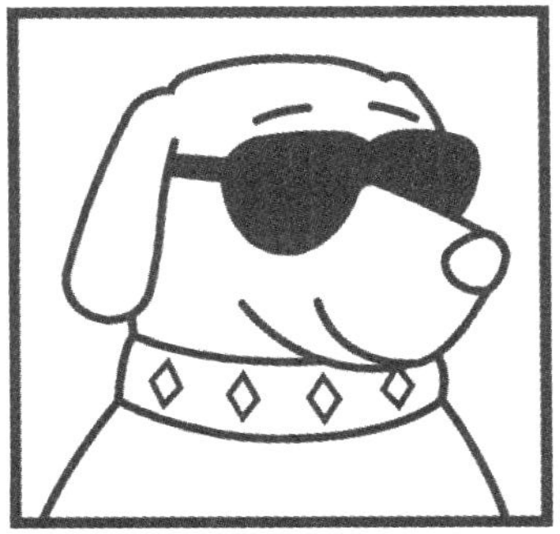

Presented to:

____

by

____

The

LOUDEST

Stuttering Award

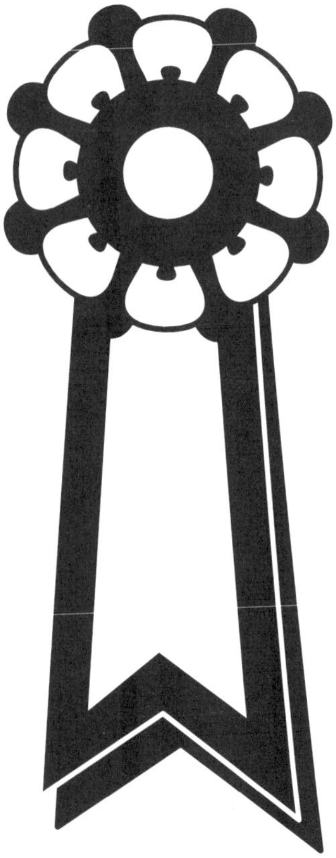

Presented to:

____

by

____

THE STRONGEST STUTTERING AWARD

Presented to:

____

by

____

The

WEIRDEST

Stuttering Award

Presented to: ______________________

by ______________________

THE BEST SPANISH STUTTERING AWARD

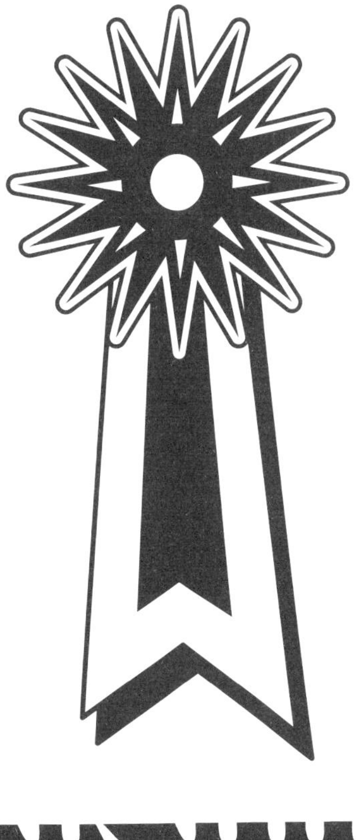

Presented to:

____

by

____

THE

BEST

Stretching

STUTTERING

AWARD

Presented to:

____

by

____

The Best

Bou- Bou- Bou-

BOUNCING

Stuttering Award

Presented to:

____

by

____

THE

BEST

• • • PAUSING

AWARD

Presented to:

____

by

____

The
Best

STUTTERING-ON-PURPOSE

AWARD

Presented to:

____

by

____

THE

Best Eye Contact

Stuttering Award

Presented to:

____

by

____

THE

Worst Eye Contact

Stuttering Award

Presented to:

____

by

____

THE

STUTTERING AWARD

Presented to:

---

by

THE

STUTTERING
AWARD

Presented to:

by

Speech Class Permission Form

Dear ______________________________,

During speech class, students first learn to use their "speech tools" (speaking strategies) in the speech room. Then it becomes helpful to take students to public locations, such as stores and restaurants, to practice their speaking strategies in the real world. Please complete this form if you would like your child to have the opportunity to use his or her speaking strategies in public locations in the nearby area.

I, ______________________________, give permission for ______________________________

to be taken by ______________________ to public locations, such as stores and restaurants, to practice using speech tools. If you have questions about these visits, please

contact me at ______________________________________

.

Sincerely,

Parent or guardian signature ______________________________ Date________________

B
Handout for Teachers

The Child Who Stutters: Notes to the Teacher

Note. This material is from *The Child Who Stutters: Notes to the Teacher* by L. Scott and D. E. Williams, 2005, Memphis, TN: The Stuttering Foundation. Copyright 2005 by the Stuttering Foundation of America; 800/992-9392; www.stutteringhelp.org. Adapted with permission.

Teachers often report difficulty knowing what to do about a child who stutters in the classroom. For example . . .

- Should he be expected to give oral reports, read out loud, or answer questions?
- Should you talk to him about his speech or ignore it?
- What should you do if other children tease the child?

These are only a few of the questions often asked by teachers.

The Preschool and Kindergarten Child

All children in this age group are busily learning to talk. As such, they make speech mistakes. We call these "mistakes" disfluencies. Some children have more than others, and this is normal. There are certain children, however, who have many disfluencies—particularly repetition and prolongation of sounds. These are quite noticeable to listeners.

If you are concerned that a child may be stuttering, do not pay any special attention to the child at this point. Rather, talk to a speech pathologist for suggestions.

Also, talk to the parents about their opinion of the problem so that you know whether this is typical speech behavior for the child. In most instances, if parents, teachers, and others listen to and answer the child in a patient, calm, and unemotional way, the child's speech returns to normal as his language abilities and his adjustments to school improve. If the child continues to have disfluencies, however, you may want to ask a speech pathologist to observe him.

The Elementary School Child

There are children in this age group who not only repeat and prolong sounds markedly but also struggle and become tense and frustrated in their efforts to talk. They need help. Without it their stuttering problem will probably adversely affect their classroom performance. As suggested with the preschool child, consult with a speech pathologist as well as with the parents and discuss your observations with them. If you, the parents, and the speech pathologist agree that this child's disfluencies are different from other children in your classroom, you may decide as a team to evaluate the child for stuttering.

A major concern for most teachers is the child's reaction to his stuttering in the classroom. How should the child be expected to participate in class? The answer to this question depends on the individual child. At one extreme is the child who may be quite unconcerned and happy to participate like any other child; at the other extreme is the child who will cry and refuse to talk. Most are somewhere in between. If the child is being seen by a speech pathologist, find out what she believes are reasonable expectations. Also, ask the child how he would like to participate. Sometimes participation requirements become part of the child's IEP.

Talk with the Child: Show Your Support

Usually it is advisable for you to talk with the child privately. Explain to him that when talking—just like when learning other skills—we sometimes bobble or repeat or get tangled up on words. With practice we improve. Explain that you are his teacher and that his stuttering is okay with you.

By talking to the child in this way, you help him learn that you are aware of his stuttering and that you accept it—and him.

Answering Questions

As you are asking questions in the classroom, you can do certain things to make it easier for a child who stutters.

- Initially, until she adjusts to the class, ask her questions that can be answered with relatively few words.
- If every child is going to be asked a question, find out if the child who stutters prefers to be called on early or later. Tension and worry can build up in some children when they have to wait their turn or, in others, when they know they have to answer sooner than other children. It is important to ask each child.
- Assure the whole class that (1) they will have as much time as they need to answer questions, and (2) you are interested in having them take time and think through their answers, not just answer quickly.

Reading Aloud in Class

Many children who stutter are able to handle oral reading tasks in the classroom satisfactorily, particularly if they are encouraged to practice at home. There will be some, however, who will stutter severely while reading aloud in class. The following suggestions may help these children.

Most children who stutter are fluent when reading in unison with someone else. Rather than not calling on the child who stutters, let her have her turn with one of the other children. Let the whole class read in pairs sometimes so that the child who stutters does not feel "special." Gradually she may become more confident and be able to manage reading out loud on her own.

Teasing

Teasing can be very painful for the student who stutters, and it should be eliminated as much as possible.

- If the child has obviously been upset by teasing, talk with her one-on-one. Help the child understand why others tease and brainstorm ideas for how to respond.
- If certain children are picking on the child, talk to these children alone and explain that teasing is unacceptable.
- Try to enlist the teasing children's help. Most want the approval of the teacher.
- If the problem persists, you may want to consult a guidance counselor or social worker if one is available in your building. They often have good suggestions for managing teasing.

Speech Therapy

If you are unsure whether a speech pathologist is available in your school, talk with your building administrator. Also, suggest to the parents that they seek one out who specializes in stuttering and who has a Certificate of Clinical Competence from the American Speech-Language-Hearing Association. The Stuttering Foundation of American offers free referrals at www.stutteringhelp.org and www.tartamudez.org or call 800/992-9392.

We have listed a few general points here. Always keep in mind that each child is different, and your caring positive attitude will make a big difference.

Tips for Talking with the Child Who Stutters

1. Do not tell the child to slow down or "relax."
2. Speak with the child in an unhurried way, pausing frequently. Wait a few seconds after the child finishes speaking before you begin to speak. This slows down the overall pace of conversation.
3. Help all members of the class learn to take turns talking and listening. All children—and especially those who stutter—find it much easier to talk when there are few interruptions, and they have the listener's attention.
4. Use your facial expressions, eye contact, and other body language to convey to the child that you are listening to the content of her message and not how she is talking.
5. Expect the same quality and quantity of work from the student who stutters as from the one who does not.
6. Try to decrease criticisms, rapid speech patterns, and interruptions.
7. Do not complete words for the child or talk for her.
8. Have a one-on-one conversation with the student who stutters about needed accommodations in the classroom. Be respectful of his needs but not enabling.
9. Do not make stuttering something to be ashamed of. Talk about stuttering just like any other matter.

C
Stories and Poems by People Who Stutter

The stories and poems contained in this section were written specifically for this manual. Contributors were asked to write a story or poem about a personal experience they thought would engage school-age children in talking openly about stuttering. These writings discuss experiences related to school and home and include teasing, empowerment, avoidance, relationships, and humorous situations. This collection of stories and poems were written at a higher reading level than those offered in the activities. They include language and content specifically geared to mature and older school-age children.

The material may be used to engage students with particular interests or needs. For example, if a student is interested in sports, you may want to assign Nora O'Connor's story titled "Taking the Ball Hard to the Basket—and in Life!" O'Connor's story compares stuttering to playing basketball, which many students will relate to. If a student likes poetry, then Elizabeth Kapstein's poem titled "Why Speak?" may help this student open up and talk about stuttering. If a student is uncomfortable with being teased, John Coakley's story "The Summer Before Sixth Grade" will offer him a way to consider how another person dealt with being teased.

You may use the stories and poems with many of the activities in this book, such as You Feel That Way Too?–Activity 31, Dear Abby–Activity 34, Big News–Activity 36, and Post It–Activity 37. For example, when using the activity You Feel That Way Too? you may have mature students choose a story or poem from this section. Students may also use these stories and poems to practice any speech tool.

Taking the Ball Hard to the Basket—and in Life!

by Nora A. O'Connor

My speech has always been very rocky. I don't feel that I have a lot of grace in my voice. When I was a kid, I dreamed of smooth, clean speech. I would watch other people speak and wonder why it was so easy for them. My mouth would move with lots of stumbling and hard blocks as I tried to get my words out. But when I put my foot on the basketball court, my moves were slick, quick, and full of style. I handled the ball like no other girl (or boy) my age. The kids used to call me "Cool Breeze." I would breeze right by the defenders without them knowing who passed them. My shot was nothing but "all net." Kids always wanted me on their team and didn't care that I stuttered. I knew I was in control on the basketball court and people respected me. I liked that feeling, but I didn't like how I felt about my stutter. I wanted to be as smooth with my speech as I was with handling the basketball. I wanted to feel the same amount of confidence as I did dribbling the ball.

It took some time to stand up to my stutter and face it off the way I did with the opponents on the basketball court. Slowly I started to feel that I could be a confident speaker even if I stuttered. I could look someone in the eye and believe that my words were going to be heard. I could drive my point across the same way I drove the ball hard to the basket. I won a lot of medals playing basketball and received many standing ovations. I lost a lot of games, too, and made mistakes on the court. I've had a lot of successes in my life as a person who stutters and have received a lot of praise. I also have felt very sad and frustrated with my stutter. But I continue to take that ball hard to the basket. I know if I don't try, then I won't ever know how it feels to win or lose.

Why Speak?

by Elizabeth Kapstein

sit down, speak to me.

don't speak till spoken to,
when spoken to, speak loudly.

don't speak when others are speaking,
speak softly, others are sleeping.

don't speak so loud, speak softly,
speak up, speak loud.

you speak so much,
you rarely speak,
you speak so softly I can hardly hear you.

no, no, don't speak yet,
okay, speak now.

you spoke? speak again.

Refusing a Stuttering Translator

by Gregory Snyder

It was a Sunday evening when my friend Matt and I showed up at the fast food restaurant. It was my turn to pay that time, so we walked up to the counter and began to place our orders. My friend placed his order with ease, but I did not. I was struggling to get my words out, so the guy behind the counter began to look to my friend and asked him to translate my broken words.

I felt shame because of my stuttered speech, but I also felt angry because the restaurant employee chose to give up on me and turn to my friend instead.

Something clicked inside of me because I immediately thought "no more!" After shooing my friend away, I forced the employee to listen to my order and my stuttering. Sure it may have taken a little longer than usual, and the restaurant employee sure did look nervous, but I got exactly what I wanted. If living my life to its fullest involves stuttering, then that's what I'll do.

Playground Justice

by Barry Yeoman

When I was 10 there was a bully who teased me all the time for stuttering. Peter would imitate my stutter and then laugh, and it upset me every day. I dreaded recess because I knew Peter would do this on the playground.

When I told my speech therapist, he had an idea: "Pretend Peter is auditioning for a play about stuttering, and tell him how good he sounds." I was skeptical, but I followed his suggestion. Next time Peter made fun of me, I said, "That sounds just like me! You should be in the movies. You're such a great actor!"

After two or three times, Peter changed completely. He saw that his teasing wasn't ruffling me anymore. He liked my approval and wanted to keep it. While we never really became friends, at least I no longer had an enemy, and I was no longer afraid of the playground.

Reasons

by Ken St. Louis

When I was a kid, I lived on a sheep ranch in Colorado. I went to a one-room school with four to six of my cousins, and I was the only one in my grade through the fifth grade. My aunt was our teacher. I don't remember ever being teased about my stuttering at school. I guess I was lucky for that. What I do remember is 4-H, which was our main social activity. When I was older, about 12 to 14 years old, I was on the 4-H livestock judging team. My biggest problem was not judging the classes of four animals (like four lambs or four steers) but in giving "reasons" afterward. Giving reasons was really a formal speech to the main judge, where we had to go individually to this adult judge and, in 5 minutes, explain exactly why we judged the animals from best to worst in the order that we did. I found that I could not predict how much my stuttering would occur on the reasons; it was sometimes just a minor nuisance, but sometimes it was severe (for me!) and prevented me from thinking clearly and doing my best. I'm sure I substituted words and reorganized my thoughts to minimize stuttering, which no doubt ended up in lower scores on my reasons.

Sharing a Problem

by Alan Badmington

When I was young I developed a stutter. I had difficulty at school when reading aloud. I avoided asking and answering questions in class because I was afraid of becoming tongue-tied. I was afraid that I might stutter.

I never really talked about it with my friends or family—I guess I felt too embarrassed. Besides, I didn't think that they really understood.

When I grew older everything changed. I started to talk about my stutter with everyone—even strangers. I didn't hide it anymore. I realized it wasn't something to be ashamed of.

And do you know what? I found that people didn't really care about my stutter—they were more interested in me as a person. They admired my sporting skills—they enjoyed my jokes and sense of humor—they liked being in my company. And above all they could see that my stutter was only a small part of me. I was Alan the athlete, Alan the poet, Alan the coin collector, and (way down their list) Alan who also just happened to stutter.

It wasn't a big deal to them. We are all unique. I just happened to talk a little differently from most. So what?

Looking back, I only wish I had been more open about my stutter at a much earlier age. I didn't need to bottle it up inside. If you share a problem with someone, then it never seems quite so bad. I now realize that if I'd talked about it with others, I wouldn't have felt so alone and isolated. Why don't you try it?

The Time Game

by Junior Tereva

"Hey what's the time?" I was asked. Suddenly everyone's eyes are focused on me. How silly not to be anticipating that I was going to be the only person in the room wearing a watch.

My thoughts are, "Oh, no! It's 8:35 p.m.—**danger**! I'm going to have problems saying this one." At the same time I feel panic and fear and confusion beginning to build.

Quickly I respond: "Well the big hand is pointing this way, and the little hand is pointing in this direction, and it's nighttime"—my arms imitating a clock. Finally someone shouts out, "Ah ha . . . 8:35 p.m. . . . cool game!" I think to myself, "Phew! That was a close one." Pretending to be a clock saved me from stuttering.

If I could go back and change my way of thinking toward my stutter during childhood, I would be more open and not avoid challenging words or situations. It's taken me 30 years to understand that it's okay to stutter, and it's okay to show the world who you really are. People accept you regardless.

The Fear of a Word

by Jason W. Pearson

Not many know just how I feel,
The fear, doubt, anger, not knowing how to deal.
What is the right word?
What can I say?
Just some thoughts that pass this way.

How will they look at me; what will they think?
If they laugh at my speech, surely my spirit will sink.
If I could just say what I wanted to say
I would do so much more each and every day.
I could act on stage, run for office, or just be me.
I can achieve what I dreamed to be.

I like to laugh, play, and compete;
I like good friends and going out to eat.
I have a part of me that I don't like to show;
People have made fun of and treated me kind of low.

I may say things differently,
But my message is still the same;
I will never give up,
I won't give in to shame.

I won't keep my mouth and thoughts on a mental shelf;
I will be ambitious, true, and I will like myself.
I cannot change the way I speak;
I will climb to the top of this enormous peak.
There is only I that stands in my way
Of thinking and speaking what I choose to say.

I will not be defeated by a word,
A person, a situation, or even a verb.
I will look my fears in the eye
And say what I want; I know I won't die.

The Summer Before Sixth Grade

by John Coakley

The summer before sixth grade I went to a 5-week speech therapy program in upstate New York. It took a lot of very hard work but it seemed to pay off. The program finished in early August, and I had never been so fluent. My family couldn't shut me up!

On the first day of school, some of my friends were curious about the program—and stuttering in general—so I was answering their questions. Nobody was making fun of me, and it felt good to be able to talk about a subject few of them knew much about. Even the really popular kids had a few questions. Sometimes popular kids can be cool. Jason was not that kind of popular kid. By the end of the conversation that we'd all been enjoying, he said, "Well, I don't have to worry about speech class. I've got a clean mouth." "That's got nothing to do with it, Jason," I replied. Fortunately, everybody else seemed to understand that Jason was the one who should have been embarrassed and not the kid who stuttered.

By the way, my month of "perfect" fluency ended during my first French class. I found that it was a lot harder to use my speech tools in a different language. That didn't mean that the speech tools had failed me. It just meant that using them would take more work than I had thought.

Remain Who You Are!

by Yelena Averbukh

When I was 7 years old, I did not know that I stuttered. But apparently that was the fact because my mother called a strange guy called a speech pathologist. He wanted me to sing when I talked or whistle before every phrase I said. I remember that I did not mind spending time with him, but would have rather played with my friends in the park.

I had always had some friends to play with because I could think of new games to play, and I was always in the center of action. Even if I stuttered then, it did not matter to me because I paid it no mind, and frankly my friends were too involved in the games I designed to notice me stutter.

When I got a little bit older and turned 12, I became more self-conscious and my stuttering started to bother me. I started to avoid all possible speaking situations, such as phone conversations and chatting with my friends. I did not return phone calls and did not respond to birthday party invitations. I was feeling very lonely and wished to be with my friends.

My friends thought that I became a snob and that I did not like their company anymore. They stopped approaching me and started teasing me for the silence that I carried with me as a protective shield from stuttering.

It took me a long, long time—almost 15 years—to figure out that no one but me cared about my stuttering. My friends did not care about my speech. All they wanted was for me to remain their friend and not a silent outsider.

I hope this story will remind you to always be the nice and friendly person that you are, even if you stutter at times.

Revenge Doesn't Make You Feel Better

by Jason W. Pearson

When I was in middle school, I never wanted to go to school. I would be teased by most other kids because I could not speak the same way they could. I would stutter on most of my words, especially "hello" and people's names.

They would make up names to call me. They would laugh and imitate the way I stuttered. I was never the most athletic of the kids; I would say I was average. I was very thin, not the fastest, but I would never give up. I never quit. Most times when we would pick teams for games, I was usually in the middle or close to last.

There would be times I would daydream that I was a superhero—the Hulk or Spider-man were some of my favorites. And the kids that teased me were the enemies. Of course the superhero always won and did everything perfectly. Everybody liked the superhero.

Most times when I was teased, I would ignore it and do something I enjoyed: play on a computer, read a book, or play basketball. When they saw I was not going to get mad and react, they lost interest, and we would play a game of tag or kickball or some other group game.

One day in seventh grade, a group of kids—David, Brett, and Maurice—were teasing me. I had enough, and I was going to get revenge and show them that I was tough. I was going to play the part of the superhero and not take being teased anymore.

I chased them as they taunted me, and I finally caught each one and punched them in the stomach as hard as I could—first Brett, who was bigger than I was; then David, who was slower than I was; and then Maurice. Except with Maurice—I wrestled him to the ground and sat on his chest and punched him in both arms repeatedly until he cried. It was a bad feeling. I had just wanted them to stop. I wanted them to accept me, but from then on they were afraid of me. I got in trouble with the teacher, the principal, and my parents. I was given detention, I had to write a letter of apology, and I lost all computer privileges. I was not included in any of the group games for a long time, and I had this bad feeling in my stomach for hurting Maurice. I still have that feeling in my stomach when I think about what I did. I made someone feel as bad as I felt when they teased me. I did not feel better like I thought I would; I felt worse.

I did not want to hurt anyone that bad. I had just wanted to make them stop. It did not stop. The pain I felt from causing pain to another person was just as bad as the pain I felt when I was being teased. I found out later, when we all became friends, it was better to find common interests and show them I liked the same things they did.

Fortunately we became good friends the next year and had sleepovers at each other's house and had a lot of fun. I still think about when I hurt Maurice, and that same twang of pain from hurting someone else sits in my stomach. Revenge was not a good feeling—acceptance was.

Registration Day
by David Brandau

I remember it like yesterday, though it is now almost 20 years ago. It was registration day for the second year of high school. My stuttering had shown its ugly head during the first year. I could no longer hide, control, and dance around this monster like I did in elementary school. Now I was at the great city high school where I was to follow my father, the great track star, and the great man whom I could never please. I walked in the giant front doors, happy after a nice restful summer. I had almost forgotten about the monster that had shown his big and ugly face last year. But there was Balser to remind me: "Hey look, there's BBBBBBBBBBBBBBBBBrandau." For me the world stopped, and all I could see were 100 or perhaps one million of my classmates staring at me, the class dummy. Yes, summer was over, yet the terrible high school years were only just beginning.

Was there something that I could have said or done to make it better? I chose to keep silent, hoping it would go away. Three years later the silence was deafening, and all that I had to say I had said to myself. I hated myself. It took years to recover, and only now am I a happy stuttering fool, having the time of my life, doing anything and going anywhere that I want. I am a free man. But I think I could have been a free teenager, if only I could have found someone to talk to—a therapist, a fellow stutterer, anyone. Please talk, say anything, don't silence your voice—it's beautiful; rejoice in your stutter, for it is you, truly you.

Stuttering Can Be Funny
by Bernie Weiner

Most of you who read this must think that there cannot be anything funny about stuttering. How can something that hurts so bad make you laugh even a little bit? Well, believe it or not, you will sometimes have something happen because you stutter that makes you want to bust out laughing. Hopefully, people will be laughing with you and not at you.

One time when I was at a meeting in Boston for people who stutter, a bunch of us decided to go see some of the interesting places in the city. We also wanted to have dinner at a nice restaurant that was right on the water. In Boston people ride the trains to go to a lot of different places, so we also took the train. Everything went well until we took the train back to our hotel. Not all of us could fit on the first train. A few of us squeezed into the first train while others had to wait for the next train to come. As the train car door was closing, I tried to tell the rest of the people where to get off to get back to our hotel. At that moment I had the most gigantic speech block that you can imagine. I tried everything to say the name of the stop where they should get off, but I just couldn't do it. I have the bad habit of tapping my cheek when I get caught in a stuttering block. As the door to the train car closed, I was still tapping my cheek, trying to get the word out, and the train started to leave. I was worried that the rest of the people would not know where to get off.

When we got off the train, we waited for the rest of our group to get back to see if they had gotten lost. As my friends got off the second train, they were all tapping their cheeks like I had been doing. This made me laugh so hard that I was almost crying. We all saw that stuttering can sometimes result in something funny. It is okay to laugh and not always feel sad because we talk differently. Try to keep a smile on your face when things get real hard and your stuttering is at its worst. It will get better—you will see.

What Is Your Name?

by Anthony Troiano

I remember my school years very vividly. Unfortunately, much of what I remember about school was the constant fear that I might stutter. My stutter was severe, and I never met anyone else who stuttered. Fluent people were forever telling me how they "used" to stutter or how they knew another person who stuttered, but I never seemed to meet up with this army of stutterers. I was embarrassed by my stutter and went to great lengths to hide it. I would carefully pick and choose my words to answer questions others might pose and would answer using as few as possible. If I started to block on a sound, I would use different words or stop talking altogether. Anything not to stutter! But there was one word I could never avoid, my own name—Anthony!

What could I do, tell others my name was Joe or Bob when they asked? At the time I wished it was a simple one-syllable name, but, no, I was blessed with three! If you count my last name there were six syllables for me to block on, and I would agonize over the possibility of doing just that. One day my most feared humiliation would come true. One day in the schoolyard I ran into another student whom I had seen a few times when changing classes. He was with a group of friends, and he asked me, "What is your name?" I could feel my throat tighten before he finished his question, and I immediately hesitated before attempting to say anything. He looked at me for a second before joking with his friends, "This guy does not even know his own name!" I wished a trap door would open below me providing a quick escape from my tormenters. My fear and embarrassment of stuttering was so strong that it never occurred to me to be open about my stuttering and to educate others.

Today I have learned so much about myself as a person who stutters, and I talk freely without fear. And about my name: The name that caused me so much anxiety all those years ago now fits me like a glove. I am self-employed, and the name of my company contains my own name, compelling me to announce it every time the telephone rings. Imagine—not only saying my name but doing it on the telephone! Sometimes I answer fluently, sometimes not, but the joy is in the doing. Also, I have since met many other stutterers and have come to realize that I am not alone.

Getting Married

by Andy Floyd

When I was a teenager growing up with stuttering, a weight problem, and thick glasses, I never imagined myself dating, let alone getting married. But in my late teens, I lost some weight, got contacts, and most importantly, gained self-esteem and confidence.

So, there it was—I was in my early 20s and I was getting married. From a year before the wedding to the moment itself, I never thought twice about my decision to marry the most beautiful, smartest, and nicest girl I had ever met. What I did worry about were the vows and the ring ceremony. My wife-to-be had the habit of watching "The Wedding Story" on TLC, and I watched some of them with her. Every time I saw it, my mind focused on all the speaking parts of the ceremony. I had a hard time talking in front of one other person sometimes, let alone the 150 expected at our wedding. I thought of all the things I could do to help myself—I had gone through a bunch of speech therapy, I had gone to National Stuttering Association meetings and conventions, and I was a speech–language pathologist myself for goodness sake! I must be able to come up with something to calm myself down enough to be able to use some tools. Right? Well, no, not really.

There we were at my wedding, in front of those 150 people on top of a mountain, and we had to speak into microphones that just added to my fright. My wife had informed the minister about my stuttering, but he was not very understanding. For example, I blocked on my wife's name during the ceremony, and the minister actually whispered her name to me like I had forgotten it! I wanted to punch him; but everything went on with no problems. Because we videotaped our wedding, I've gone back and counted that I stuttered about seven times during the ceremony. Did it ruin my wedding? Did my wife immediately divorce me? Nothing can be further from the truth. The whole time I was looking into the eyes of the one person who really mattered and who understands and loves me—my wife.

I'm writing this because when I was a teenager, I thought that stuttering during my wedding was a huge deal, and I would do anything to speak fluently. Now I realize that the words in the vows and ring ceremony are what's important—not how you say them.

Class Presentations

by Mark De Biasio

Throughout grade school and high school I would always hate having to give presentations in front of the class. It was bad enough being called upon by the teacher to answer a question or read a paragraph out of a book, but I couldn't imagine how I would be able to do a presentation in front of the class while having all eyes on me. While waiting for my my turn to present, I would have butterflies in my stomach and sweaty hands. I would be silently reading over my presentation while looking for words that I knew would give me trouble and trying to change them with other words that would be easier to say. I would hope that the students presenting before me would take up all of the time for the day so my turn would be put off until the next day. When my turn finally came to present, I would keep my head down and read from my papers rather than looking at my audience. I was afraid to make eye contact with anyone. Some other things I would do would be to stomp my foot on words that I might get stuck on. I would also leave out parts of my presentation and would often have points taken away from my grade due to my presentation being too short and for reading from the paper.

Now that I am grown up, I sometimes have to go to meetings and speak in front of small groups of people. I still get nervous but try not to think about it as much as when I was younger. I have found that by keeping my mind on what I have to say, rather than worrying about if I am going to stutter, has allowed me to get through my speaking a lot easier. I still have blocks from time to time but try not to let it bother me.

As an adult I never really experienced anyone making fun of me like I sometimes did as a child. I found that children notice stuttering more than adults do and react to it more by teasing. I notice now that people are more interested in what I have to say rather than how I say it.

The Power of Humor

by Lee Reeves

I've always had a pretty good sense of humor. I could make a joke or say something funny about just about anything. Anything, that is, except for my stuttering. My stuttering was always something I tried to hide. It was humiliating and embarrassing. It was certainly not funny.

That all changed though when I was 12. It happened in the seventh grade one day in science class. We had to give an oral report—the most dreaded event for a kid who stutters. My report was on "matter." During my presentation I wanted to say that all matter is made up of molecules. But when I got to the word molecule I found myself in one of those humdinger stuttering blocks. It was the kind of block where you're just stuck.

As I stood in front of the class, all I could get out was "mmmmmmm-a-mmmmmm-mmmmm-a-mmmmmmm . . ." A crowbar couldn't have pried my lips apart. And then it happened. I blurted out "atoms!" Everyone just cracked up including the teacher and me. I had changed the word but was still technically correct because matter is made up of molecules, and molecules are composed of atoms. What was remarkable though was that everyone was laughing *with* me and not *at* me. I wasn't trying to be funny, but what came out was very humorous. Everyone, including me, became pretty relaxed over my stutter, and I went ahead and finished my speech without too much more trouble.

At home that evening at dinner, I told my parents what had happened, and we all laughed again. It was then that I realized that using humor to break the tension about my stuttering could be a very useful tool. I'm not suggesting that you avoid fearful words by switching to another one. It just happened that way that day, and I have since learned other tools to help me get through troublesome words or sounds.

Since then I have often used humor to help me, as well as those I'm speaking with, to "break the silence" about stuttering. Using phrases like, "Wow! I'm having a bad word day!" or "I'm a professional stutterer—don't try this at home!" or "That was a good one—wanna try it?" are great ways to get stuttering out in the open and be less mysterious. Although stuttering is not always funny, being able to laugh *about* a stuttering event and not *at* the person who stutters can help all of us be better communicators.

D

Altered Speech Feedback

Altered Speech Feedback's (ASF) most notable forms, Delayed Auditory Feedback (DAF) and Frequency Altered Feedback (FAF), are now available in portable and wearable prosthetic devices. The cost for these modern units is approximately $5,000 plus additional evaluation and fitting costs. Altered speech feedback devices are typically worn in one ear. These prosthetic devices work by capturing the speaker's speech signal, altering this signal digitally, and then reintroducing the speech signal into the speaker's ear. The most technologically advanced altered speech feedback devices fit neatly in the ear or behind the ear, utilize both DAF and FAF technology, and are indistinguishable from miniature, state-of-the-art digital hearing aids. Such devices are designed to promote forward-moving speech in those who stutter. In other words, altered speech feedback devices are used in an attempt to reduce the frequency of stuttering. These prosthetic devices have received a lot of public attention and have been featured on television talk shows, such as "The Oprah Winfrey Show," on radio news programs, in newspapers, and throughout the Internet.

DAF units capture the speech signal and then digitally return it to the stutterer's ear with a delay time of varying lengths. Although it remains unknown exactly how DAF reduces stuttering, one interpretation suggests that the DAF requires users to slow their speech, thus reducing stuttering (Bloodstein, 1995; Starkweather, 1987). Others feel that DAF may promote forward-moving speech simply as a result of auditory feedback and not as a result of slowed speech (Ingham & Andrews, 1971; Sparks, Grant, Millay, Walker-Batsen, & Hynan, 2002). It has been demonstrated that the delay may be set as short as 50 milliseconds to reduce stuttering (Kalinowski, Stuart, Sark, & Armson, 1996; Stuart & Kalinowski, 1996), and thus speech rate reduction resulting from DAF may not play a significant role in the decrease of stuttering. Others have noted that DAF also increases fluency when people who stutter speak at fast rates (Armson & Stuart, 1998; Kalinowski, Stuart, Wamsley, & Rastatter, 1999). This would indicate that DAF might reduce stuttering for reasons other than slowed or prolonged speech.

FAF units alter the frequency or pitch of the client's voice (the speech signal) that is digitally returned to the stutterer's ear. The wearer of an FAF device usually chooses to hear his own voice at a slightly higher pitch, but lower pitch settings are available as well. Some have reported that FAF has fewer noticeable side effects on the speech of stutterers than DAF (Starkweather & Givens-Ackerman, 1997), and others have noted that FAF may reduce stuttering, in some situations, by up to 80 to 90% (Kalinowski, Stuart, Wamsley, & Rastatter, 1999).

Some researchers believe that DAF and FAF facilitate forward-moving speech because these devices emulate choral speech (Andrews et al., 1983; Armson & Stuart, 1998; Kalinowski, Armson, & Stuart, 1995; Kalinowski & Saltuklaroglu, 2004). When stutterers speak in chorus or in unison, such as when reading the same passage or reciting the Pledge of Allegiance, most do not stutter (Kalinowski & Saltuklaroglu, 2003).

Regardless of the numerous rationales or theories that attempt to explain the effects of altered speech feedback on the speech of stutterers, Andrews et al. (1983) found that the various forms of altered speech feedback have been reported initially to reduce the stuttering behaviors of nearly all, if not all, stutterers. Because DAF and FAF devices are prosthetic, once the stutterer takes the device off, the reduction in stuttering behaviors stops (Snyder, 2002; Starkweather & Givens-Ackerman, 1997). In other words, as of yet there is no research to suggest that these devices offer any significant carryover effect. For some, DAF and FAF may even lose their effectiveness while being used (Starkweather & Givens-Ackerman). Significantly though, clinicians are noticing that some users of altered speech feedback devices are experiencing increased speaking confidence once the device is removed. When discussing a particular altered speech feedback device that uses both DAF and FAF, Bartles & Ramig (2004) suggested that the DAF and FAF technology in the device "may not affect overt stuttering behaviors, but instead supply some wearers with greater confidence" (p. 66). Carryover effects regarding speaker confidence is an area ripe for future research.

DAF (Starkweather, 1987; Van Riper, 1973) and FAF (Armson & Stuart, 1998) technologies have been reported to be highly variable among users. One study reported that FAF (the authors used the term *frequency-shifted feedback*) offered only a minor reduction of stuttering behaviors in children, whereas it offered a much greater reduction of stuttering behaviors in adults (Howell, Sackin, & Williams, 1999).

Having met many users of altered speech feedback devices, it is safe to say that some stutterers offer positive comments and experiences with DAF and FAF devices. Others offer mixed reports, whereas others offer negative experiences. This type of individualized feedback is very similar to the varied reports that people who stutter offer toward any other type of therapy or treatment. Mackesey (2003) warns, "For some, DAF is a godsend; for others, the results are not nearly as dramatic. So before you purchase, it will pay to do a little homework" (p. 3).

When discussing a specific unit that combines DAF and FAF technology, Ramig (2003) recommends that before purchasing the device, the client participate in a 3-hour fitting with a licensed provider. The cost of this fitting may be as much as $400 (Mackesey, 2003; Ramig, 2003).

Altered speech feedback devices may be used in various ways. Whereas wearers may choose to use the device during most speaking situations, some stutterers find DAF and FAF units to be useful during specific speaking situations, such as when giving a presentation or on difficult stuttering days. These devices may also offer immediate relief for stutterers who have not found relief elsewhere. For example, Jezer (1998) explained that at the age of 57 he felt able to communicate effectively only by using an electronic altered speech feedback device.

On the negative side, it is commonly reported that many school-age children feel stigmatized when wearing an altered speech feedback device. It is important to note, however, that many children who stutter also feel stigmatized by attending speech class. Mackesey (2003) has offered caution about fitting a child with a portable altered speech feedback device and has warned, "The child may end up believing that he or she must permanently rely on an external speech aid" (p. 3).

At this point in the development of altered speech feedback devices, poor signal-to-noise ratio is a common complaint. Microphones on the units pick up and alter not only the speech signal but environmental sounds as well (Skotko, 2004). Environmental noise remains a problem—one that can be both distracting and annoying. Put simply, altered speech feedback devices may help the stutterer speak, but may impede certain listening tasks and listening situations. For example, a child or adult using a DAF device in a classroom situation would currently hear many environmental noises through a delay. To avoid this, the student would have to keep the unit off until ready to speak and then turn it on before speaking. One popular device has also been reported to produce a hissing noise that emanates from the device itself (Skotko). Considering that the predominant time spent in most classes is spent listening, the use of altered speech feedback may prove to be distracting for students. Also, because the devices are typically worn in one ear, many clients may demonstrate a functional, monaural hearing loss while the device is being worn.

An adult woman who stutters described her experience using altered speech feedback. These comments speak to the complexity of the issue. She explained that as a doctor she often presents to dozens and sometimes hundreds of her colleagues at medical meetings. Several times over the years she has felt completely unable to speak without the use of her altered speech feedback unit during these meetings. She described the use of altered speech feedback during these difficult speaking situations as a "miracle." She also discovered that wearing her device afforded her a comfortable and practical way to explain to her colleagues that she was a stutterer and was using the device to help her talk. She found this form of advertising her stuttering to be beneficial and rewarding. Occasionally, she even wore her unit turned off simply to give herself an excuse to talk openly about stuttering.

Although at times this doctor felt her altered speech feedback unit offered her tremendous relief, she also felt defeated by her reliance on it and labeled her device the "stealer of the soul." She found the environmental noise that her microphone picked up to be highly distracting during these public-speaking situations. She felt that wearing her altered speech feedback unit removed her from the interaction aspect of communication by making it difficult to focus on her audience.

In discussing the therapeutic ramifications of altered speech feedback (ASF) devices, Snyder stated:

> A prosthetic device is nothing more than appliance. It's not designed to "cure" stuttering, only to reduce the frequency of stuttering. While ASF prosthetic devices could be used as the sole component in stuttering management, they can also be incorporated with other strategies, such as stuttering modification and anti-avoidance strategies. How an ASF device is incorporated into treatment (or if it is incorporated at all) depends on the personal therapeutic goals of each individual client. (G. Snyder, personal communication, August 16, 2004)

Starkweather and Givens-Ackerman (1997) suggest that some school-age children who are difficult to treat may derive some benefit from DAF or FAF units. The clinician might consider keeping an altered speech feedback unit in her office and use it, on occasion, simply as a way of demonstrating to clients that they are physically capable of speaking in a modified, less-struggled manner (Van Riper, 1973). Of course, the clinician may also engage students in choral-speaking activities to demonstrate that they are capable of producing forward-moving speech. Either way, *it would be inaccurate to suggest to students that because they may speak for a short period of time without stuttering (using these devices or techniques), that they would be able to speak like this at all times.* Clinicians need to keep in mind that DAF and FAF units cease to reduce stuttering once the devices are removed or turned off. By allowing students to use an altered speech feedback device on occasion during therapy, the clinician is merely demonstrating that their bodies are physically capable of speaking in a forward-moving, less struggled way.

Parents who hear about altered speech feedback devices may call a speech pathologist's office and ask, "I just saw a device on television that cures stuttering—can you get my son (or daughter) one?" Parents often feel desperate and guilty about not being able to rid their child of stuttering and may rush quickly into purchasing an altered speech feedback device. And, as many people in the stuttering community know, decisions made out of fear and desperation are often poor decisions. The clinician needs to be well informed about altered speech feedback and protect parents from any claims that insinuate or imply a stuttering cure.

Because of recent technological advances and the advent of portable altered speech feedback units, research on these matters is both ongoing and eagerly awaited. Snyder (2003) offers a realistic summation. He writes, "We should inform clients that the compelling fluency enhancement via speech feedback is not a panacea, and its prosthetic implementation continues to be tested and improved" (p. 35).

E

Resources for People Who Stutter

FRIENDS: The National Association of Young People Who Stutter

Web address: www.friendswhostutter.org
Phone: 866/866-8335
Co-founder and director: Lee Caggiano
Mailing and e-mail addresses for Lee Caggiano: 145 Hayrick Lane, Commack, NY 11725-1520; LCaggiano@aol.com
Co-founder and newsletter editor: John Ahlbach
Mailing and e-mail addresses for John Ahlbach: 1220 Rosita Road, Pacifica, CA 94044-4223; jtahlbach@aol.com

Founded in 1998, FRIENDS is a nonprofit, volunteer organization that provides a network of support for children and teens who stutter, their families, adults who stutter, and professionals. FRIENDS publishes a monthly newsletter titled *Reaching Out,* that includes articles and material for parents, clinicians, and people of all ages who stutter. FRIENDS offers an annual convention, regional workshops, and an Internet discussion forum for teens who stutter. The organization publishes a number of books and posters.

National Stuttering Association (NSA)

Web address: www.WeStutter.org
Phone: 800/WE STUTTER (937-8888)
E-mail address: info@westutter.org
Mailing address: 119 W. 40th Street, 14th Floor, New York, NY, 10018
Director of operations: Tammy Flores
National spokesperson: Lee Reeves

The National Stuttering Association (formerly the National Stuttering Project) is a nonprofit self-help organization for adults, teens, children, families, and professionals with over 80 local chapters. The NSA publishes a bimonthly newsletter titled *Letting Go* and a quarterly publication called *CARE* for parents of children who stutter, edited by Robert Quesal. The NSA offers many books, posters, and publications on its Web site, runs an on-line teen chat room, and has an annual convention. Several stories and poems published by the NSA are included in this book.

Our Time Theatre Company

Web address: www.ourtimetheatre.org
Phone: 212/414-9696
E-mail address: moreinfo@ourtimetheatre.org
Mailing address: One Union Square West, Suite 810A, New York, NY 10003
Founder and artistic director: Taro Alexander

Our Time Theatre Company is a nonprofit organization dedicated to providing an artistic home for people who stutter. Based in New York City, Our Time provides an environment free from ridicule where young people who stutter discover the joy of creating and performing original theater. Our Time company members study acting, singing, playwriting, drumming, and dance with plays that are performed in New York City theaters, at speech–language–hearing conferences, for the greater stuttering community, at conventions, in schools, and for the general public. Our Time has two companies, one for children who stutter (ages 9–12) and one for teens who stutter (ages 13–19), and serves all its members free of charge.

Stuttering Foundation of America (SFA)

English Web address: www.stutteringhelp.org
Spanish Web address: www.tartamudez.org
Phone: 800/992-9392, 800/967-7700
Fax: 901/452-3931
E-mail address: stutter@stutteringhelp.org
Mailing address: 3100 Walnut Grove, Suite 603, P.O. Box 11749, Memphis, TN 38111-0749
President: Jane Fraser

The Stuttering Foundation of America (SFA) is a nonprofit organization that publishes many low-cost books, videos, DVDs, posters, and other materials for professionals, stutterers, and family members. The SFA sponsors conferences, seminars, and training workshops for speech–language pathologists. The SFA also offers various brochures and publications on its Web site. Many of the SFA materials, including the Web site, are available in Spanish.

Stuttering Home Page

Web address: www.stutteringhomepage.com
Site maintained by: Judith Maginnis Kuster
E-mail address: judith.kuster@mnsu.edu

The Stuttering Home Page is a valuable Internet resource for people who stutter and for professionals because of its thorough content and endless links to other stuttering resources. This Web site offers information about stuttering for children, teens, and adults who stutter; families; and professionals. For children, there are kid- and teen-friendly sections that offer activities. For professionals, there is a plethora of information, including the complete catalog of the International Stuttering Awareness Day (ISAD) online conferences, papers and research articles about stuttering and other fluency disorders, and information on therapy and support groups from around the world.

References

Ainsworth, S. (1968). A clinical success: Lynne. In J. Fraser (Ed.), *Stuttering: Successes and failures in therapy* (Publication No. 6, pp. 11–20). Memphis, TN: Stuttering Foundation of America.

Ainsworth, S., & Fraser, J. (2002). *If your child stutters: A guide for parents* (Publication No. 11). Memphis, TN: Stuttering Foundation of America.

American Speech-Language-Hearing Association (2000). *Schools survey 2000.* Rockville, MD: Author.

Amster, B. J., & Starkweather, C. W. (2000). Comments on "utterance length, syntactic complexity, and childhood stuttering" by Yaruss. *Journal of Speech, Language, and Hearing Research, 43,* 810–813.

Amy (1999). Climbing to the top. In A. Bradberry & N. Reardon (Eds.), *Our Voices: Inspirational insight from young people who stutter* (p. 26). Anaheim Hills, CA: National Stuttering Association.

Anderson, J. D., & Conture, E. G. (2000). Language abilities of children who stutter: A preliminary study. *Journal of Fluency Disorder, 25,* 283–304.

Andrews, G., Craig, A., Feyer, A. M., Hoddinott, S., Howie, P., & Neilson, M. (1983). Stuttering: A review of research findings and theories circa 1982. *Journal of Speech and Hearing Disorders, 48,* 226–246.

Andrews, G., & Cutler, J. (1974). Guilt, shame, and family socialization. *Journal of Family Issues, 18,* 99–123.

Armson, J., & Stuart, A. (1998). Effect of extended exposure to frequency altered feedback on stuttering during reading and spontaneous speech. *Journal of Speech, Language, and Hearing Research, 41,* 479–490.

Arndt, J., & Healey, E. C. (2001). Concomitant disorders in school-aged children who stutter. *Language, Speech, and Hearing Services in Schools, 32,* 68–78.

Bartles, S., & Ramig, P. (2004, April). Clinical research into the use of the SpeechEasy® device. *Stammering Research, 1,* p. 66. Retrieved August 11, 2005, from http://www.stamres.psychol.ucl.ac.uk/Vol1-Issue1.pdf

Bergmann, G. (1987). Stuttering as a prosodic disturbance: A link between speech execution and emotional processes. In H. F. M. Peters and W. Hulstijin (Eds.), *Speech motor dynamics in stuttering* (pp. 393–407). New York: Springer-Verlag.

Blood, G. W., Ridenour, V. J., Jr., Qualls, C. D., & Hammer, C. S. (2003). Co-occurring disorders in children who stutter. *Journal of Communication Disorders, 36,* 427–448.

Blood, G., & Seider, R. (1981). The concomitant problems of young stutterers. *Journal of Speech and Hearing Research, 46,* 31–33.

Bloodstein, O. (1995) *A handbook on stuttering* (5th ed.). San Diego, CA: Singular Publishing Group.

Bloodstein, O. (2002). Early stuttering as a type of language difficulty. *Journal of Fluency Disorders, 27,* 163–167.

Breitenfeldt, D. H. (2003, October 1). *A stutterer's odyssey through life.* Paper presented at the 2003 International Stuttering Awareness Day Online Conference. Retrieved March 7, 2005, from http://www.mnsu.edu/comdis/isad6/papers/breitenfeldt6.html

Breitenfeldt, D. H., & Lorenz, D. R. (2000). *Successful stuttering management program (SSMP) for adolescent and adult stutterers* (2nd ed.). Cheney: Eastern Washington University.

Brisk, D. J., Healey, E. C., & Hux, K. A. (1997). Clinician's training and confidence associated with treating school-age children who stutter: A national survey. *Language, Speech, & Hearing Services in Schools, 28,* 164–175.

Bryngelson, B., Chapman, M. E., & Hanson, O. K. (1950). *Know yourself: A workbook for those who stutter.* Minneapolis, MN: Bruges Publishing.

Cable, R. M., Colcord, R. D., & Petrosino, L. (2002). Self-reported anxiety of adults who do and do not stutter. *Perceptual and Motor Skill, 94,* 775–784.

Caggiano, L. (1998, October 1). *Adolescents who stutter: The urgent need for support groups (a parent's perspective).* Paper presented at the 1998 International Stuttering Awareness Day Online Conference. Retrieved March 7, 2005, from http://www.mnsu.edu/dept/comdis/isad/papers/caggiano.html

Caggiano, M. (1998). Stutter. In J. Westbrook & J. Ahlbach (Eds.), *Listen with your heart: Reflections on growing up with stuttering* (pp. 42–43). Pacifica, CA: FRIENDS.

Caggiano, L., Kapstein, E., & Reitzes, P. (2003, September 23). *Overview of stuttering, treatment, and the stuttering self-help community.* Presentation at the New York Academy of Traumatic Brain Injury's Seminar on Speech and Language Disorders: Biological Basis and Clinical Manifestations, New York, NY.

Campbell J. H. (2003). Therapy for elementary school-age children who stutter. In H. H. Gregory, J. H. Campbell, D. G. Hill, & C. B. Gregory (Eds.), *Stuttering therapy: Rationale and procedures* (pp. 217–262). Needham Heights, MA: Allyn & Bacon.

Carabetta, M. (1999). Living as a broken record. In A. Bradberry & N. Reardon (Eds.), *Our Voices: Inspirational insight from young people who stutter* (pp. 55–56). Anaheim Hills, CA: National Stuttering Association.

Carlisle, J. A. (1985). *Tangled tongue: Living with a stutter.* Canada: University of Toronto Press.

Caseman, L. F. (2001). No more constant dread. In K. O. St. Louis (Ed.), *Living with stuttering: Stories, basics, resources, and hope* (pp. 117–119). Morgantown, WV: Populore.

Cepler, M. (2003). From that day forward. In J. Ahlbach & L. Caggiano (Eds.), *The best of reaching out* (pp. 3–4). Pacifica, CA: FRIENDS.

Chmela, C. A., & Reardon, N. A. (1997). *The school-age child who stutters: Working effectively with attitudes and emotions.* Handout to be used in conjunction with video presentation. Memphis, TN: Stuttering Foundation of America.

Chmela, C. A., & Reardon, N. A. (2001). *The school-age child who stutters: Working effectively with attitudes and emotions* (Publication No. 5). Memphis, TN: Stuttering Foundation of America.

Christian. (2002, September–October). My name is Christian and I wish it wasn't. *Reaching Out.* (Available from FRIENDS, 1220 Rosita Rd., Pacifica, CA 94044-4223), p. 4.

Cochran, C. (1998). Am I the only one? In J. Westbrook & J. Ahlbach (Eds.), *Listen with your heart: Reflections on growing up with stuttering* (pp. 33–34). Pacifica, CA: FRIENDS.

Conture, E. G., (2001). *Stuttering: Its nature, diagnosis, and treatment* (2nd ed.). Needham Heights, MA: Allyn & Bacon.

Conture, E. G. (2003). Why does my child stutter? In. E. G. Conture (Ed.), *Stuttering and your child: Questions and answers* (3rd ed., Publication No. 22, pp. 9–19). Memphis, TN: Stuttering Foundation of America.

Conture, E. G., & Guitar, B. (1993). Evaluating efficacy of treatment of stuttering: School-age children. *Journal of Fluency Disorders, 18,* 253–287.

Conture, E. G., Louko, L. J., & Edwards, M. L. (1993). Simultaneously treating stuttering and disordered phonology in children: Experimental treatment, preliminary findings. *American Journal of Speech Language Pathology,* 2(3), 72–81.

Cooper, C. (2000, October 1). *School-based strategies for working with children who stutter: A positive team approach.* Paper presented at the 2000 International Stuttering Awareness Day Online Conference. Retrieved March 7, 2005, from http://www.mnsu.edu/dept/comdis/ISAD3/papers/ccooper.html

Cooper, E. B. (1979). Intervention procedures for the young stutterer. In Gregory, H. H. (Ed.), *Controversies about stuttering therapy* (pp. 63–96). Baltimore, MD: University Park Press.

Cooper, E. B., & Cooper, C. S. (1985). *Cooper personalized fluency control therapy–revised.* Allen, TX: DLM Teaching Resources.

Craig, A. (1990). An investigation into the relationship between anxiety and stuttering. *Journal of Speech and Hearing Disorders, 55,* 290–294.

Culatta, R., & Goldberg, S. A. (1995). *Stuttering therapy: An integrated approach to theory and practice.* Needham Heights, MA: Allyn & Bacon.

Dartnell, T. (2003, October 1). *Passing as fluent.* Paper presented at the 2003 International Stuttering Awareness Day Online Conference. Retrieved September 7, 2005, http://www.mnsu.edu/comdis/isad6/papers/dartnall6.html

Davis, S., Howell, P., & Cooke, F., (2002). Sociodynamic relationships between children who stutter and their non-stuttering classmates. *Journal of Child Psychology and Psychiatry and Allied Disciplines, 43,* 939–947.

Dell, C. W. (1993). Treating school-age stutterers. In R. F. Curlee. (Ed.), *Stuttering and related disorders of fluency* (pp. 45–67). New York: Thieme.

Dell, C. W. (2000). *Treating the school age stutterer: A guide for clinicians* (2nd ed., Publication No. 14). Memphis, TN: Stuttering Foundation of America.

DeNil, L. F., & Bruten, G. J. (1991). Speech-associated attitudes of stuttering and non-stuttering children. *Journal of Speech and Hearing Research, 34,* 60–66.

Donaher, J. (2001). Letting it out. [Handout]. In L. Caggiano, J. Donaher, J. Givens, & C. W. Starkweather, *New trends in stuttering therapy.* Presentation at the meeting of the New Jersey Speech-Language-Hearing Association, Atlantic City, NJ.

Donaher, J. (2003a, November–December). Encouraging clients to take risks in therapy. In *Reaching Out.* (Available from FRIENDS, 1220 Rosita Rd., Pacifica, CA 94044-4223), p. 1, 6.

Donaher, J. (Speaker). (2003b, November). In J. G. Donaher, L. S. Trautman, R. Shine, L. Caggiano, & B. Murphy, Effective therapy techniques for school-aged children who stutter. Panel discussion at the American Speech-Language-Hearing Association. Chicago, IL.

Donohue, C. (2003, July 7). Feelings when stuttering in front of a group. Essay posted to the Stuttering Homepage. Retrieved May 28, 2005, from http://www.mnsu.edu/comdis/kuster/PWSspeak/donohue.html

Floyd, A. (1999). Jumping at the chance. In A. Bradberry & N. Reardon (Eds.), *Our Voices: Inspirational insight from young people who stutter* (pp. 128–131). Anaheim Hills, CA: National Stuttering Association.

Fucci, D., Leach, E., Mckenzie, J., & Gonzales, M. D. (1998). Comparison of listener's judgments of simulated and authentic stuttering using magnitude estimation scaling. *Perceptual and Motor Skills, 87,* 1103–1106.

Gaines, N. D., Runyan, C. M., & Meyers, S. C. (1991). A comparison of young stutterer's fluent versus stuttered utterances on measures of length of complexity. *Journal of Speech and Hearing Research, 34,* 37–42.

Gottwald, S. R., & Starkweather, C. W. (1995). Fluency intervention for preschoolers and their families in public schools. *Language, Speech, and Hearing Services in Schools, 26,* 117–126.

Gregory, H. H. (1986). *Stuttering: Differential evaluation and therapy.* Austin, TX: PRO-ED.

Gregory, H. H. (1995). Analysis and commentary. *Language, Speech, and Hearing Services in Schools, 26* (2), 196–200.

Gregory, H. H. (2002). What is involved in therapy? In. E. G. Conture (Ed.), *Stuttering and your child: Questions and answers* (3rd ed., Publication No. 22, pp. 39–50). Memphis, TN: Stuttering Foundation of America.

Gregory, H. H., & Gregory, C. B. (1999). Counseling children who stutter and their parents. In R. F. Curlee (Ed.), *Stuttering and related disorders of fluency* (2nd ed., pp. 43–64). New York: Thieme.

Guerin, C. (2003, April 21). Stuttering chat: Online support for people who stutter [Msg. 18543]. Message posted to Ref-Links electronic mailing list, archived at http://groups.yahoo.com/group/stutteringchat/message/18543

Guitar, B. (1998). *Stuttering: An integrated approach to its nature and treatment.* Baltimore, MD: Lippincott Williams & Wilkins.

Guitar, B. (2000). Starting to help yourself. In J. Fraser (Ed.), *Do you stutter: A guide for teens* (Publication 21, pp. 53–63). Memphis, TN: Stuttering Foundation of America.

Guitar, B. (Speaker). (2005). In E. Conture, B. Guitar, & J. Fraser (Co-Producers), *Therapy in action: The school-age child who stutters* [Video Recording No. 79]. Memphis, TN: Stuttering Foundation of America.

Guitar, B., & Peters, T. J. (2003). *Stuttering: An integration of contemporary therapies* (3rd ed., Publication No. 16). Memphis, TN: Stuttering Foundation of America.

Guitar, B. & Reville, J. (2003). Counseling school-age children in group therapy. In J. Fraser (Ed.), *Effective counseling in stuttering therapy* (Publication No. 18, pp. 71–84). Memphis, TN: Stuttering Foundation of America.

Harkavy, W. (2002, September 25). Stutt-L: Stuttering: Research and clinical practice [Msg. 001885]. Message posted to Ref-Links electronic mailing list, archived at http://listserv.temple.edu/archives/stutt-l.html

Hatahet, S. (1999). I know how you feel. In A. Bradberry & N. Reardon (Eds.), *Our Voices: Inspirational insight from young people who stutter* (p. 28). Anaheim Hills, CA: National Stuttering Association.

Hayhow, R., Cray, A. M., & Enderby, P. (2002). Stammering and therapy views of people who stammer. *Journal of Fluency Disorders, 27,* 1–18.

Healey, C. E., Scott, L. A., & Ellis, G. (1995). Decision making in the treatment of school-age children who stutter. *Journal of Communicative Disorders, 28,* 107–124.

Heite, L. B. (2001, October 1). *La petite mort: Dissociation and the subjective experience of stuttering.* Paper presented at the 2001 International Stuttering Awareness Day Online Conference. Retrieved March 7, 2005, from http://www.mnsu.edu/dept/comdis/isad4/papers/heite4.html

Hicks, R. (2002, October, 10). Beneath the waterline of the stuttering iceberg [Discussion forum for a paper presented at the 2002 International Stuttering Awareness Day Online Conference]. Message posted to http://cahn.mnsu.edu/5foer/_disc44/00000011.htm

Hicks, R. (2003, October 1). *The iceberg analogy of stuttering.* Paper presented at the 2003 International Stuttering Awareness Day Online Conference. Retrieved March 7, 2005, from http://www.mnsu.edu/comdis/isad6/papers/hicks6.html

Hill, D. G. (2003). Counseling parents of children who stutter. In J. Fraser (Ed.), *Effective counseling in stuttering therapy* (Publication No. 18, pp. 37–52). Memphis, TN: Stuttering Foundation of America.

Hood, S. B. (1975). Effect of communicative stress on the frequency and form—Types of disfluent behavior in adult stutterers. *Journal of Fluency Disorders, 1,* 36–47.

Hopewell, B. (2000). How I turned an education obstacle into an opportunity. *Journal of College Admission, 166,* p. 3.

Howell, P., Sackin, S., & Williams, R. (1999). Differential effects of frequency-shifted feedback between child and adult stutterers. *Journal of Fluency Disorders, 24,* 127–136.

Hugh-Jones, S., Smith, P. K. (1999). Self-reports of short- and long-term effects of bullying on children who stammer. *British Journal of Educational Psychology, 69,* 141–158.

Ingham, R. J., & Andrews, G. (1971). Stuttering: The quality of fluency after treatment. *Journal of Communicative Disorders, 4,* 279–288.

James, S. E., Brumfitt, S. M., & Cudd, P. A. (1999). Telephone: Views of a group of people with stuttering impairment. *Journal of Fluency Disorders, 24,* 299–317.

Jezer, M. (1997). *Stuttering: A life bound up in words.* New York: Basic Books.

Jezer, M. (1998, October 1). *Speaking is my challenge—And I'm facing up to it.* Paper presented at the 1998 International Stuttering Awareness Day Online Conference. Retrieved March 7, 2005, from http://www.mnsu.edu/dept/comdis/isad/papers/jezer.html

Johnson, R. (2003, July–September). Taking the plunge. In *Letting Go.* (Available from the National Stuttering Association, 119 W. 40th Street, 14th Floor, New York, NY 10018), pp. 1, 7.

Kalinowski, J., Armson, J., & Stuart, A. (1995). Effect of normal and fast articulatory rates on stuttering frequency. *Journal of Fluency Disorders, 20,* 293–302.

Kalinowski, J., & Saltuklaroglu, T. (2003). Choral speech: The amelioration of stuttering via imitation and the mirror neuronal system. *Neuroscience and Biobehavioral Reviews. 27,* 339–347.

Kalinowski, J., & Saltuklaroglu, T. (2004). The road to efficient and effective stuttering management: information for physicians. *Current Medical Research and Opinion, 20*(4), 509–515.

Kalinowski, J., Stuart, A., Sark, S., & Armson, J. (1996). Stuttering amelioration at various auditory feedback delays and speech rates. *European Journal of Disorders of Communication, 31,* 259–269.

Kalinowski, J., Stuart, A., Wamsley, L., & Rastatter, M. (1999). Effects of monitoring and frequency-altered feedback on stuttering frequency. *Journal of Speech, Language, and Hearing Research, 42,* 1347–1354.

Klumb, G. (2002, December). Who would have thought? Talking to students turned out to be fun. In *Letting Go.* (Available from the National Stuttering Association, 119 W. 40th Street, 14th Floor, New York, NY 10018), p. 7.

Kraaimaat, F. W., Vanryckeghem, M., & Van Dam-Baggenc, R. (2002). Stuttering and social anxiety. *Journal of Fluency Disorders, 27,* 319–331.

Kuster, J. (2004). Internet treasures for kids and teens who stutter. *The Asha Leader, 9*(17), 14–15.

Langevin, M. (2001, October 1). *Helping children deal with teasing and bullying.* Paper presented at the 2001 International Stuttering Awareness Day Online Conference. Retrieved March 7, 2005, from http://www.mnsu.edu/dept/comdis/isad4/papers/langevin.html

Langevin, M., Bortnick, K., Hammer, T., & Wiebe, E. (1998). Teasing/bullying experienced by children who stutter: Toward development of a questionnaire. *Contemporary Issues in Communication Science and Disorders, 23,* 12–24.

Linton, E. (2003, Summer). The challenge and gift of speech at symposium XXII. *The Speak Easy Newsletter, 23,* 2.

Logan, K. J., & Conture, E. G. (1995). Length, grammatical complexity, and rate differences in stuttered and fluent conversational utterances in children who stutter. *Journal of Fluency Disorders, 20,* 35–61.

Logan, K. J., & Lasalle, L. R. (2003). Developing an intervention program for children with stuttering and concomitant impairments. *Seminars in Speech and Language, 24,* 13–20.

Louko, L., Conture, E., & Edwards, M. E. (1999). Treating children who exhibit co-occurring stuttering and disordered phonology. In R. F. Curlee (Ed.), *Stuttering and related disorders of fluency* (2nd ed., pp. 124–138). New York: Thieme.

Lukong, J. (2003, October–November). A story from Africa. In *Letting Go.* (Available from the National Stuttering Association, 119 W. 40th Street, 14th Floor, New York, NY 10018), pp. 1, 5.

Luper, H. L., & Mulder, R. L. (1964). *Stuttering therapy for children.* Englewood Cliffs. NJ: Prentice-Hall.

Luterman, D. M. (2001). *Counseling the communicatively disordered and their families* (4th ed.). Austin, TX: PRO-ED.

Mackesey, T. (2003, June). Straight talk on portable delayed auditory feedback devices. In *Letting Go.* (Available from the National Stuttering Association, 119 W. 40th Street, 14th Floor, New York, NY 10018), p 3.

Manning, W. H. (1996). *Clinical decision making in the diagnosis and treatment of fluency disorders.* Albany, NY: Delmar.

Manning, W. H. (1999a, October 1). *Creating your own map for change.* Paper presented at the 1999 International Stuttering Awareness Day Online Conference. Retrieved March 7, 2005, from http://www.mnsu.edu/dept/comdis/isad2/papers/manning2.html

Manning, W. H. (1999b). Sports analogies in the treatment of stuttering: Taking the field with your client. In A. Bradberry & N. Reardon (Eds.), *Our Voices: Inspirational insight from young people who stutter* (pp. 156–163). Anaheim Hills, CA: National Stuttering Association.

Manning, W. H. (2000). *Clinical decision making in fluency disorders.* San Diego, CA: Singular Publishing.

McClure, J. (2003, January). Attitude-changing therapy is most effective. In *Letting Go.* (Available from the National Stuttering Association, 119 W. 40th Street, 14th Floor, New York, NY 10018), pp. 1, 7.

McClure, J., & Yaruss, J. S. (2003). Stuttering survey suggests success of attitude-changing treatment. *The Asha Leader, 8*(9), pp. 3, 19.

Messenger, M., Onslow, M., Packman, A., & Menzies, R. (2004). Social anxiety in stuttering: measuring negative social expectancies. *Journal of Fluency Disorders, 29,* 201–212.

Moran, W. R., & Shoop, S. A. (2001, May 15). Nicholas Brendon faces down stuttering demon. *USA Today.* Health section. Retrieved July 7, 2005, from http://www.usatoday.com/news/health/spotlight/2001-05-15-brendon-stuttering.htm

Murphy, B. (1996, November). *Empowering children who stutter: Reducing shame, guilt, and anxiety.* Handout presented at the National Speech-Language-Hearing Association's annual convention, Seattle, WA. Retrieved March 7, 2005, from http://www.mnsu.edu/comdis/kuster/TherapyWWW/murphy.html

Murphy, B. (1997a). Old fart face (part of a featured speech at the 1991 National Stuttering Project convention in Dallas, Texas). Retrieved March 7, 2005, from http://www.mnsu.edu/dept/comdis/kuster/PWSspeak/bmurphy.html

Murphy, B. (1997b, June). *Helping school-aged children who stutter: Working with emotions.* Paper presented at the meeting of the Stuttering Foundation of America and the Department of Audiology & Speech Pathology at the University of Memphis, TN.

Murphy, B. (1999). A preliminary look at shame, guilt, and stuttering. In N. B. Ratner & E. C. Healey (Eds.), *Stuttering research and practice: Bridging the gap* (pp. 131–143). Hillsdale, NJ: Erlbaum.

Murphy, B. (2000, October 1). *Speech pathologists can help children who are teased because they stutter.* Paper presented at the 2000 International Stuttering Awareness Day Online Confer ence. Retrieved March 7, 2005, from http://www.mnsu.edu/dept/comdis/ISAD3/papers/murphy.html

Murphy, B. (Speaker). (2003, November). In Donaher, J. G, Trautman, L. S., Shine, R., Caggiano, & Murphy, B., *Effective therapy techniques for school-aged children who stutter.* Panel discussion at the meeting of the American Speech-Language-Hearing Association, Chicago, IL.

Murphy, W. P., & Quesal, R. W. (2002). Strategies for addressing bullying with the school-age child who stutters. *Seminars in Speech and Language, 23,* 205–212.

Natke, U., Sandrieser, P., van Ark, M., Pietrowsky, R., & Kalveram, K. T. (2004). Linguistic stress, within-word position, and grammatical class in relation to early childhood stuttering. *Journal of Fluency Disorders, 29,* 109–122.

Nippold, M. A. (1990). Concomitant speech and language disorders in stuttering children. *Journal of Speech and Hearing Disorders, 55,* 51–60.

Nippold, M. A. (2001). Phonological disorders and stuttering in children: What is the frequency of co-occurrence? *Clinical Linguistics and Phonetics, 15,* 219–228.

Nippold, M. A. (2002). Stuttering and phonology: Is there an interaction? *American Journal of Speech–Language Pathology, 11,* 99–110.

Nippold, M. A. (2004a). Phonological and language disorders in children who stutter: Impact on treatment recommendations. *Clinical Linguistics and Phonetics, 18,* 145–159.

Nippold, M. A. (2004b). Why we should consider pragmatics when planning treatment for children who stutter. *Language, Speech, and Hearing Services in Schools, 35,* 34–45.

Paden, E. G. (2005). Development of phonological ability. In E. Yairi & N. G. Ambrose. (Eds.), *Early childhood stuttering: For clinicians by clinicians* (pp. 197–234). Austin, TX: PRO-ED.

Peters, H. F. M., & Hulstijn, W. (1987). Programming and initiation of speech utterances in stuttering. In H. F. M. Peters & W. Hulstijn (Eds.), *Speech motor dynamics in stuttering* (pp. 185–195). New York: Springer-Verlag.

Peters, H. F. M., Hulstijin, W., & Starkweather, C. W. (1989). Acoustic and physiological reaction times of stutterers and nonstutterers. *Journal of Speech and Hearing Research. 32,* 668–680.

Polak, T. J. (1999). Stuttering Poem. In A. Bradberry & N. Reardon (Eds.), *Our Voices: Inspirational insight from young people who stutter* (p. 21). Anaheim Hills, CA: National Stuttering Association.

Quesal, B. (1999). Basic truths about stuttering therapy. In A. Bradberry & N. Reardon (Eds.) *Our Voices: Inspirational insight from young people who stutter* (pp. 163–166). Anaheim Hills, CA: National Stuttering Association.

Ramig, P. (1993). Parent–clinician–child partnership in the therapeutic process of the preschool- and elementary-aged child who stutters. *Seminars in Speech and Language, 14,* 226–237.

Ramig, P. (1997, August 25). Factors responsible for my change. Seminar presented at the Second World Congress on Fluency Disorders, San Francisco, California. Retrieved March 7, 2005, from http://www.mnsu.edu/dept/comdis/kuster/casestudy/path/pramig.html

Ramig, P. (2003, October 2). Office hours: The professor is in [Discussion forum at the 2003 International Stuttering Awareness Day Online Conference]. Message posted to http://cahn.mnsu.edu/6profin/_disc22/00000015.htm

Ramig, P. R., & Bennett, E. M. (1995). Working with 7- to 12-year-old children who stutter: Ideas for intervention in the public schools. *Language, Speech, and Hearing Services in Schools, 26,* 138–150.

Ramig, P. R., & Bennett, E. M. (1997). Clinical management of children: Direct management strategies. In R. F. Curlee and G. M. Siegel (Eds.), *Nature and treatment of stuttering: New directions* (2nd ed., pp. 294–312). Needham Heights, MA: Allyn & Bacon.

Ratner, N. B. (1995). Treating the child who stutters with concomitant language or phonological impairment. *Language, Speech, and Hearing Services in Schools, 26,* 180–186.

Ratner, N. B., & Sih, C. (1987). The effects of gradual increases in sentence length and complexity on children's dysfluency. *Journal of Speech and Hearing Disorders, 52,* 278–287.

Ratner, N. B., & Hakim, H. B. (2004). Nonword repetition abilities of children who stutter: An exploratory study. *Journal of Fluency Disorders, 29,* 179–199.

Reardon, N. A. (2000). Succeeding with school-based therapy. *Advance for Speech–Language Pathologists and Audiologist, 10,* 19.

Reed, L. (1999, December 2). Celebrating me: Taming the speech monster workshop. Workshop presented at the 1999 New Jersey Youth Day Workshop. Paper retrieved on March 7, 2005, from http://www.mnsu.edu/dept/comdis/kuster/TherapyWWW/reedworkshop.html.

Reitzes, P. (2002). Stutter across America: Summer trek takes FRIENDS message on the road. *Advance for Speech–Language Pathologists and Audiologists, 12,* 11.

Reitzes, P. (2005, October 1). *The why and the how of voluntary stuttering.* Paper presented at the 2005 International Stuttering Awareness Day Online Conference. Retrieved October 1, 2005, from http://www.mnsu.edu/comdis/isad8/papers/reitzes8.html

Reitzes, P., & Caggiano, L. (2003). FRIENDS convention to be held in New York metro area. *Advance for Speech–Language Pathologists and Audiologists, 13,* 26–27.

Reitzes, P., & Starkweather, C. W. (1999). Stutter-free policy: NYU requirement was in direct opposition to ASHA standards and practices. *Advance for Speech–Language Pathologists and Audiologists, 9,* 10–11.

Rentschler, G. J. (2004, November). *Developing clinical tools for stuttering therapy: Building effective activities.* Short course presented at the annual convention of the American Speech-Language-Hearing Association, Philadelphia, PA.

Riley, G. D., & Riley, J. (1983). Evaluation as a basis for intervention. In D. Prins & R. J. Ingham (Eds.), *Treatment of stuttering in early childhood: Methods and issues* (pp. 128–152). San Diego, CA: College–Hill Press.

Roach, C. J. (2003). Covert-S [Msg. 547]. Message posted to Ref-Links electronic mailing list, archived at http://health.groups.yahoo.com/group/Covert-S/message/547

Schneider, P. (1994). A self-adjustment approach to fluency enhancement. *Proceedings of the First World Congress on Fluency Disorders, Germany, 1,* 334–337.

Schneider, P. (1998). Self-adjusting fluency therapy. *Journal of Children's Communication Development, 19,* 57–63.

Schneider, P. (2003). Counseling school-age children who stutter. *Perspectives on Fluency and Fluency Disorders, 13*(2), 14–17.

Schofield, R. (2001). When the words won't come. [Electronic Version]. *Speaking Out.* Retrieved on August 12, 2004, from http://www.stammering.org/whenthewords.html

Scott, L., & Williams, D. E. (2005). *The child who stutters: Notes to the teacher.* [Brochure]. Memphis, TN.

Shaina. (1999). What letting go means to me. In A. Bradberry & N. Reardon (Eds.), *Our Voices: Inspirational insight from young people who stutter* (p. 29). Anaheim Hills, CA: National Stuttering Association.

Shapiro, D. A. (1999). *Stuttering intervention: A collaborative journey to fluency freedom.* Austin, TX: PRO-ED.

Sheehan, J. G. (1968). A clinical success: Leonard. In J. Fraser (Ed.), *Stuttering: Successes and failures in therapy* (Publication No. 6, pp. 77–86). Memphis, TN: Stuttering Foundation of America.

Sheehan, J. G. (1970). *Stuttering Research and Therapy.* New York: Harper & Row.

Sheehan, J. G. (1975). Conflict theory and avoidance-reduction therapy. In J. Eisenson (Ed.), *Stuttering: A second symposium* (pp. 97–148). New York: Harper & Row.

Sheehan, J. G. (2003). Principals of counseling people who stutter. In J. Fraser (Ed.), *Effective counseling in stuttering therapy* (Publication No. 18, pp. 27–36). Memphis, TN: Stuttering Foundation of America.

Silverman, F. H. (2004). *Stuttering and other fluency disorders* (3rd ed.). Long Grove, IL: Waveland Press.

Sisskin, V. (2002). Therapy planning for school-age children who stutter. *Seminars in Speech and Language, 23,* 173–180.

Skotko, J. (2004, April). Experience of a speech pathologist providing clients with the SpeechEasy® device. *Stammering Research, 1,* 63–65. Retrieved August 11, 2005, from http://www.stamres.psychol.ucl.ac.uk/Vol1-Issue1.pdf

Sliger, A. F. (2001). I thought I was the only one. In K. O. St. Louis (Ed.), *Living with stuttering: Stories, basics, resources, and hope* (pp. 74–77). Morgantown, WV: Populore.

Snyder, G. (2002, October 1). *The use of altered speech feedback in stuttering management.* Paper presented at the 2002 International Stuttering Awareness Day Online Conference. Retrieved March 7, 2005, from http://www.mnsu.edu/comdis/isad5/papers/snyder.html

Snyder, G. (2003, July 22). Prosthetic stuttering management [Letter to the editor]. *The Asha Leader, 8,* 35.

Sparks, G., Grant, D. E., Millay, K., Walker-Batsen, D., & Hynan, L. S. (2002). The effect of fast speech rate on stuttering frequency during delayed auditory feedback. *Journal of Fluency Disorders, 27,* 187–201.

Starkweather, C. W. (1987). *Fluency and stuttering.* Englewood Cliffs, NJ: Prentice Hall.

Starkweather, C. W. (1999). The effectiveness of stuttering therapy: An issue for science? In N. B. Ratner & E. C. Healey (Eds.), *Stuttering research and practice: Bridging the gap* (pp. 231–244). Mahwah, NJ: Erlbaum.

Starkweather, C. W. (2002, March). Gestalt workshop—Woody's response. *Speaking Out.* Retrieved July 23, 2004, from http://www.stammering.org/gestaltworkshop_woodysresponse.html

Starkweather, C. W. (2003, June 9). Stutt-L: Stuttering: Research and clinical practice [Msg. 004275]. Message posted to Ref-Links electronic mailing list, archived at http://listserv.temple.edu/archives/stutt-l.html

Starkweather, C. W., & Givens-Ackerman, J. (1997). *Stuttering.* Austin, TX: PRO-ED.

Starkweather, C. W., & Givens, J. (2003, October 1). *Stuttering as a variant of post traumatic stress disorder: What we can learn.* Paper presented at the 2003 International Stuttering Awareness Day Online Conference. Retrieved March 7, 2005, from http://www.mnsu.edu/comdis/isad6/papers/starkweather6.html

Starkweather, C. W., & Gottwald, S. R. (1990). The demands and capacities model II: Clinical implications. *Journal of Fluency Disorders, 15,* 143–157.

Steiner, D. (2002, September 22). Stutt-L: Stuttering: Research and clinical practice [Msg. 001845]. Message posted to Ref-Links electronic mailing list, archived at http://listserv.temple.edu/archives/stutt-l.html

Stewart, T. (1997). The use of drawings in the management of adults who stammer. *Journal of Fluency Disorders, 22,* 35–50.

St. Louis, K. O. (1999). Person-first labeling and stuttering. *Journal of Fluency Disorders, 24,* 1–24.

St. Louis, K. O. (2001). *Living with stuttering: Stories, basics, resources, and hope.* Morgantown, WV: Populore.

Stuart, A., & Kalinowski, J. (1996). Fluent speech, fast articulatory rate, and delayed auditory feedback: Creating a crisis for a scientific revolution? *Perceptual and Motor Skills, 82,* 211–218.

Stuttering Foundation of America. (2005). *16 Famous People Who Stutter* [Brochure]. Memphis, TN: Author.

Stuttering Homepage (2005). *Some ways I have been teased about my stuttering.* Retrieved July 17, 2005, from http://www.mnsu.edu/comdis/kuster/kids/teasing/howteased.html

Sugerman, M. (2001). I didn't want to be different. In K. O. St. Louis (Ed.), *Living with stuttering: Stories, basics, resources, and hope* (pp. 78-81). Morgantown, WV: Populore.

Summerlin, T. D. (2001). Working now for a new attitude, In K. O. St. Louis (Ed.), *Living with stuttering: Stories, basics, resources, and hope* (pp. 31–35). Morgantown, WV: Populore.

Tatarniuk, R. (1998). Cerena. In J. Westbrook & J. Ahlbach (Eds.), *Listen with your heart: Reflections on growing up with stuttering* (p. 11). Pacifica, CA: FRIENDS.

Trautman, L. S., Healey, C. E., & Norris, J. A. (2001). The effects of contextualization on fluency in three groups of children. *Journal of Speech, Language, and Hearing Research, 44,* 564–576.

Troiano, T. (2002, July 18). Stutt-L: Stuttering: Research and clinical practice [Msg. 001375]. Message posted to Ref-Links electronic mailing list, archived at http://listserv.temple.edu/archives/stutt-l.html

Troiano, T. (2004, March 4). Stutt-L: Stuttering: Research and clinical practice [Msg. 006752]. Message posted to Ref-Links electronic mailing list, archived at http://listserv.temple .eduarchives/stutt-l.html

van Lieshout, P. H. H. M., Peter, H. F. M., Starkweather, C. W., & Hulstijin, W. (1993). Physiological differences between stutterers and nonstutterers in perceptually fluent speech: EMG amplitude and duration. *Journal of Speech and Hearing Research, 36,* 55–63.

Van Riper, C. (1948). *Stuttering.* Chicago: The National Society for Crippled Children and Adults.

Van Riper, C. (1973). *The treatment of stuttering* (2nd ed.). Englewood Cliffs, NJ: Prentice Hall.

Van Riper, C. (1975). The stutterer's clinician. In J. Eisenson (Ed.), *Stuttering: A second symposium* (pp. 453–492). New York: Harper & Row.

Van Riper, C. (1982). *The nature of stuttering* (2nd ed.). Englewood Cliffs, NJ: Prentice Hall.

Vinjamoori, A. (2004, November–December). One step at a time. *Literary Cavalcade. 57,* 24–25.

Wall, M. J., & Meyers, F. L., (1995). *Clinical management of childhood stuttering* (2nd ed.). Austin, TX: PRO-ED.

Walton, P., & Wallace, M. (1998). *Fun with fluency: Direct therapy with the young child.* Austin, TX: PRO-ED.

Williams, D. E. (1979). A perspective on approaches to stuttering therapy. In Gregory, H. H. (Ed.), *Controversies about stuttering therapy* (pp. 241–268). Baltimore, MD: University Park Press.

Williams, D. E., (2003). Talking with children who stutter. In J. Fraser (Ed.), *Effective counseling in stuttering therapy* (Publication No. 18, pp. 53–64). Memphis, TN: Stuttering Foundation of America.

Williams, D. E, & Scott, L. (2005). *The child who stutters: Notes to the teacher.* [Brochure]. Memphis, TN: Stuttering Foundation of America.

Williams, D. F., & Dugan, P. M. (2002). Administering stuttering modification therapy in school settings. *Seminars in Speech and Language, 23,* 187–194.

Wilson, K. P. (2004). *Proactive alternative assessment of emotion in children who stutter.* Florida State University D–Scholarship Repository, Article No. 2. Retrieved August 21, 2004, from http://dscholarship.lib.fsu.edu/undergrad/2

Wingate, M. E. (1997). *Stuttering: A short history of a curious disorder.* Westport, CT: Bergin & Garvey.

Wolk, L. (1998). Intervention strategies for children who exhibit coexisting phonological and fluency disorders: A clinical note. *Child Language Teaching and Therapy, 14*(1), 69–82.

Yairi, E., & Ambrose, N. G. (2005). *Early childhood stuttering: For clinicians by clinicians.* Austin, TX: PRO-ED.

Yaruss, J. S. (1999). Utterance length, syntactic complexity, and childhood stuttering. *Journal of Speech, Language, and Hearing Research, 42,* 329–344.

Yaruss, J. S. (2002). Facing the challenge of treating stuttering in the schools. *Seminars in Speech and Language, 23,* 153–158.

Yaruss, J. S., Murphy, B., Quesal, R. W., & Reardon, N. A. (2004). *Bullying and Teasing: Helping Children Who Stutter.* Clifton Park, NY: National Stuttering Association.

Yaruss, J. S., & Reardon, N. A. (2002). Successful communication for children who stutter: Finding the balance. *Seminars in Speech and Language, 23,* 195–204.

Yaruss, J. S., & Reardon, N. A. (2003). Fostering generalization and maintenance in school settings. *Seminars in Speech and Language, 24,* 33–40.

Yeoman, B. (2003, August). *Proud stuttering men.* Workshop conducted at the Sixth Annual convention of FRIENDS: The National Association of Young People Who Stutter, Secaucus, NJ.

Young, A. (1998). A speech to fifth grade. In J. Westbrook & J. Ahlbach (Eds.), *Listen with your heart: Reflections on growing up with stuttering* (pp. 14–15). Pacifica, CA: FRIENDS.

Zackheim, C. T., & Conture, E. G. (2003). Childhood stuttering and speech disfluencies in relation to children's mean length of utterance: A preliminary study. *Journal of Fluency Disorders, 28,* 115–142.

Zebrowski, P. M. (2003). Understanding and coping with emotions: Counseling teenagers who stutter. In J. Fraser (Ed.), *Effective counseling in stuttering therapy* (Publication No. 18, pp. 85–104). Memphis, TN: Stuttering Foundation of America.

About the Author

Peter Reitzes, MA, CCC-SLP, is a person who stutters and a certified and licensed speech–language pathologist working in an elementary school and in private practice in Brooklyn, New York. Reitzes has presented at speech–language pathology conferences and conventions, including the American Speech-Language-Hearing Association's annual convention, the New York and New Jersey Speech-Language-Hearing Association's annual conventions, the Speak Easy annual convention, and an *Advance* magazine conference. Reitzes has facilitated workshops for FRIENDS: The National Association of Young People Who Stutter and other stuttering self-help organizations. In July, 2002, Reitzes co-facilitated "Stutter Across America"—a FRIENDS project. Stutter Across America was an eight-stop mobile workshop that brought stuttering support to cities and towns across the United States. Reitzes has been interviewed about stuttering by the *New York Times, The Chicago Tribune,* National Public Radio, and Fox News. He has written articles for the International Stuttering Awareness Day (ISAD) Online Conference, *Advance for Speech–Language Pathologists and Audiologists,* the National Stuttering Association, and FRIENDS. Reitzes is co-founder and co-editor of the online journal *Journal of Stuttering Therapy: Advocacy and Research* at www.journalofstuttering.com. Visit Reitzes at his homepage: www.stuttering.com